MCQs in Anaesthesia

I.V Fluid
ant calm
meitaning

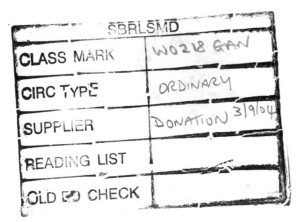
For Churchill Livingstone:

Publisher: Michael Parkinson
Project Editor: Barbara Simmons
Copy Editor: Susan Beasley
Project Controller: Kay Hunston
Design Direction: Erik Bigland

MCQs in Anaesthesia

A. Ganado FRCA

Consultant Anaesthetist, Birmingham Heartlands Hospital, Birmingham, UK

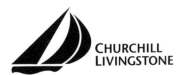

CHURCHILL
LIVINGSTONE

EDINBURGH LONDON NEW YORK PHILADELPHIA SAN FRANCISCO SYDNEY
TORONTO 1998

CHURCHILL LIVINGSTONE
A Division of Harcourt Brace and Company Limited

Churchill Livingstone, 1–3 Baxter's Place,
Leith Walk, Edinburgh EH1 3AF

First published 1998

ISBN 0443 05915 2

British Library of Cataloguing in Publication Data
A catalogue record for this book is available from the British
Library.

Library of Congress Cataloging in Publication Data
A catalog record for this book is available from the Library of
Congress.

Medical knowledge is constantly changing. As information
becomes available, changes in treatment, procedures,
equipment and the use of drugs become necessary. The
author and publisher have, as far as it is possible, taken care
to ensure that the information given in the text is accurate
and up-to-date. However, readers are strongly advised to
confirm that the information, especially with regard to drug
usage, complies with current legislation and standard of
practice.

The
publisher's
policy is to use
**paper manufactured
from sustainable forests**

Produced by Addison Wesley Longman Singapore Pte Ltd
Printed in Singapore

Preface

There are a number of publications of anaesthetic multiple choice questions, but most of them give no, or very brief, explanation of the answers to the questions. For the last ten years or so, Heartlands Hospital has been running a twice yearly anaesthetic course primarily aimed at the Primary FRCA, and I have been setting MCQs for this course. After scoring the candidates' paper, I gave them a copy of the correct answers to the MCQs, together with a detailed explanation of the topic covered in the questions. These explanations were thought to be very useful as a learning tool, and therefore I got the idea of making a book of them – hence *MCQs in Anaesthesia*. The MCQs are targeted principally at anaesthetists preparing for the final anaesthetic fellowship examination, and all the questions are original. The explanations are very factual, in 'lecture notes' format, cover wide aspects of anaesthetic practice, and are aimed to impart maximal knowledge with the least number of words.

I would like to thank the publisher's editors for helping me with the text, and especially Mrs Ann Amos, the anaesthetic secretary at Heartlands Hospital, who had the unenviable task of typing out my hand-written notes, which were so illegible that I could hardly read them myself.

Birmingham 1997   A. Ganado

Contents

5- 3

1.1 **With regard to lower limb local anaesthetic blocks:**

a) Operations anywhere on the thigh can be performed with a 3 in 1 block
b) Operations anywhere on the leg can be performed with a sciatic nerve block
c) The femoral nerve arises from lumbar nerves L1–L3
d) The sciatic nerve arises solely from the sacral plexus
e) At L4 level, the femoral nerve lies between the quadratus lumborum and the psoas major

1.2 **Uterine tone during pregnancy is reduced by:**

a) PGE_2 and PGF_2 prostaglandins
b) Methoxamine and noradrenaline
c) Histamine and serotonin (5-hydroxytryptamine)
d) Neuromuscular blocking drugs
e) Alcohol

1.3 **When drugs are used in combination:**

a) Two drugs are synergistic when their combined effect is greater than the sum of the parts
b) There is usually an increased risk of reactions at receptor sites and an increase in the adverse effects caused by the agents
c) Combination of midazolam and propofol for induction of anaesthesia reduces the ED_{50} of the drugs
d) Addition of alfentanil to propofol for induction of anaesthesia antagonizes the effects of propofol
e) Recovery from anaesthesia is generally prolonged following induction with propofol/midazolam compared with propofol alone

1.4 **In septic shock:**

a) The cause is always generalized infection
b) Hypovolaemia is due to reduced systemic vascular resistance, and plasma leakage into the extravascular space because of increased vascular permeability
c) Lactic acidosis should be treated with bicarbonate
d) FiO_2 should be increased if necessary to 100% to keep SaO_2 above 90%
e) Renal damage usually occurs first, followed by intestinal and finally pulmonary failure

1.5 **With regard to the caudal (sacral) epidural space:**

a) It is confined to the sacral hiatus
b) Intrathecal puncture is not possible with a 19-gauge needle because the dural sac does not reach the sacral hiatus $S_2 - S_3$
c) Its contents include dural sac, sacral and coccygeal nerve roots and venous plexuses
d) Infection is more likely with caudal block than with extradural lumbar block
e) A circumcision can be started 5 minutes following a successful caudal block

1.6 **With regard to perioperative myocardial ischaemia:**

a) Myocardial ischaemia is more likely intraoperatively than postoperatively in susceptible patients
b) Myocardial ischaemia is more likely to cause ST elevation on the electrocardiogram (ECG) than ST depression
c) Preoperative ischaemic changes on an ECG are less predictive of postoperative myocardial ischaemia than preoperative arrhythmias
d) It is more likely to be caused by tachycardia than bradycardia
e) High lactate dehydrogenase levels are more diagnostic of myocardial ischaemia than high creatinine phosphokinase levels

1.7 **Advantages of epidural postoperative analgesia using local anaesthetic include:**

a) Reduction in stress response
b) Improved myocardial blood flow with thoracic epidural
c) Improved pulmonary function which is superior to the improvement obtained with patient-controlled analgesia
d) Reduction in the immunosuppression caused by surgery
e) Reduction in incidence of deep vein thrombosis

1.8 **Clonidine:**

a) Is an alpha-2 adrenergic agonist
b) Increases sympathetic tone
c) Reduces the minimum alveolar concentration (MAC) of anaesthetic agents
d) Has analgesic properties
e) Dilates coronary and cerebral arteries

1.9 **Drug actions on the cardiovascular system include:**

a) Adrenaline causes alpha and beta-1 and beta-2 stimulation, while noradrenaline stimulates alpha and beta-1 but not beta-2 activity
b) Methoxamine has inotropic and chronotropic effects on the heart
c) Dopamine increases peripheral resistance; dobutamine reduces it
d) Dopexamine causes dilatation of renal, cerebral, coronary and mesenteric vascular beds
e) Nitroglycerine causes mainly arterial vasodilatation, nitroprusside mainly venous dilatation

1.10 **Oxygen consumption:**

a) Equals available oxygen in a fit patient
b) Is increased in neonates
c) Is reflected in mixed venous oxygen tensions
d) Is reflected in haemoglobin saturation values
e) Equals an average of 5 ml or every 100 ml of blood flow

2

1.11 **Cerebral blood flow:**

a) Corresponds to 15% of cardiac output in an adult
b) Varies little within the range of autoregulation (mean systemic blood pressure between 60 and 160 mmHg)
c) Is significantly reduced with high PaO_2
d) Is increased more with isoflurane than with halothane
e) Is reduced with ketamine

1.12 **With regard to hepatitis C:**

a) Infection can follow blood transfusions
b) Chronic liver disease is uncommon following infection
c) Carrier states are uncommon
d) Hepatitis B vaccine protects against hepatitis C
e) Infection is common after needle-sticks

1.13 **Comparing midazolam and diazepam:**

a) Midazolam does not cause any cardiovascular or respiratory depression
b) Midazolam is unlikely to cause thrombosis or thrombophlebitis
c) The metabolites of midazolam have negligible sedative effects unlike the metabolites of diazepam
d) Both cause retrograde amnesia
e) Day cases can be allowed to drive home if the effects of midazolam or diazepam are reversed with flumazenil

1.14 **With regard to drugs affecting coagulation:**

a) After the drugs are stopped, platelet dysfunction with aspirin lasts longer than with non-steroidal anti-inflammatory drugs
b) Low molecular weight heparin is less likely to induce bleeding than unfractionated heparin, while maintaining the same efficacy on deep vein prophylaxis
c) When it is necessary to stop bleeding caused by heparin, ever increasing doses of protamine should be administered until the bleeding stops
d) For elective surgery, warfarin should be stopped 24 hours before surgery to reduce the risk of bleeding
e) Aprotonin is a useful drug to administer in disseminated intravascular coagulation because it increases fibrinogen levels

1.15 **With regard to disseminated intravascular coagulation:**

a) Thrombocytopenia is a common feature
b) Heparin is a prime indication because of microvascular thrombosis
c) Hypofibrinoginaemia should be treated with fresh frozen plasma
d) It may be a feature of amniotic fluid embolism
e) The condition usually only occurs in critically ill patients

1.16 **With regard to anaesthetic agents in epileptics:**

a) Patients on anticonvulsant drugs are relatively resistant to vecuronium and atracurium
b) Pethidine is a preferable analgesic to morphine
c) Methohexitone is preferable to thiopentone as an induction agent
d) Propofol and etomidate should be avoided
e) Ketamine is contraindicated

1.17 **Uteroplacental perfusion is reduced by:**

a) Aortocaval compression
b) Inhalation of 1–1.5 MAC halothane or isoflurane
c) Large doses of ketamine
d) Sympathomimetic drugs with predominantly alpha effects
e) Respiratory alkalosis

1.18 **With regard to day case anaesthesia:**

a) High-risk patients in physical status groups III and IV should always be excluded
b) It is not suitable for morbidly obese patients without systemic disease
c) It is not suitable for patients over 70 without systemic disease
d) Ondansetron is preferable to droperidol as an antiemetic
e) Recovery is quicker with desflurane than with isoflurane

1.19 **Problems with eclampsia/pre-eclampsia may include:**

a) Thrombocytopenia
b) Laryngeal oedema
c) Mimicry of acute cocaine intoxication
d) Reduction in uteroplacental blood flow
e) Contraindication of epidural analgesia

1.20 **In ophthalmic local anaesthesia:**

a) The oculomotor nerves are the third, fourth and sixth cranial nerves
b) Orbital regional anaesthesia requires block of the ophthalmic nerve and oculomotor nerves
c) The facial nerve is normally blocked with a retrobulbar block, but not with a periorbital block
d) Oculocardiac reflex is maintained during a successful retrobulbar/peribulbar block
e) Sudden loss of vision may be due to globe perforation

1.1   a) False   b) False   c) True   d) False   e) True

EXPLANATION

The lumbar plexus is formed from the anterior primary roots of the first four lumbar nerves, each of which receives a grey communicating root from the lumbar sympathetic ganglia. The sacral plexus is formed from the anterior primary roots of the fourth and fifth lumbar nerves, and the five sacral and coccygeal nerves, and receives grey communicating roots from the sympathetic trunk. Branches from S2, S3 and S4 form the sacral parasympathetic outflow (Table 1.1).

Table 1.1   Anatomy of the lumbar plexus

Nerve	Origin	Anatomy	Sensory innervation
Iliohypogastric	L1	Crosses quadratus lumborum to divide into lateral and anterior branches	Lateral gluteal region and pubic area
Ilioinguinal	L1	Just below anterior iliac spine, it pierces internal oblique, and passes into the inguinal canal with the spermatic cord	Upper medial thigh and external genital organs
Genitofemoral	L1–L2	Divides into genital and femoral branches	Genital – scrotum/labia. Femoral – central area of upper thigh, both anteriorly and posteriorly
Lateral cutaneous nerve of thigh	Posterior divisions L2–L3	Passes behind inguinal ligament just medial to anterior superior iliac spine	Anterolateral aspect of thigh as far as knee anteriorly
Femoral	Posterior divisions of L2–L4	Descends behind psoas and deep to inguinal ligament just lateral to femoral artery. Gives off medial and intermediate nerves of thigh and ends as saphenous nerve	Medial and intermediate nerves of thigh – medial thigh. Saphenous – medial part of leg, anteriorly and posteriorly
Obturator	Anterior divisions of L2–L4	Emerges from medial border of psoas to run in lateral wall of pelvis, and enters the obturator canal	Medial thigh up to knee joint
Sciatic	L4, L5 S1–S3	Leaves pelvis through greater sciatic foramen, descends between ischial tuberosity and greater trochanter; and at popliteal fossa divides into the tibial and common peroneal nerves. The latter subdivides into the superficial peroneal and deep peroneal nerve. The sural arises from tibial and common peroneal nerves; posterior cutaneous nerve of thigh is also a branch of sciatic	Posterior cutaneous – posterior thigh and leg, anterior and posterior. Common peroneal – lateral areas of calf and leg. Superior peroneal – lateral leg and lateral dorsum of foot. Deep peroneal – medial margin of dorsum of foot. Sural – lateral margin of foot and leg. Tibial – divides into medial and lateral planters – sole, heel
Pudendal	S2–4	Leaves pelvis through greater and lesser sciatic foramen to pass along lateral wall of ischiorectal fossa and gives rise to peroneal nerve which divides into superficial and deep branches	Scrotal/labial area

5

Common blocks

A nerve tracer should be used to elicit paraesthesiae before local anaesthetic infiltration.

Ilioinguinal/iliohypogastric. A spinal needle is inserted one finger's breadth medial to and below the anterior superior iliac spine, directed laterally to strike the ileum, and 10 ml local anaesthetic injected between point of entry and ileum; from the same point, the needle is directed inferomedially to pierce the aponeurosis of the external oblique, and a further 10 ml injected in a fan-like fashion.

Lateral cutaneous nerve of thigh. The needle is inserted 1 cm medial to and 2 cm below the anterior superior iliac spine. When the needle pierces the fascia lata with a click, 2 ml local anaesthetic are injected, and a further 2 ml injected deep to the fascia lata both medially and laterally to the point of insertion.

Femoral nerve block. This provides useful analgesia after knee surgery. The needle is inserted 1 cm lateral to the femoral artery, just below the inguinal ligament, and directed slightly upwards, and 10–20 ml of local anaesthetic injected at a depth of 3–4 cm.

Saphenous nerve block. The saphenous nerve is the terminal branch of the femoral nerve, which becomes subcutaneous at the medial side of the knee. It is blocked by a subcutaneous injection just below the knee joint.

Sciatic nerve block. In combination with a 3 in 1 block, this can provide analgesia in all operations on the lower limb.

Anterior sciatic nerve block. Two lines are drawn—one along the inguinal ligament, and a lower parallel line at the level of the greater trochanter. A vertical line is then drawn from the junction of the middle and medial third of the inguinal line to meet the trochanteric line, and the point of intersection is the site of needle insertion. The needle is inserted in a slightly lateral direction to make contact with the femur; the needle is then withdrawn and directed medially to glide off the femur, advanced another 0.5 cm, and 20-30 ml 0.5% bupivacaine injected.

Posterior sciatic nerve block. A line is drawn between the posterior superior iliac spine and greater trochanter; the needle is inserted 3 cm below the midpoint of this line, advanced vertically to the skin for 6-8 cm, and 20-30 ml 0.5% bupivacaine injected.

3 in 1 block. The lumbar plexus lies between the quadratus lumborum posteriorly and psoas muscle anteriorly, and is enveloped by the fasciae of these two muscles (Fig. 1.1). The femoral nerve descends posterior to and in close proximity to the psoas, and emerges lateral to it at the junction of the middle and lower third of the muscle. Above the inguinal ligament, the femoral nerve is bounded laterally by the fascia of the iliac muscle, medially by the psoas fascia, and anteriorly by the transversalis fascia. As the nerve passes under the inguinal ligament into the thigh, it is still enveloped by the fused iliopsoas fascia posteriorly and laterally, fascia lata anteriorly, and iliopectineal fascia medially. This fascial sheet enables a single injection of local anaesthetic below the inguinal ligament around the femoral nerve to spread upwards along the fascial envelope to block not only the femoral nerve but also the lateral cutaneous nerve of thigh and the obturator nerve (this latter nerve is difficult to block on its own). With the help of a nerve tracer the needle is inserted one finger's breadth lateral to the femoral artery, and aimed upwards until paraesthesiae are elicited, or the femoral nerve activated. Paraesthesiae indicate that the tip of the needle is in the fascial envelope. 20-30 ml of 0.5% bupivacaine are injected, with firm finger pressure behind the needle to prevent retrograde flow. Following the injection, the finger pressure is maintained for a few minutes.

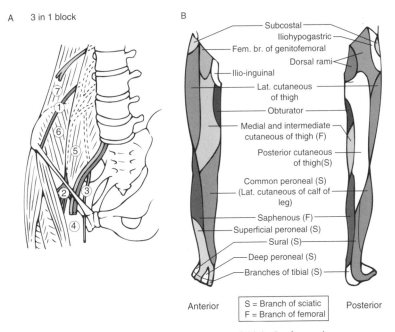

A   3 in 1 block

B

Subcostal
Iliohypogastric
Fem. br. of genitofemoral
Dorsal rami
Ilio-inguinal
Lat. cutaneous of thigh
Obturator
Medial and intermediate cutaneous of thigh (F)
Posterior cutaneous of thigh(S)
Common peroneal (S)
(Lat. cutaneous of calf of leg)
Saphenous (F)
Superficial peroneal (S)
Sural (S)
Deep peroneal (S)
Branches of tibial (S)

Anterior   Posterior

| S = Branch of sciatic |
| F = Branch of femoral |

Fig 1.1 *3 in 1 block: 1 – lateral cutaneous nerve of thigh; 2 – femoral nerve; 3 – obturator nerve; 4 – femoral artery; 5 – psoas muscle; 6 – iliac muscle; 7 – quadratus lumborum muscle.*

Combined lumbosacral plexus block. Operations on the lower limb cannot be performed solely with a 3 in 1 block; a further sciatic block is required. Alternatively, a combined lumbosacral plexus block, as described by Winnie (1991) using a single injection technique can be administered for any lower limb surgery. As with the 3 in 1 block, a lumbosacral plexus block relies on the fascial spread upwards and caudally, as the lumbar plexus is blocked by a paravertebral approach at L4 between the quadratus lumborum and psoas major. The patient lies in the lateral position. A line is drawn between the iliac crests, while a second line is drawn from the posterior superior iliac spine to intersect the intercrestal line. A 3.5-inch 22-gauge needle is inserted at the intersection point at right angles to the skin, and slightly medially. If the needle strikes the transverse process of L4, it is directed slightly more caudally and advanced until paraesthesiae are elicited (5–6 cm below skin surface). 40 ml of local anaesthetic are then injected.

Reference
Winnie A P 1991 Regional anaesthesia of the extremities. American Society of Anesthesiologists, Annual Refresher Course Lectures, J B Lippincott, USA

7

1.2   a) False   b) False   c) False   d) False   e) True

EXPLANATION

Nerve supply to the uterus:

Motor: sympathetic from T1–L2   } via paracervical plexus
parasympathetic from S2–S4

Sensory: sympathetic pathways via hypogastric plexus to T11-T12.

There are a number of agents which affect uterine tone:

1. Alpha-adrenergic receptor agonists increase tone and contraction, e.g. noradrenaline, methoxamine, metaraminol.
2. Beta-adrenergic receptor agonists, especially beta-2 agonists, decrease tone and contraction, e.g. adrenaline, salbutamol.
3. Oxytocin and ergometrine increase uterine contraction. Alcohol suppresses oxytocin secretion from the posterior portion of the pituitary gland.
4. Prostaglandins PGE_2 and PGF_2 increase uterine contractions.
5. Anaesthetic agents: volatile agents reduce uterine tone, the effect being dose related; intravenous agents, analgesics, neuromuscular blocking drugs and acetylcholinesterase inhibitors have no effect.
6. Other agents: acetylcholine, bradykinin, histamine and serotonin increase contraction; smooth muscle relaxants, e.g. nitrate and papaverine, cause cervical relaxation.

1.3   a) True   b) False   c) True   d) False   e) True

EXPLANATION

Definitions:

Coinduction. Use of two or more drugs to induce general anaesthesia.
Additive interaction. When the action of two drugs is equal to the sum of their effects (i.e. 1 + 1 = 2).

Synergistic interaction. When the combined effect of two drugs is greater than the sum of their effects (i.e. 1 + 1 > 2).

Antagonistic interaction. When the combined effect of two drugs is less than the sum of their effects (i.e. 1 + 1 < 2).

ED_{50}. The dose of drug that cures (in this case, dose that induces anaesthesia in) 50% of animals (as opposed to LD_{50}—the dose that kills 50% of animals).

Drug interactions can be studied by making isobolographic plots of drug potency. When two drugs are combined, the ED_{50} of one drug is plotted on the x-axis, the other drug on the y-axis and a line drawn between them. This line represents the combination of the two drugs if their effects are additive. Different combinations of the two drugs are given, the ED_{50} calculated, and lines plotted. If the resulting plot is below the additive line there is synergy; if it is above there is antagonism.

There is at present a trend of combining two or more drugs for induction of anaesthesia. Contrary to previous views, drug combination is not associated with increased risks of interactions at receptor sites, or delay in drug elimination. On the contrary, there may be advantages to drug combination. The most popular combination is propofol and midazolam. The advantages of combining these two drugs compared with using propofol as the sole induction agent are: improved pharmacodynamic effect; synergism of drugs, i.e. small dose of midazolam (or analgesic, e.g. alfentanil) reduces disproportionately the amount of propofol required; reduction in adverse reactions to the drugs because smaller doses are used, prevention of awareness in absence of premedication; and reduced costs because less propofol is used. The only disadvantage is that recovery is prolonged, but if no more than 2 mg of midazolam is administered in an adult, the delay in recovery is minimal and the combination of 2 mg of midazolam and propofol has been used successfully for day case anaesthesia. When midazolam and propofol are used for induction, a dose of 0.2 mg/kg of midazolam reduces the ED_{90} for propofol from 1.88 to 1.03 mg/kg.

1.4	a) False	b) True	c) False	d) False	e) False

EXPLANATION

Aetiology. Traditionally considered to be due to Gram-negative organisms, septic shock can also be caused by Gram-positive organisms, fungi, viruses or parasites. It can also follow non-infectious conditions, e.g. trauma, pancreatitis.

Pathogenesis. Endotoxin is released from Gram-negative bacteria, leading to numerous events. The hypovolaemia is due to arterial and venous dilatation and leakage of plasma into the extravascular space owing to increased vascular permeability. There is also platelet aggregation and granulocyte activation. Moreover, there is release of kinins, prostaglandins, endorphins and myocardial depressant agents. These agents affect the vasculature, plus a number of vital organs such as heart, kidneys, liver, lung and brain, resulting in multiple organ failure. The course of multiple organ failure is usually predictable, starting with lung damage, followed by hepatic, then intestinal and finally renal failure. Apart from granulocyte activation and release of kinins, prostaglandins, etc., multiple organ failure may be related to diminished tissue oxygenation, because the activated neutrophils cause cell damage so that oxygen delivery and consumption are abnormal. Furthermore, there may be a breakdown of the intestinal barrier causing intestinal bacteria to release endotoxins which contribute to multiple organ failure. Coagulation is also abnormal.

Clinical features. Hypovolaemia causes a refractory drop in blood pressure, and tachycardia. There is also peripheral vasodilatation and signs of infection: rapid respiration; high temperature; leucocytosis; and eventually multiple organ failure, usually commencing with lung damage (possibly adult respiratory distress syndrome) followed by hepatic, intestinal and renal failure. The myocardium is depressed with dilatation of ventricles, tachycardia, reduction in blood pressure (BP) and vascular resistance and increase in cardiac index. The haemopoietic system is also affected and coagulopathies are common.

Treatment. This involves treating the infection, plus respiratory and cardiovascular support, and treating metabolic changes and organ failure. The aims of treatment should be: to achieve a mean arterial pressure not less than 60 mmHg; pulmonary wedge pressure between 14 and 18 mmHg; haemoglobin above 16 g/100 ml; oxygen saturation above 92%; cardiac index above 4 l/min/m²; normal blood lactate (lactic acidosis should not be treated with bicarbonate; instead the cause of the acidosis should be treated).

Respiratory. In mild cases, hypoxaemia, hypocarbia and mild alkalosis may be treated with supplementary oxygen. In many cases intermittent positive-pressure ventilation (IPPV) is required, possibly with positive end-expiratory pressure (PEEP). Increasing FiO_2 levels may be required to increase SaO_2 above 90% but increasing FiO_2 towards 100% to achieve this can cause lung damage.

Cardiovascular. Reductions in left ventricular preload, vasodilatation and myocardial depression are all indications for use of vasopressors (e.g. dopamine, adrenaline, noradrenaline). Probably the best vasopressors to use are noradrenaline and dobutamine. A slow heart rate at the early stages carries a good prognosis, while a persistent hyperdynamic state is a bad sign.

Any renal/hepatic failure must also be treated, together with coagulation problems.

The use of phosphodiesterase inhibitors (e.g. enoximone), monoclonal antibodies, kinin antagonists or oxpentifylline, which reduces blood viscosity, is controversial.

Prognosis. Mortality 20–50%.

1.5 a) False b) False c) True d) True e) False

EXPLANATION

The caudal (sacral) epidural space is a triangular space which runs the length of the sacrum. The sacral hiatus is a triangular opening formed by the absence of the 5th, and possibly 4th, laminar arch and enables access to the sacral epidural space. The caudal space is bordered superiorly by the lumbar vertebral bodies, posteriorly by the laminae and laterally by the anterior and posterior sacral foramina. The contents include dural sac, filum terminale, sacral and coccygeal nerve roots, venous plexuses, fibrous and fatty tissue.

The sacral hiatus (volume 34 ml in the adult male) is covered by the sacrococcygeal ligament which is pierced by the 5th sacral and coccygeal nerves. It usually has a sacral cornu on each side. It is located at the apex of the equilateral triangle where the other two points of the triangle are the posterior superior iliac spines. Another way of locating the sacral hiatus is to place the tip of the index finger at the end of the coccyx; the sacral hiatus is 4–5 cm from this, usually at the level of the proximal interphalangeal joint.

A caudal block is easy to perform in children and is very useful for postoperative pain relief in circumcisions, hernias and orchidopexies. It is also relatively safe, but both intravenous injection causing acute local anaesthetic toxicity and intrathecal injection are possible; therefore aspiration is vital while injecting the local anaesthetic. In adults, caudals are much more difficult (obesity, unpredictable anatomy) but they are still useful for perineal operations (e.g. haemorrhoidectomy, transurethral resection of the prostate) and obstetrics-forceps delivery, episiotomies, continuous caudal block for labour, although this might block the perineal muscles and may delay labour.

Advantages of caudals are the relative safety and lack of hypotension. Disadvantages include the length of time for analgesia to develop (about 20 min with bupivacaine) and technical difficulty. Caudals are not very useful for operations above L1, because very high volumes are required for high blocks; infection is also more likely because of rectal proximity (it is possible to place the needle in the rectum and then redirect and inject into the caudal space).

1.6   a) False   b) False   c) True   d) True   e) False

EXPLANATION
Perioperative myocardial ischaemia causes a significant morbidity and mortality. Ischaemia is detected in about 20% of patients intraoperatively, compared to 40% postoperatively. It is therefore very important to detect the patients who are at risk and reduce the incidence, if possible. Perioperative risks include:

- A history of ischaemic heart disease.
- Congestive heart failure and left ventricular hypertrophy.
- Severe hypertension.
- Peripheral vascular disease.
- Patients having vascular operations.
- Advanced age.
- Limited exercise tolerance.
- Chronic renal failure.
- Digoxin therapy – digoxin and left ventricular hypertrophy can cause ECG changes which may obscure ischaemic changes.
- Stress – elevated adrenaline and noradrenaline levels cause coronary vasoconstriction; therefore any factors causing stress should be avoided, i.e. inadequate analgesia, postoperative shivering due to hypothermia, etc. Catecholamines also predispose to platelet aggregation and vasoconstriction, which can further lead to coronary thrombosis.
- Anaemia should also be avoided; haematocrit levels most protective against thrombosis are around 30%.

Detection of myocardial ischaemia
Electrocardiography
Preoperative changes. Preoperative ECG changes associated with myocardial ischaemia include arrhythmias, Q waves, ST elevation, or more likely depression, and T wave changes. A dysrhythmia on a preoperative ECG is a better indicator of postoperative myocardial ischaemia than the presence of ischaemic changes, i.e. ST, Q and T wave changes. A normal resting preoperative ECG does not exclude coronary artery disease, but it is likely that patients who do not develop ischaemic changes with an exercise ECG will not develop cardiac ischaemia postoperatively.
Intraoperative changes. Intraoperatively, ST depression does not necessarily indicate myocardial ischaemia. ST segment depression is quite common in intraoperative ECG monitors, where the frequency response is reduced to filter out distortion from muscle movement and electrical equipment.
Postoperative changes. T wave changes are not uncommon even in the absence of myocardial ischaemia, therefore ECG diagnosis will have to depend on ST/Q wave changes.
Pulmonary pressures. Myocardial ischaemia causes rises in pulmonary artery pressures, but these rises can occur with increases in afterload; so increases in pulmonary capillary wedge pressures are not valuable in diagnosing myocardial ischaemia.
Enzyme changes. Lactate dehydrogenase (LDH) and creatinine phosphokinase (CPK) are used frequently to diagnose myocardial infraction, but postoperatively LDH levels are raised after biliary surgery and red cell haemolysis, while CPK rises after muscle trauma. CPK is more diagnostic than LDH, and if CPK remains elevated 18 hours after surgery, myocardial infarction is likely.

Measures to reduce perioperative ischaemia

1. Antianginal drugs: prophylactic use of nitrates, calcium blockers or beta blockers to reduce cardiac work and perioperative tachycardia; also reduction of use of potent vasoactive drugs.
2. Adequate analgesia/avoidance of stress: i.e. high-dose narcotics (patient-controlled analgesia or infusions) but especially epidural analgesia which also has the advantage of reducing the hypercoaguable state induced by surgery.
3. Others:
- Non-steroidal anti-inflammatory agents, besides providing effective analgesia, reduce thrombosis by their antiplatelet effect.
- Alpha-2 agonists (e.g. clonidine) cause a reduction in noradrenaline release from presynaptic terminals, producing sedation and analgesia. Clonidine also suppresses the normal increase in postoperative fibrinogen levels, and reverses platelet aggregation. All these effects are likely to be associated with a reduced incidence of myocardial ischaemia.
- Avoidance of anaemia and hypothermia.

1.7   a) True   b) True   c) True   d) True   e) True

EXPLANATION

Postoperative relief with epidural analgesia is superior to any other form of postoperative analgesia and is accompanied by a reduction in postoperative complications, namely:

1. *Stress*. Stress stimulates the sympathetic system, and surgical trauma releases stress response mediators (cytokines) into the circulation. Both these factors can have disastrous effects on cardiac, coagulation and immune systems. Epidural analgesia with local anaesthetics (less so with epidural opiates) reduces considerably the changes associated with stress.

2. *Cardiac*. Cardiac problems account for a significant amount of postoperative morbidity and mortality. Postoperative pain activates the sympathetic system causing coronary vasoconstriction and increases myocardial oxygen demand, thus predisposing to myocardial ischaemia, arrhythmias and possibly 'silent' infarcts. Thoracic epidurals block the sympathetic supply to the heart (T1–T4) and increase myocardial blood flow, thus reducing postoperative ischaemia.

3. *Coagulation*. Major surgery is associated with a hypercoaguable state which extends into the postoperative period. Epidurals and spinals with local anaesthetics reduce the incidence of deep vein thrombosis and pulmonary embolism by two to three times.

4. *Pulmonary*. Thoracic and upper abdominal operations are associated with significant postoperative pulmonary dysfunction including reduction in vital capacity, pulmonary collapse and infections. The incidence of pulmonary complications is markedly reduced with effective epidural analgesia, and more so than with patient-controlled analgesia.

5. *Gastrointestinal system*. Postoperative ileus is common, probably because abdominal pain inhibits intestinal motility. Moreover, sympathetic stimulation induced by stress further inhibits bowel activity. Postoperative thoracic epidural analgesia has been found to be associated with a reduced incidence of ileus.

6. *Immune function.* Immunity, both cellular and humoral, is suppressed for several days after surgery and can predispose to postoperative infections and possibly encourage postoperative tumour growth. The reason for the immunosuppression is unclear, but it is probably due to the fact that many mediators of the stress response suppress immunity. General anaesthesia exacerbates this by depression of the immune system. Epidural analgesia has been shown to preserve immunity.

1.8   a) True   b) False   c) True   d) True   e) False

EXPLANATION
Adrenergic receptors were originally differentiated into alpha and beta receptors. Subsequently beta receptors were subdivided into beta-1 and beta-2, while more recently alpha receptors have been divided into alpha-1 and alpha-2. Clonidine is an alpha-2 adrenergic agonist. Adrenergic agonists can be grouped into three classes: phenylethylamines (e.g. alpha-methylnoradrenaline); imidazolines (e.g. clonidine); and oxaloazephines (e.g. azepexole).

Pharmacology
Central nervous system. Alpha-2 agonists exert a central sedative effect and reduce anxiety; they are also potent analgesics. This property has been used in a number of clinical situations—in premedication to promote sedation; during induction and intubation to reduce anaesthetic requirements (because the MAC of anaesthetic agents is reduced); and for haemodynamic stability during intubation. Postoperative analgesic requirements may also be diminished by intraoperative use of these agents. Alpha-2 agonists have also been used to reduce the physiological and psychological symptoms following opiate withdrawal.

Analgesia. Alpha-2 agonists are powerful analgesics which probably exert this action at several sites including release of substance P. Every route has been tried to provide analgesia. Orally, clonidine is absorbed fully, reaches a peak plasma level within 60–90 minutes, and has a half-life of 9–12 hours. It has been used extensively for postoperative analgesia by the intrathecal and especially by the epidural route. Epidural clonidine (100–900 µg) produces dose-dependent analgesia for about 5 hours, without any sensory or motor block. The higher doses, however, are accompanied by hypotension, bradycardia and sedation. Because of this, epidural clonidine has been combined with supplements of local anaesthetic or opiates, thus reducing side-effects. Systemic clonidine has also been used for postoperative analgesia via intramuscular and intravenous routes (including intravenous infusions) but systemic alpha-2 agonists can lead to unacceptable bradycardia, hypotension and sedation.

Alpha-2 agonists have been employed in chronic pain situations especially epidurally, e.g. management of cancer pain, sympathetic dystrophy and neuropathic pain.

Cardiovascular system. Alpha-2 agonists produce both arterial and venous vasoconstriction including coronary and cerebral vasoconstriction. This is offset by reducing sympathetic outflow, and it is this latter feature which allowed clonidine to be used as an antihypertensive. The disadvantage of this is the intense sedation produced. Apart from hypotension, bradycardia is another problem. This should be treated with atropine and not ephedrine which potentiates the pressor effect of alpha-2 agonists. Clonidine has also been shown to reduce oxygen consumption and reduce postoperative shivering during anaesthetic recovery.

Coagulation. Alpha-2 blockers have also been shown to reverse platelet aggregation, and suppress the normal increase in postoperative fibrinogen levels, and may therefore reduce the incidence of postoperative thrombosis.

1.9   **a) True**   **b) False**   **c) True**   **d) True**   **e) False**

EXPLANATION
See Table 1.2.

Table 1.2   Actions of sympathomimetic drugs on the cardiovascular system

Drug	Actions*	Heart rate	Cardiac output	Blood pressure	Pulmonary artery pressure	Total peripheral resistance
Isoprenaline	Beta-1 and beta-2	++	++	−	−	− −
Dobutamine	Beta-1 and alpha	+	+	+/−	−	−
Dopamine	Beta-1, alpha and on dopamine (D) receptors	+	+	+	+	+
Adrenaline	Beta-1, beta-2 and alpha	+	++	+	+/−	+/−
Noradrenaline	Beta-1, and alpha	+/−	+0	++	++	++
Ephedrine	Beta-1, beta-2 and alpha	+	+0	+	+	+
Dopexamine	Beta-1 and beta-2 (no alpha action or on dopamine receptors)	+	+	+/−	−	−
Methoxamine	Alpha (no beta-1 or beta-2)	−	−	++	++	++
Phentolamine	Alpha blocker	+	+	− −	−	− especially arterial
Nitroglycerine		+/−		− −	+/−	− vasodilatation especially venous
Nitroprusside	Direct vasodilator	+	+	− −	− −	− especially arterial
Hydralazine	Direct vasodilator	+	+	− −	+/−	− arterial
Calcium blocker		+/−	+/−	−	+/−	− arterial
Ace inhibitors		0	+	−	−	− especially arterial
Digoxin	−	−	+/−	+/−	+/−	+/−
Calcium		0	+	+	+	+

*Beta-1 action: increase in chronotropic and inotropic action on heart; beta-2 action: peripheral vasodilatation, bronchodilatation; alpha action: peripheral vasoconstriction.

1.10   a) False   b) True   c) True   d) True   e) True

EXPLANATION

Tissue oxygenation is adequate when the oxygen supplied is at a rate sufficient to maintain aerobic metabolism. Oxygen content (CaO_2) is the volume (ml) of oxygen carried in 100 ml of blood and is normally 20 ml per 100 ml blood.

$CaO_2 = Hb \times 1.37 \times SaO_2 + (0.0034 \times PaO_2)$, i.e. dissolved oxygen level
1.37 = ml of O_2 carried by 1 g of saturated Hb
0.0034 = ml of O_2 in 100 ml blood per mmHg

The amount of dissolved oxygen is insignificantly small, but if a patient breathes hyperbaric oxygen and has a PaO_2 of 1500 mmHg (instead of the normal 90 mmHg), the dissolved oxygen would contribute significantly to the oxygen content.

Oxygen delivery is oxygen content × cardiac output = 1000 ml/min, or oxygen content × cardiac index (ml oxygen/min/m^2) = 600 ml/min/m^2.

Oxygen content is 20 ml/100 ml blood. Average tissue consumption from arterial blood is 5 ml/100 ml. Therefore venous blood is left with 15 ml/100 ml plasma, corresponding to a saturation of 75%. Body oxygen consumption = ($CaO_2 - CvO_2$) × cardiac output, which is approximately 250 ml/min, and since oxygen availability is 1000 ml/min, 750 ml/min of oxygen is not used.

Oxygen consumption is increased considerably with exercise, shivering, hyperthermia and sepsis. It is also increased in neonates, which is why babies get desaturated so rapidly. It is reduced in hypothermia and by anaesthetics. There is no single variable which will indicate adequate tissue oxygenation; however, measurements of oxygen delivery, oxygen consumption, PaO_2, haemoglobin saturation, mixed venous oxygen tension (which falls if consumption is increased) and acid-base balance (because if tissue oxygenation is inadequate lactic acidosis follows), all give good reflections of oxygen consumption.

1.11   a) True   b) True   c) False   d) False   e) False

EXPLANATION

Cerebral blood flow is 700 ml/min in a 70-kg person. The brain receives 15% of the cardiac output and consumes 20% of the oxygen. Cerebral blood flow has a direct effect on intracranial pressure. Intracranial pressure can be measured with catheters in the ventricle, subarachnoid or epidural space.

Intracranial pressure depends upon four factors: brain bulk; blood volume (i.e. cerebral blood flow); cerebrospinal fluid (CSF) volume; and intracranial pathology.

1. Brain bulk can be reduced with 20% mannitol because of osmotic dehydration. Frusemide can also be of use.

2. Blood volume, i.e. cerebral blood flow, is influenced by:
- Autoregulation – there is little change in cerebral blood flow over the mean systemic blood pressure (BP) range of 60–160 mmHg; it is reduced below these levels.
- Arterial O_2 – high PaO_2 has little effect on cerebral flow, PaO_2 below 50 mmHg causes vasodilatation.
- Arterial $PaCO_2$ – hypocapnia causes vasoconstriction and reduction in cerebral blood flow (CBF); hypercapnia causes vasodilatation and increase in CBF.

Between 25 and 55 mmHg, CBF changes by 3% per mmHg. Hypocapnia should not go beyond 25 mmHg because the accompanying cerebral vasoconstriction can lead to hypoxaemia.
- Metabolism – increase in metabolism (e.g. hyperthermia) increases CBF; reductions (e.g. hypothermia) reduce CBF.
- Drugs – barbiturates, etomidate and propofol all decrease cerebral metabolic rate and thus reduce CBF. Ketamine increases cerebral metabolism and causes sympathetic stimulation and hypertension both of which lead to increased intracranial pressure. Halothane increases CBF because of the accompanying vasodilatation and should not be used in patients with raised intracranial pressure. Isoflurane, desflurane and sevoflurane have no effects on CBF at low MACs.

3. CSF volume – hypertonic saline and mannitol reduce production of CSF.

4. Intracranial pathology – haematomas (epidural, subdural, intracerebral), tumours, abscesses, etc. causing brain compression. They should be surgically treated urgently to reduce intercranial pressure.

1.12   a) True   b) False   c) False   d) False   e) False

EXPLANATION

Apart from hepatitis A and B there is a third common form of hepatitis – hepatitis C (formerly called non-A, non-B hepatitis). Like hepatitis B, it is blood-borne and hepatitis C now accounts for about 90% of post-transfusion hepatitis. In the past, diagnosis was made by exclusion in a patient who has abnormal liver function tests. Now, however, a hepatitis C virus has been identified and antibodies to this virus have been developed; therefore screening for hepatitis C is now available in modern transfusion departments. Vaccination with hepatitis B vaccine does not protect against hepatitis C; hepatitis C vaccine has recently been developed.

The incubation period varies from 2–26 weeks and, as mentioned above, most cases follow transfusion of blood or blood products. Sexual transmission is less common with hepatitis C than with B and it is very rare to contract it from needle-sticks. The clinical features are similar to other forms of hepatitis, but it is usually not a severe form and jaundice is less common. Carrier states of hepatitis C are frequent and infection with the virus can lead to chronic hepatitis and cirrhosis.

The risk of theatre personnel contracting hepatitis C is much less than with hepatitis B, but precautions (wearing of gloves etc.) to avoid blood contamination should be undertaken.

1.13   a) False   b) True   c) True   d) False   e) False

EXPLANATION
See Table 1.3.

Table 1.3   Comparisons between midazolam and diazepam

	Midazolam	Diazepam
Action	Acts on benzodiazepine receptors. Anxiolytic, sedative and anticonvulsant. Anterograde amnesia (i.e. amnesia after administration) but no retrograde amnesia	Same but more prolonged action
Intravenous injection	Thrombosis/thrombophlebitis unlikely	Thrombosis/thrombophlebitis; large vein should be used
Duration	Elimination half-life 2.4 h in fit adults; 5.6 h in elderly. Dose should be reduced in aged	Elimination half-life 20 h in fit adults; 80–90 h in elderly. Dose reduced in aged
Metabolism	Liver 50% and extra-hepatic. Metabolites cause no sedation	Liver metabolism, into desmethyldiazepam which has sedative action
Side-effects	Cardiovascular, respiratory and psychomotor depression	Same but more prolonged
Reversal	Flumazenil by a competitive inhibition at benzodiazepine receptors	Flumazenil. Especially with diazepam, re-sedation may occur because the duration of action of flumazenil is much shorter than that of diazepam

1.14   a) True   b) True   c) False   d) False   e) False

EXPLANATION

Drugs that influence coagulation can be divided into a number of groups:

1. Drugs that inhibit coagulation:
- Warfarin prevents vitamin K production so that factors II, VII, IX and X are not produced. For effective anticoagulation prothrombin time (PT) should be 1.5-2 times normal level; INR (international normalized ratio) 2-3 times normal for elective surgery. Warfarin should be stopped 48-72 hours prior to surgery. It can be reversed with vitamin K.
- Heparin binds to platelets and inhibits coagulation factors II, IX, X, XI and XII. Its clinical effects are measured by the thrombin time (TT), activated partial thromboplastin time (APPT) or activated clotting time (ACT). For adequate anticoagulation for vascular surgery etc., ACT should be twice baseline values. Heparin can be in the unfractionated or low molecular form. Compared to unfractionated heparin, low molecular weight heparin binds less to platelets and selectively inhibits factor X. It is less likely to induce bleeding, but maintains the same efficacy on deep vein thrombosis prophylaxis. It is also more resistant to reversal with protamine. Heparin can be reversed with protamine, but the

protamine dose should not exceed 1 mg for every 100 units of heparin because over-neutralization can increase bleeding.

2. Finbrinolytic (thrombolytic) drugs used to break down thrombi or emboli, e.g. streptokinase. These drugs stimulate breakdown of plasminogen into plasmin and can lead to hypofibrinoginaemia; if the fibrinogen level is below 100 mg/100 ml, 10–20 units of cryoprecipitate should be given.

3. Platelet inhibitors – aspirin and non-steroidal anti-inflammatory drugs (NSAIDs) both impair platelet aggregation. However, when aspirin is stopped this effect lasts for a further 10 days, while with NSAIDs the effect ceases once the drug is cleared. Therefore aspirin is more likely to cause protracted surgical bleeding than NSAIDs. There are a number of drugs that cause platelet function abnormalities but are rarely significant. These include aspirin and NSAIDs, betalactam antibiotics, calcium channel blockers, beta blockers (propranolol), quinidine, vasodilators (e.g. nitroprusside, nitroglycerine), anticoagulants and antifibrinolytics, local anaesthetics, psychotropic drugs.

4. Drugs that cause thrombocytopenia. Thrombocytopenia rarely causes problematical surgical bleeding until the platelet count drops below 50 000/ml. Drugs that can cause thrombocytopenia include antibiotics, diuretics, gold salts, heparin, protamine, quinidine.

5. Drugs that enhance clotting – antifibrinolytic drugs. These inhibit conversion of plasminogen into plasmin, e.g. aprotonin, which is a natural antifibrinolytic, and epsilon-aminocaproic acid and tranexamic acid, which are synthetic antifibrinolytics. These agents have been used with variable success in operations where excessive bleeding can be a problem, e.g. prostatectomies, liver transplants, on haemophiliacs, etc. They have also been used in cardiopulmonary bypass where they appear to protect platelets and reduce postoperative bleeding. Although these agents increase fibrinogen levels and hypofibrinoginaemia is one of the features in disseminated intravascular coagulation (DIC), they should not be used in this condition as they can cause widespread thrombosis.

| 1.15 | a) True | b) False | c) False | d) True | e) True |

EXPLANATION

Disseminated intravascular coagulation (DIC) is a coagulation disorder occurring in critically ill patients where activation of the clotting system results in consumption of coagulation factors including platelets and overactivation of the fibrinolytic system. In the past, it was felt that microvascular thrombosis was a predominant feature, but in most cases thrombosis does not occur, and heparin should not be administered, as it may increase the bleeding. Predisposing illnesses include Gram-negative septicaemia, trauma, malignancy, burns, transfusion reactions, embolism, drug interactions, and a number of conditions in pregnancy (pre-eclampsia, amniotic fluid embolism, abortions, placental abruption). Clinically there is widespread oozing from wounds and in severe cases bleeding from gut or lung. The patient is shocked, hypoxic and acidotic. Coagulation screening shows increased prothrombin time, thrombocytopenia, and reduced fibrinogen levels. The coagulation problems are treated with fresh frozen plasma, platelets if thrombocytopenia is present, and cryoprecipitate when fibrinogen levels are low. The underlying cause of the DIC should be treated (e.g. infection, placental retention), while supportive measures are instituted, e.g. treatment of respiratory problems, electrolyte and acid-base imbalance, etc.

1.16   a) True   b) False   c) False   d) True   e) False

EXPLANATION

In epileptics it is wise to avoid drugs which cause clinical excitatory movements or increased EEG activity. Of the induction agents, both thiopentone and ketamine have anticonvulsant properties. Methohexitone and etomidate produce excitatory movements in some cases, and fits have occurred with their use. Propofol has been associated with odd incidents of myoclonus, convulsions, opisthotonus, though no cortical excitatory changes occur on the EEG. It probably should therefore not be used in epileptics.

As regards volatile agents, enflurane should be avoided because it increases EEG activity, especially with deep anaesthesia, and a number of cases of convulsions have been reported.

High-dose opioids can occasionally cause rigidity, fits and myoclonic movements. Pethidine is probably the worst, especially in renal failure, because it is broken down into norpethidine which has convulsant properties.

Problems associated with long-term antiepileptic therapy

1. Patients on long-term anticonvulsant therapy have been shown to be resistant to a number of non-depolarizing relaxants including vecuronium, atracurium and pancuronium.

2. Side-effects of anticonvulsants. Many anticonvulsants cause liver enzyme induction, and can therefore accelerate the metabolism of other drugs. Antiepileptics may also be associated with platelet abnormalities, causing thrombocytopenia and excessive bleeding, megaloblastic anaemias, and liver dysfunction.

1.17   a) True   b) False   c) True   d) True   e) True

EXPLANATION

The major risk to the fetus during surgery on a pregnant woman is intrauterine hypoxia or asphyxia. Since fetal oxygenation is dependent on maternal oxygen levels, it is important that anaesthesia should not prejudice maternal oxygenation or uteroplacental perfusion.

Maternal oxygenation. Mild maternal hypoxia is well tolerated by the fetus because fetal haemoglobin has a high affinity for oxygen; however, severe maternal hypoxia can cause fetal hypoxia and brain damage.

Uteroplacental perfusion. During anaesthesia reduction of uteroplacental perfusion can occur from:

1. Maternal hypotension:

- Haemorrhage and hypovolaemia.
- Deep levels of anaesthesia. Low-dose volatile agents maintain uterine perfusion because although there may be some hypotension this is compensated by the uterine vasodilator effects of the agents. However higher concentrations (2 MAC) for prolonged periods can cause marked hypotension and decreased placental flow.
- High spinals or epidurals causing sympathetic blockade.
- Acid-base changes. Mild respiratory acidosis is unimportant, but severe respiratory acidosis causes myocardial depression and hypotension.
- Respiratory (and metabolic) alkalosis shifts the maternal dissociation curve to the left and causes umbilical artery constriction. Moreover, the positive pressure ventilation causing the alkalosis can reduce venous return and thus cause hypotension. Therefore hyperventilation should be avoided during pregnancy.

2. Alpha-acting sympathomimetics. Sympathomimetic drugs with predominantly alpha effects cause uterine vasoconstriction (e.g. phenylephrine; high-dose dopamine); likewise light anaesthesia and preoperative anxiety increase circulating catecholamines which impair uterine flow. Ketamine is a sympathomimetic agent which increases uterine tone and causes uterine vasoconstriction. Toxic doses of local anaesthetics have the same effect.

1.18   a) False   b) False   c) False   d) True   e) True

EXPLANATION

Selecting appropriate patients for day case anaesthesia can be difficult. For ASA I and II physical status, patients are often asked to fill in a written questionnaire to identify risk factors. In many hospitals, the preoperative evaluation is done on the day of surgery and relies on the surgeon to 'screen' patients when seen in surgical clinic. This system can lead to a high percentage of postponements with problem patients. For ASA III and IV patients preoperative anaesthetic clinics are probably the best option. In healthy patients minimal preoperative laboratory screening is necessary (e.g. Hb, urinalysis) but patients with systemic disease will need further tests (ECG, CXR, electrolytes).

Day patient surgery need not be restricted to young healthy patients. Geriatric patients and patients in ASA group III and IV may be considered so long as their systemic disease is well controlled preoperatively. The same rule applies to morbidly obese patients without systemic disease. Patients who should not be done as day cases include unstable ASA groups III and IV, the morbidly obese with systemic disease, patients with a history of severe anaesthetic problems (e.g. malignant hyperpyrexia), insulin-dependent diabetics, patients with coagulopathies or haemoglobinopathies, and patients with social problems (e.g. nobody to look after them at home).

In the last 10 years a number of anaesthetic agents have been introduced which shorten the recovery period and reduce the incidence of nausea and vomiting postoperatively. Propofol is the best induction agent available because of its rapid elimination and low incidence of nausea, vomiting and drowsiness, compared for example with thiopentone where these side-effects can be significant even 5 hours after induction. Nausea and vomiting should be avoided if possible in day cases because these symptoms might prevent them going home. Avoidance of long-acting opiates and use of ondansetron will reduce postoperative emesis. Ondansetron is preferable to droperidol because the incidence of drowsiness and extrapyramidal symptoms is less. Isoflurane is associated with a fairly rapid recovery, but desflurane and sevoflurane are even better. If a muscle relaxant is required, mivacurium has been found to be very effective. A dose of 0.08 mg/kg produces a maximal block in 4 minutes with full recovery in 25 minutes. Mivacurium infusion gives a more predictable and rapid recovery than suxamethonium infusion.

1.19   a) True   b) True   c) True   d) True   e) False

EXPLANATION
Pre-eclampsia occurs in about 5% of pregnancies; eclampsia in about 0.5% and accounts for 20–30% of maternal mortalities. Once affected by severe pre-eclampsia, each succeeding pregnancy increases the risk of complications.

Pre-eclampsia is the development of hypertension with proteinuria, oedema or both occurring after the 20th week of pregnancy. There is hypertension if the systolic pressure rises by 30 mmHg or the diastolic by 15 mmHg or there is a systolic/diastolic of 140/90. Proteinuria is significant if it is greater than 300 mg/l in 24 hours. Oedema is a collection of fluid in the non-dependent parts of the body including laryngeal oedema, and is due to water and salt retention. Eclampsia implies organ damage and occurs when blood pressure is 160/110 while at bed rest; there may also be renal damage, cerebral manifestations with EEG changes due to cerebral oedema (visual problems, headache, fits), liver damage, haemolysis, increased bleeding time, thrombocytopenia (increased platelet adherence), pulmonary oedema. Severe pre-eclampsia and eclampsia are associated with high maternal and fetal mortality. The problems with eclampsia are due to the presence of circulating vasoconstricting agents (angiotensin, thromboxane) causing uterine vasospasm, and vasodilating substances (prostaglandins).

The standard treatment of pre-eclampsia/eclampsia is hydralazine/labetolol to lower the blood pressure or magnesium sulphate which attenuates uterine vascular response to vasopressors. Phenytoin can also be employed as an anticonvulsant and has the added advantage of causing uterine vasodilatation. Some practitioners believe that epidural analgesia is hazardous because of the possible coagulation problems in eclampsia and, moreover, if epidural hypotension requires the use of vasopressors, maternal and fetal mortality may be increased. In practice, epidural analgesia is acceptable if there are no bleeding problems, and blood volume and blood pressure are controlled. If general anaesthesia is employed, intubation may be difficult because of laryngeal oedema and may be accompanied by severe hypertension. This can be attenuated with hydralazine; nitroprusside or labetolol.

EXPLANATION

Orbital regional anaesthesia requires block of the ophthalmic branch of the trigeminal nerve (IV) to produce globe and medial conjunctiva anaesthesia, and block of the oculomotor nerves (III, IV, VI) to block the eye muscles. Suitable local anaesthesia can be achieved with a peribulbar or retrobulbar block. A retrobulbar block (but not peribulbar) misses the peripheral conjunctiva which is supplied by the lacrimal, frontal and infraorbital nerves. The retrobulbar or peribulbar block is achieved with local anaesthetic and hyaluronidase which helps the local anaesthetic to spread along the connective tissue to reach the oculomotor nerves. (This is easier to achieve in the elderly than the young because of more dense connective tissue in the latter.)

Before conducting the retrobulbar/peribulbar block an injection of 1 ml local anaesthetic is required in the inferotemporal quadrant (i.e. below and lateral to the lateral orbit). The injection is made via either the transconjunctival route or the transcutaneous (through the eyelid) route. With the former technique, the lower eyelid is retracted with a finger and the needle enters the conjunctiva tangentially to the globe. The landmark for the transcutaneous route is the same, but the eyelid does not need to be retracted.

Retrobulbar block

A retrobulbar block requires only one injection of a small volume of local anaesthetic, has a quick onset of action, and gives satisfactory motor and sensory blockade. However, the facial nerve is not anaesthetized, and this may be required to achieve akinesia of the eyelids.

The eye should be looking straight ahead, because the optic nerve is safest in this position. The conjunctiva is first anaesthetized with a few drops of 1% amethocaine or 2% lignocaine. A 3.5-cm, 25-gauge needle is inserted at the lower temporal orbit rim, very close to the bone. It is directed backwards and parallel to the orbit floor for a distance of 1.5 cm when the tip of the needle should be just past half of the anteroposterior length of the globe. If the needle is advanced further, it should hit the lateral wall of the orbital bone. The needle is then directed slightly upwards and medially, aiming for an imaginary point behind the globe on a line formed by the pupil and macula. The globe should be watched all the time to detect globe rotation if the sclera is punctured by the needle. The needle should not be inserted for more than 2.5 cm and 4 ml of local anaesthetic with hyaluronidase are injected very slowly.

If the facial nerve needs to be blocked, this is best done as it exits the skull through the stylomastoid foramen. In the O'Brien method, the patient is asked to open and close the mouth to identify the condyle of the mandible in front of the ear. The needle is inserted perpendicularly until it strikes bone, and 2 ml of local anaesthetic injected, with a further 1 ml as the needle is withdrawn. In the Van Lint method, the needle is inserted 1 cm lateral to the lateral canthus of the eye, and 4 ml anaesthetic injected towards the upper and lower eyelids.

Peribulbar block

A peribulbar block requires at least two injections, but a facial block is not required. It takes longer to have effect (thus bicarbonate is sometimes added to speed onset), and requires larger volumes than a retrobulbar block; however, incidence of complications is less.

The technique is the same but the local anaesthetic is not injected behind the globe, but around it. The needle (25 gauge, 2.5 cm) is inserted at the same inferotemporal site, and 10 ml of local anaesthetic is injected slowly around the globe, just anterior to the point where the needle strikes the lateral wall of the orbit, at a depth of 2.5 cm. The globe should be soft, move freely and there should be no proptosis. If there is increased tension in the orbit or globe, one should stop the injection. A second injection will almost certainly be necessary on the nasal side medial to the caruncle, where a further 5 ml are injected at a depth of 1.5-2 cm, with the needle pointing straight backwards parallel to the medial wall. Further injections may be required through the upper eyelid at the nasal and temporal sites at the level of the medial and lateral margins of the iris.

Complications
Peribulbar block is safer than retrobulbar.

1. Globe penetration or perforation. This is the most serious complication and is more likely in myopic eyes as they are thinner and longer. The incidence is about 0.1% or less. If perforation occurs, there is resistance, pain, loss of vision, hypotonia or vitreous haemorrhage. Perforation can be avoided by directing the needle towards the orbital margin.

2. Retrobulbar haemorrhage – about 1–3% incidence with retrobulbar blocks. It is more likely in the elderly and if the patient is on anticoagulants or aspirin and NSAIDs. Retrobulbar haemorrhage causes increasing intraocular pressure with tight eyelids and proptosis and periorbital haematoma. The retinal artery or optic nerve may be compressed, in which case decompression surgery is required.

3. Optic nerve damage. This can be due to direct needle damage or retrobulbar haemorrhage and can lead to partial or total loss of vision. The local anaesthetic is injected into the optic sheath into the CSF. There may be loss of vision, drowsiness, vomiting, respiratory depression, cardiac arrest. Correct retrobulbar injection can block the optic nerve leading to a loss in light perception.

4. The oculocardiac reflex is abolished by a successful block; therefore the patient should be monitored for bradycardia.

5. Minor haemorrhage and conjunctival oedema.

Sub-Tenon's injection
This blocks the long and short ciliary nerves and the ciliary ganglion and provides anaesthesia to the cornea, iris and ciliary body, while preserving the optic nerve, and avoiding the complications associated with retrobulbar/peribulbar blocks. It can be used for cataract surgery, corneal transplantation, adult squint repair and retinal and glaucoma surgery. A 30-gauge, 1.25-cm needle is inserted in the superotemporal quadrant of the globe 5-15 mm from the limbal margin into the sub-Tenon's space, and 2 ml local anaesthetic with hyaluronidase injected.

2.1 In the flow-volume loop in Figure 2.1:

a) Point 'A' represents peak expiratory flow rate
b) The 'loop' below the horizontal volume line represents inspiration
c) Point 'B' represents the residual volume
d) Line 'C' represents forced vital capacity
e) The dashed loop is characteristic of upper airway obstruction

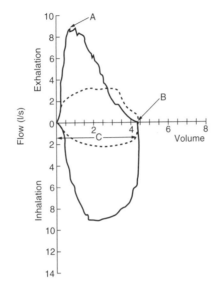

Fig 2.1 Flow–volume loop.

2.2 When deciding upon preoperative tests:

a) A preoperative chest X-ray should be done on an asymptomatic patient of 50
b) Routine 6-monthly X-rays in smokers over the age of 50 are very useful in detecting early carcinoma of the bronchus
c) Preoperative electrocardiography should be done on a asymptomatic patient above the age of 70
d) Serum electrolytes and blood glucose should be measured preoperatively on a patient on prolonged steroid therapy
e) Haemoglobin levels should be done on all females of child-bearing age

2.3 Drugs which produce elevated levels of the following cause analgesia:

a) 5-hydroxytryptamine (serotonin)
b) Substance P
c) Noradrenaline
d) Gamma-aminobutyric acid
e) Prostaglandins

25

2.4 Prostaglandins:

a) Are long chain fatty acids
b) Have anti-inflammatory action and reduce platelet aggregation
c) Usually cause vasoconstriction
d) Can be used to suppress premature uterine contractions in labour
e) May be useful in treating asthma

2.5 In the autonomic system:

a) The parasympathetic system is transmitted in cranial nerves and sacral fibres from the spinal cord
b) Parasympathetic effects are identical to those of acetylcholine
c) Postganglionic sympathetic fibres release catecholamines, except at sweat and adrenal glands, where acetylcholine is released
d) Sympathetic effects are more localized than parasympathetic actions
e) Parasympathetic stimulation increases bladder emptying; sympathetic stimulation reduces it

2.6 With regard to histamine and allergy:

a) Histamine (H_1) receptors are limited to the skin and respiratory mucosa, while H_2 receptors are limited to the gut
b) The decrease in peripheral vascular resistance seen in allergic reactions is due to activation of H_1 receptors but not of H_2 receptors
c) Histamine causes chronotropic and inotropic effects on the heart
d) An allergic reaction is more likely to manifest itself as bronchospasm than cardiovascular collapse
e) Morphine is more likely to cause histamine release than fentanyl

2.7 With regard to blood glucose:

a) Increasing the level by administration of glucose is beneficial in patients with cerebral damage
b) Prolonged hypoglycaemia in neonates can lead to neurological damage
c) Hypoglycaemia is common after major surgery if no intravenous glucose is given during the operation
d) Levels rise during pregnancy
e) Levels are increased with prolonged steroid therapy

2.8 Of the intravenous induction agents:

a) Ketamine is contraindicated in asthma
b) The pain on injection of propofol is due to the propylene glycol in its formulation
c) Propofol is an alkylphenol agent in water with soya oil, glycerol and egg extract
d) Apart from the barbiturates all the other induction agents are safe in porphyria
e) Cardiovascular depression is less with midazolam induction than with ketamine induction

2.9 Features of etomidate include:

a) The induction agent least likely to cause allergic reaction because it causes no histamine release
b) Incidence of nausea and vomiting very low
c) Inhibits steroid synthesis and increases antidiuretic hormone release
d) Hangover on recovery is almost as bad as with thiopentone
e) Causes minimal venous irritation

2.10 Premalignant conditions/factors include:

a) Oesophagitis for carcinoma of the oesophagus
b) Colonic polyps for carcinoma of the colon
c) Smoking for adenocarcinoma of the bronchus
d) Liver cirrhosis for primary liver cell carcinoma (hepatoma)
e) Crohn's disease of the colon for carcinoma of the colon

2.11 Metabolic responses to stress are such that:

a) An initial decrease in energy metabolism is followed by increased energy expenditure
b) There is an initial decrease in insulin levels followed by increased levels
c) Cortisol, catecholamines, glycogen and growth hormone are increased
d) Metabolic acidosis occurs
e) Large amounts of glucose should be given in the acute stages of trauma

2.12 In a critically ill patient the parameters used to determine the APACHE II score include:

a) Alveolar-arterial oxygen gradient
b) Intracranial pressure
c) Glasgow coma score
d) Haemoglobin
e) Serum sodium and potassium

2.13 A chest X-ray:

a) Should be performed preoperatively on every patient above 50
b) Taken with inadequate inflation can cause increased opacity of the lung fields
c) Which is normal, shows the right lobe of the diaphragm lying at the 6th rib anteriorly and about 2 cm higher than the left
d) Is useful in assessing lung function
e) Of a normal-sized heart shows it occupying less than 50% of the chest width

2.14 **Antihypertensive drug actions include:**

a) Clonidine reduces blood pressure by its agonist activity on alpha-1 adrenoceptors
b) Diltiazem is an angiotensin converting enzyme (ACE) inhibitor
c) ACE inhibitors are most useful in treating hypertensives when the renin levels are elevated
d) Nifedipine drops blood pressure by acting as a calcium channel entry blocker
e) Hydralazine reduces blood pressure by a direct action on vascular smooth muscle

2.15 **Minimum alveolar concentration:**

a) Is a reflection of the potency of the anaesthetic agent
b) Is increased with obesity
c) Is increased in pregnancy
d) Is decreased with hypoxia, hypercarbia and acidosis
e) Is higher in males than in females

2.16 **The administration of sodium bicarbonate to treat metabolic acidosis:**

a) Is imperative in resuscitation during all cardiac arrests
b) Can cause intraventricular haemorrhage in a neonate
c) Produces an increase in blood pH that mirrors the rise in cerebrospinal fluid pH
d) Improves tissue oxygenation
e) Can cause hypernatraemia and hypokalaemia

2.17 **In diabetic ketoacidosis:**

a) Presentation may be as an acute abdomen
b) Bicarbonate is a prime indication to treat the metabolic acidosis
c) Intravenous fluids should be almost exclusively normal saline
d) Hyperkalaemia is a common cause of death
e) 1 litre of 5% dextrose contains 5 g of dextrose

2.18 **In vitamin deficiency:**

a) Vitamin B_{12} deficiency may cause megaloblastic anaemia, peripheral neuropathy and cord degeneration
b) Pernicious anaemia is treatable with folic acid
c) Vitamin D deficiency can lead to rickets in children and osteomalacia in adults
d) Vitamin K deficiency and hypoprothrombinaemia are likely when there is a failure of fat absorption
e) Nicotinic acid deficiency can cause scurvy

2.19 In one-lung ventilation with a patient in the lateral position:

a) There is increased perfusion and ventilation in the dependent lung when both lungs are ventilated
b) If the non-dependent lung is deflated the PaO_2 will drop by about 50% in a patient with normal respiratory function
c) Vasodilators reduce shunting from the deflated non-dependent lung to the inflated dependent lung
d) The $PaCO_2$ rises considerably
e) The application of positive end-expiratory pressure (PEEP) to the ventilated dependent lung considerably improves PaO_2

2.20 Potentiation of non-depolarizing relaxants occurs with:

a) Hypernatraemia
b) Myasthenic syndrome
c) Aminoglycoside antibiotics
d) Tacrine hydrochloride
e) Metabolic acidosis

2.1   a) True   b) True   c) True   d) True   e) True

EXPLANATION

The recording of respiratory flow plotted against time produces a spirogram; if flow is plotted against volume, instead of time, a flow-volume loop is obtained. The expiratory peak represents the peak expiratory flow rate, following which, expiratory flow rates diminish progressively as the airways narrow until zero flow is obtained at the residual volume. As in spirometry, the forced vital capacity (FVC) and forced expiratory volume in 1 second (FEV_1) can be determined from the loop and thus any element of restrictive or obstructive lung disease (FEV_1/FVC less than 80%) determined. The 'dashed' loop is typical of an obstructive pattern in the upper airway, larynx or trachea. A flow-volume loop is more sensitive in detecting obstruction than FEV_1/FVC ratios because decreased flows occur before changes in FEV_1 or FEV_1/FVC ratios. When the obstruction is extrathoracic (inspiratory stridor) the changes are more marked during inspiration. In intrathoracic obstruction, expiration is mainly affected; while fixed obstruction in the upper airway affects the whole loop.

2.2   a) False   b) False   c) True   d) True   e) True

EXPLANATION

See Table 2.1, page 32–33.

2.3   a) True   b) False   c) True   d) True   e) False

EXPLANATION

Analgesia has been dominated in the past by two main classes of analgesic: opioids which exert analgesia by acting on opiate receptors, mainly mu receptors and non-steroidal anti-inflammatory drugs (NSAIDs) which are prostaglandin inhibitors. Then came the partial agonists with action on mu or kappa receptors. There are now newly discovered physiological mechanisms involved in transmitting/inhibiting pain, and a number of new analgesics are being introduced taking this into account.

Opioids/NSAIDs are ineffective in neurogenic pain, but drugs that act at sodium channels (sodium-blocking drugs) are quite effective in neuropathic pain by reducing membrane excitability (e.g. mexiletene used for diabetic neuropathy). Apart from prostaglandins, inflammatory processes release bradykinins and it is possible that bradykinin antagonists may have a useful role as analgesic and anti-inflammatory agents.

Neuropeptides, such as substance P act on specific receptors, and are believed to play a major role in pain transmission. Therefore, substance P inhibitors (e.g. capsaicin) may have a place as analgesics. Capsaicin is a pepper derivative and a substance P inhibitor which has been used for a number of conditions, especially trigeminal and post-herpetic neuralgia, diabetic neuropathy and cluster headaches.

A further method of achieving analgesia is to influence the neurotransmitters in the spinal cord (i.e. serotonin, gamma-aminobutyric acid (GABA), noradrenaline and endogenous opioids, and possibly acetylcholine) which have a role in inhibiting pain transmission.

This descending inhibitory control arises from cortex, thalamus and brain stem. Thus acupuncture/TENS (transcutaneous electrical nerve stimulation) may produce analgesia by stimulating the release of endogenous opiates, while the new analgesic tramadol exerts some of its action by increasing serotonin release and also levels of noradrenaline by preventing noradrenaline re-uptake. Similarly, tricyclic antidepressants are useful analgesic adjuvants because they increase noradrenaline levels.

There are then the alpha-2 agonists which produce a strong analgesic response and their potency is syngergistically enhanced by concomitant treatment with opioids. Their mode of action of analgesia is unclear but they definitely inhibit release of substance P and act at both supraspinal and spinal levels.

Summary
Some examples of the actions of analgesic drugs:

1. Opioids: primarily at mu receptors to produce analgesia and respiratory depression.
2. Agonist-antagonist type analgesics (partial agonists): an example is buprenorphine which acts at mu receptors, but less so than morphine, and behaves as an antagonist by competing for receptor sites. Pentazocine and nalbuphine are agonists at kappa receptors (which mediate analgesia and respiratory depression but less so than mu receptors) and antagonists at mu receptors.
3. Non-steroidal anti-inflammatory drugs: reduce pain and inflammation by prostaglandin inhibition.
4. Bradykinin inhibitors: effective because bradykinins cause pain and inflammation.
5. Sodium channel blocking drugs: useful in neurogenic pain, and act by reducing membrane excitability, e.g. anticonvulsants, lignocaine and antiarrhythmics.
6. Substance P inhibitors: substance P is a neurotransmitter in pain pathways and therefore inhibitors have analgesic properties, e.g. capsaicin, alpha-2 agonists.
7. Drugs that stimulate the release of pain inhibitory substances in the descending spinal cord pathways (serotonin, GABA, noradrenaline, endogenous opiates); TENS/acupuncture which release endogenous endorphins; tramadol increasing levels of serotonin and noradrenaline; tricyclic antidepressants which produce analgesia by increasing noradrenaline levels.

2.4   a) True   b) True   c) False   d) False   e) True

EXPLANATION
Prostaglandins are present in many human organs especially in seminal fluid; but the blood concentration is very low.

They are synthesized from fatty acids present in the phospholipids of cell membranes. Their main precursor is arachidonic acid. There are a number of groups and subgroups of prostaglandins, i.e. PGA, PGB, PGC, PGD, PGE, PGF and PGI (prostacyclin). They are inactivated during passage in the pulmonary circulation. Prostaglandins have diverse actions and prostaglandins in different groups may have opposite effects.

31

Table 2.1   Recommended preoperative tests

	Hb	WBC	PT/PTT	Platelets	Electrolytes
Asymptomatic	M > 65 F > 14				> 65
Neonates	Y				
Age:					
<40	F				
40–50	F				
50–65	F				
65–75	M/F				
>75	M/F				
CVS disease					
Pulmonary disease					
Liver disease			Y		
Renal disease	Y				Y
Diabetes					Y
Bleeding disorder			Y	Y	
CNS disorder		Y			Y
Malignancy	Y				
Drugs:					
Radiation		Y			
Smoking	Y				
Diuretics					Y
Digoxin					Y
Steroids					Y
Anticoagulants	Y		Y		
Operation with blood loss	Y				

Key: M = male; F = female; Y = yes – should be done; +/– = debatable

1. *Anti-inflammatory action.* Prostaglandins are released in physiological insults, i.e. chronic inflammation, especially ophthalmic and bony inflammation. Aspirin and NSAIDs exert their anti-inflammatory action by inhibiting prostaglandin synthesis.

2. *Platelets.* Most prostaglandins (especially prostacyclin) inhibit platelet aggregation and may be useful to prevent or treat thrombotic episodes, especially since most of them are also vasodilators.

3. *Blood vessels.* Prostaglandins are usually potent vasodilators and increase capillary permeability, causing a fall in blood pressure. However, prostaglandins in the PGF group can cause vasoconstriction of pulmonary artery and veins.

Creatinine	Glucose	SGOT alkaline phosphate	Chest X-ray	ECG	Blood groups and antibodies
> 65	> 65		Perhaps > 75	M > 40 F > 50	
				M	
				M	
Y	Y			Y	
Y	Y		+/−	Y	
Y			Y	Y	
			Y	Y	
		Y			
Y					
Y	Y			Y	
Y	Y			Y	
			Y		
			Y	Y	
			Y		
Y					
Y					
	Y			Y	
					Y

4. *Bronchial muscle.* Prostaglandins in the 'E' group (PGE) are bronchodilators and can be used as aerosols in asthmatics. In the 'F' group (PGF) prostaglandins cause bronchoconstriction.

5. *Uterine muscle.* PGEs and PGFs increase uterine contraction and are used for induction of abortion.

6. *Gut secretions.* Gastric, pancreatic and intestinal secretions are inhibited by PGE and PGA prostaglandins, which may be of some therapeutic use, e.g. misoprostol is a PGE analogue used in the prevention and treatment of peptic ulceration induced by NSAIDs.

EXPLANATION

The characteristic feature of the autonomic system is that its efferent fibres emerge from the spinal cord or brain as medullated fibres, are interrupted in their course by a synapse in a peripheral ganglion, and then relayed for distribution as fine non-medullated fibres. The autonomic system is divided into sympathetic and parasympathetic systems.

Sympathetic system

Sympathetic afferents. Afferents from visceral organs and body wall ascend in the autonomic plexuses and spinal nerves, synapsing in the dorsal ganglion of the spinal nerve, eventually reaching the hypothalamus and frontal cerebral cortex. They travel with the corresponding efferent autonomic fibres. Normally, one is unaware of these afferent impulses except when they are great enough to exceed the pain threshold, e.g. renal colic, angina.

Sympathetic efferents. Sympathetic efferents arise from the intermediolateral horn of the spinal cord from T1 to L2. Preganglionic axons exit the spinal cord and together with the anterior nerve roots form the anterior primary ramus, and then as the white communicating ramus join a ganglion on the sympathetic chain (not necessarily the ganglion at the level of spinal cord exit). The sympathetic chain is a trunk of ganglia (3 cervical, 11 thoracic, 3 lumbar and 4 sacral) lying 2.5 cm lateral to the vertebral column. A synapse may occur at the ganglion in the chain producing postganglionic axons, or else the preganglionic fibre may pass through the sympathetic ganglion and synapse with peripheral ganglia. Each preganglionic fibre diverges into seven or eight postganglionic axons. The postganglionic fibres are divided into somatic and visceral groups.

Somatic. Each spinal nerve receives a grey communicating ramus carrying postganglionic fibres from the sympathetic chain to be distributed to the segmental skin areas supplied by the spinal nerve.

Visceral. Postganglionic fibres to the head and neck and thoracic viscera arise from ganglia in the cervical sympathetic chain (stellate ganglia). The abdominal and pelvic viscera are supplied by postganglionic axons, which, however, arise from peripheral ganglia; the ganglia receive preganglionic fibres from the splanchnic nerves, while the postganglionic fibres form plexuses – coeliac, hypogastric, pelvic.

- Head and neck: supplied by postganglionic axons from T1–T2 (from stellate and cervical ganglia)
- Upper limb: T2–T7 (from stellate and thoracic ganglia)
- Thoracic viscera: T1–T4 (from cervical and thoracic ganglia)
- Abdominal viscera: T4–L2 (from coeliac plexus)
- Lower limb: T11–L2 (preganglionic fibres from T11–T2 synapse with lumbar ganglia L1–L3, from which postganglionic axons supply the upper leg, and with lumbar ganglia L4–L5 to supply the lower leg).

Parasympathetic system

Parasympathetic afferents. There is a cranial and sacral inflow. Cranial afferents from heart, lung and gut are conveyed in the vagus nerve; sacral afferents are transmitted via pelvic splanchnic nerves (S2, 3 and 4), and are responsible for pain experienced in bladder, prostate, uterus and rectum.

Parasympathetic efferents. Again there is a cranial and sacral outflow. The cranial outflow is transmitted via the 3rd cranial (oculomotor) nerve, supplying the eye, 7th (facial) supplying lacrimal and salivary glands (except parotid), 9th (glossopharyngeal) supplying the parotid, and the 10th (vagus) which is responsible for all parasympathetic actions except on eye and salivary glands. The sacral outflow arises with the sacral nerves 2, 3 and 4 as anterior sacral rami, and passes through anterior sacral foramina to become the pelvic splanchnic nerves. These do not pass through the sympathetic chain, but synapse at hypogastric ganglia from which very short postganglionic axons are given off to supply genitalia, bladder and rectum.

Table 2.2 compares the sympathetic and parasympathetic systems.

2.6   a) False   b) False   c) True   d) False   e) True

EXPLANATION

There are two dominant histamine receptors in the body H_1 and H_2. H_1 effects are antagonized by the traditional antihistamines; while H_2 effects are counteracted by the H_2 blockers such as cimetidine and ranitidine. H_1 receptors are not limited to the skin and respiratory mucosa and H_2 receptors are not only found in the gut; both H_1 and H_2 receptors are distributed round the body. When an allergic reaction occurs the changes are mostly H_1 effects but not entirely so, and therefore if a patient is known to have had an allergic reaction, it is wise to administer prophylactic H_1 and H_2 antagonists.

The clinical signs of histamine release are cardiovascular changes, bronchospasm and rash, with cardiovascular changes being more likely than bronchoconstriction or rash, though the presence of the latter confirms the diagnosis. Cardiovascular changes are due to H_1 and H_2 effects, and are primarily a decrease in peripheral vascular resistance causing hypotension, and tachycardia due to the chronotropic effect of histamine. Histamine also causes release of adrenaline and noradrenaline from the adrenal gland and sympathetic nervous system. Histamine also increases the P-R interval on the ECG.

Of the commonly used anaesthetic agents, barbiturates can cause histamine release but cutaneous reactions are more likely than cardiovascular collapse. Of the relaxants, suxamethonium and the curare-like relaxants (curare, atracurium, mivacurium) cause histamine release, while steroidal muscle relaxants (pancuronium, vecuronium, rocuronium) do not. Morphine is well known to cause histamine release while fentanyl and its derivatives are devoid of this action. It is very important to remember that the extent of an allergic reaction is dependent on the dose and speed of administration of the drug. The reaction is much more severe if a drug is given rapidly and if a large dose is given. It is also important to remember that an allergic reaction is likely to be much more severe if a patient is given the offending agent on a second occasion. An allergic reaction should be suspected when there is an unexplained tachycardia and hypotension. The presence of a rash and bronchospasm confirms the diagnosis. Adrenaline (0.2–0.4 mg) should be administered even in the presence of tachycardia. Intravenous H_1 and H_2 blockers and steroids may also be useful, though steroids take about 6–8 hours to reach their peak effect. In the event of an allergic reaction to an anaesthetic agent, two venous blood samples are collected in EDTA bottles, as soon as possible after the reaction. One sample is sent for haemoglobin, white cell count, platelet count and haematocrit   35

Table 2.2 Comparisons between sympathetic and parasympathetic systems

	Sympathetic	**Parasympathetic**
Anatomy	Head/neck/heart: T1–T2, stellate ganglion Thoracic viscera (heart, lung, oesophagus): T1–T4 Abdominal viscera: coeliac plexus – gut up to transverse colon, liver, pancreas, spleen, adrenal, kidney Pelvis/lower limb: fibres from T11–L2 go to sympathetic chain which supplies bladder, lower colon, rectum, reproductive organs, prostate, lower limb	Cranial outflow: eye from oculomotor; lacrimal and salivary glands from facial; parotid from glossopharyngeal; all other effects from vagus Sacral: from S2, 3, 4 to supply genitalia, rectum, bladder
Physiology	Pre-ganglionic fibres release acetylcholine; postganglionic fibres release catecholamines, except at sweat glands and adrenal glands which release acetylcholine. Sympathetic stimulation causes widespread effects, and is responsible for stress response	Preganglionic fibres release acetylocholine; all postganglionic terminals release acetylcholine. Activity more localized
Tested by:	Vagal stimulation over carotid sinus	Blood pressure changes on standing
Effects:		
Eye	Dilatation	Constriction
Salivary, bronchial, lacrimal glands	Reduced secretion	Increased secretion
Bronchi	Dilatation	Constriction
Heart	Increased force, rate, contractility, excitability	Decreased force, rate, contractility
Vessels	Dilates coronary vessels; skin and splanchnic vasoconstriction	Splanchnic vasodilatation
Gut	Reduced peristalsis. No effect on gastric or pancreatic secretions	Increased peristalsis. Increased gastric and pancreatic secretions
Bladder	Increases bladder emptying	Reduces bladder emptying
Skin	Vasoconstriction (also visceral vasoconstriction); increased sweat gland secretion, piloerection	No effect
Adrenal	Increased secretion	No effect
Liver	Glycogenolysis	No effect

estimations; the second sample is sent for measurement of plasma histamine levels. Histamine has a short half-life, and levels should be estimated 10 minutes to 1 hour after the reaction, and the sample should not be haemolysed. An alternative is measurement of plasma tryptase which has a longer half-life than histamine, and remains elevated up to 6 hours after the reaction. Further samples should be taken at 3 hours, 6 hours 12 hours and 24 hours later. Subsequent management should include skin testing with low dilutions of the offending agent 6 weeks after the reaction. The RAST test involves the use of commercially prepared antigens to detect drug-specific IgE antibodies; its use is limited by a high incidence of false negatives and positives.

2.7   a) False   b) True   c) False   d) False   e) True

EXPLANATION
There is evidence to suggest that hyperglycaemia has detrimental effects on the brain during cerebral damage. This is probably because hyperglycaemia increases lactic acidosis which aggravates neuronal damage.

Hypoglycaemia occurs in neonates when the glucose level is less than 25 mg/100 ml in the first 3 days of life. After 3 days the level should be above 45 mg/100 ml. Hypoglycaemia should be treated urgently to avoid neurological damage. It can be difficult to diagnose because the symptoms are non-specific (tremors, lethargy, cardiac problems) and must be differentiated from other electrolytic abnormalities, CNS problems, congenital heart disease and sepsis.

Blood glucose levels rise considerably during surgery as part of the stress response. The hyperglycaemia is due to increased levels of adrenaline, glucagon and cortisol all of which are increased during the stress of surgery.

Blood glucose levels remain normal during pregnancy. Although there is increased secretion of insulin, which would cause hypoglycaemia, this is counteracted by increased cortisol levels which raise the blood sugar because of increased hepatic glycogen production.

2.8   a) False   b) False   c) True   d) False   e) False

EXPLANATION
See Table 2.3.

2.9   a) True   b) False   c) True   d) False   e) False

EXPLANATION
See Table 2.3.

37

Table 2.3 Actions of induction agents

	Thiopentone	Methohexitone	Etomidate
Physical	Thiobarbiturate. Precipitates in acid solution and Hartmann's	Oxybarbiturate	Imidazole 0.2% solution in 30% propylene glycol
Venous irritation	Marked irritation; less with 2.5%. Arterial injection can cause necrosis and thrombosis	Less irritant than thiopentone	Marked irritation
Pain on injection	2.5% not usually painful	Marked pain even with 1% solution	Painful because of propylene glycol
Onset and duration	Onset: less than 30 s Duration: 5–10 min	Onset: less than 30 s Duration: 5–10 min	Onset: 15–45 s Duration: 3–12 min
Recovery	Moderate to severe hangover	Moderate to severe hangover	Mild hangover
Vomiting	Moderately high	Moderately high	Very high
Excitation	Minimal	Minimal	Severe involuntary myoclonic movements
Central nervous system	Anticonvulsant; marked fall in ICP, IOP and cerebral blood flow	Can cause fits; marked fall in ICP and IOP	Can cause fits; marked fall in ICP and cerebral blood flow
Cardio-vascular system	Moderate fall in BP and CO; mild tachycardia, moderate venous dilatation	Moderate fall in BP and CO; mild tachycardia; mild venous dilatation	No change in BP, CO, heart rate or systemic vascular resistance
Respiratory depression	Moderate	Moderate	Less than barbiturates or propofol
Bronchi	No effect on bronchial tone	No effect on bronchial tone	

Propofol	Ketamine	Diazepam	Midazolam
Alkylphenol 1% in water emulsion with 10% soya oil, 2% glycerol, 1% egg extract	Arylcyclohexylamine	Insoluble in water. Contains 40% propylene glycol	Water soluble Compatible with acid
Moderate irritation	No venous irritation	Marked irritation; less with emulsion preparation – diazemuls	No venous irritation
Moderately painful; pain reduced by added lignocaine, or using a large vein	Nil	Marked pain due to propylene glycol	Nil
Onset: 15–45 s Duration: 5–10 min	Onset: 15–45 s Duration 5–20 min	Onset: 45–60 s Duration: 10–20 min	Onset: 30–60 s Duration 15–30 min
Minimal hangover; sometimes euphoria	Possible delirium and hallucinations	Prolonged sedation and hangover	Sedation; residual amnesia and rebound insomnia
Very low ? antiemetic	Moderately high	Minimal	Minimal ? antiemetic
Minimal	Minimal	Nil	Nil
Can cause fits; decreases ICP, IOP and cerebral blood flow	Anticonvulsant; increases ICP, IOP and cerebral blood flow	Anticonvulsant; decreases ICP and IOP	Anticonvulsant; decreases ICP and IOP
Marked fall in BP, CO and heart rate; no change in systemic vascular resistance	Increased BP, CO and heart rate due to sympathetic activity	Minimal changes in BP, CO and heart rate	Minimal changes in BP, CO and heart rate
Moderate	Minimal	Less than barbiturate or propofol	Less than barbiturate or propofol
No bronchial effect	Marked bronchial dilatation	No bronchial effect	No bronchial effect

Table 2.3 (Cont'd)

	Thiopentone	Methohexitone	Etomidate
Liver	Large doses increase liver enzymes	Large doses increase liver enzymes	No effect; extensively metabolized in liver
Renal perfusion	Decreased blood flow ↑ ADH	Decreased blood flow ↑ ADH	No changes
Porphyria	Not safe	Not safe	? Not safe
Comments	Antianalgesic action	Antianalgesic action	Inhibits steroid syntheses – not suitable for infusions; no histamine release and least likely to cause allergy

Key: ADH = antidiuretic hormone; BP = blood pressure; CO = cardiac output; ICP = intracranial pressure; IOP = intraocular pressure

2.10   a) False   b) True   c) True   d) True   e) False

EXPLANATION

Predisposing factors in carcinoma of the oesophagus include smoking, high alcohol intake, achalasia, Plummer-Vinson syndrome (iron deficiency anaemia and post-cricoid webb) but not oesophagitis or hiatus hernia.

Carcinoma of the large bowel accounts for 20% of all malignancies in the UK. Predisposing conditions include ulcerative colitis and polyps whether familial or not. Crohn's disease is an inflammatory process which can affect any part of the gastrointestinal tract, but unlike ulcerative colitis is not premalignant.

Carcinoma of the bronchus accounts for 35 000 deaths a year. Smoking is premalignant for squamous cell carcinoma and also for an adenocarcinoma which is much less common (about 10%); however, the association is not so strong as in squamous cancer.

One of the late complications of hepatic cirrhosis is the development of a hepatoma which may be suspected if there is a change in the size or shape of the liver.

2.11   a) True   b) True   c) True   d) True   e) False

EXPLANATION

Starvation usually accompanies the metabolic response to injury and metabolic adaptation occurs to conserve essential tissues.

Initially there is a period of decreased energy metabolism followed by increased energy expenditure.

Propofol	Ketamine	Diazepam	Midazolam
No effect; extensively metabolized in liver	No effect; extensively metabolized in liver	No effect	No effect
Marked fall in renal blood flow	Increased blood flow	Minimal changes	Minimal changes
Probably safe	Safe	Probably safe	Probably safe
Best induction agent for day case anaesthesia	'S' isomer – less delirium, shorter recovery; more analgesic than 'R' isomer. Only agent not to increase ADH secretion	Effects reversed flumenazil which is, however, shorter acting than diazepam	Effects reversed with flumenazil which is, however, shorter acting than diazepam

S and R

block Ca++ channel
in NMDA receptor
Hof anti nmn

1. *Protein metabolism.* Protein, especially muscle protein, is broken down to provide amino acids to the liver as precursors for gluconeogenesis and visceral protein synthesis. Protein breakdown leads to increased nitrogen loss. Albumin is also broken down causing hypoalbuminaemia.
2. *Carbohydrate metabolism.* Glycogen is mobilized from the liver to stimulate glycogenolysis and gluconeogenesis causing hyperglycaemia . The administration of large amounts of glucose (over 200 g/day) will reduce lipolysis, enhance fat production, reduce visceral protein synthesis and cause water retention. Additional calories are therefore best given as fat.
3. *Fat metabolism.* Lipolysis occurs, leading to increased plasma free fatty acids and glycerol which are then available for energy requirements. Fat metabolism leads to production of ketones and metabolic acidosis.
4. *Endocrine changes.* Increased cortisol, catecholamines, glycogen and growth hormone all of which stimulate glycogenolysis in liver and muscle leading to hyperglycaemia. Lipolysis is increased by catecholamines, glycogen, and growth hormone. Insulin which has the opposite effects is at first decreased and then rises.

2.12   a) True   b) False   c) True   d) False   e) True

EXPLANATION
The APACHE (acute physiology and chronic health evaluation) system was devised to determine prognosis of critically ill patients and determine success of different treatments. 12 easily measurable parameters are used and each parameter is given a score. Moreover, since age and chronic health influence outcome, these two variables are also scored.

41

1. Acute physiology score (12 parameters)
   - Rectal temperature (0 for normal temperature, + 4 for over 41°C or below 30°C)
   - Mean blood pressure (mmHg) (0 for normal, + 4 if over 160 or below 49)
   - Heart rate (0 for normal, + 4 if over 180 or below 39)
   - Respiratory rate (+ 4 if rate above 50 or below 5)
   - Alveolar-arterial oxygen gradient (A-aDO$_2$) (mmHg), score given depending on FiO$_2$
   - Arterial pH (+ 4 if over 7.7 or less than 7.15)
   - Serum sodium (+ 4 if over 180 or below 110)
   - Serum potassium (+ 4 if over 7 or below 2.5)
   - Serum creatinine (+ 4 if over 300)
   - Haematocrit (%) (+ 4 if over 60 or below 30)
   - Leucocytes (cells/ml) (+ 4 if over 40 or less than 1)
   - Neurological points: number of points from Glasgow coma score (see Table 2.4)
2. Age points: 0 (less than 44); 2 (45–54); 3 (55–64); 5 (66–74)
3. Chronic health points: 2 points for elective postoperative admission; 5 points for emergency operation or if patient has significant chronic liver, renal, respiratory, cardiovascular disease or is immunocompromised.

There are specific problems with APACHE II scoring due to different interpretation of physiological data, misdiagnosis, scoring at the wrong time and wrong scoring of chronic health points. APACHE III has therefore been introduced, which is based on five major components obtained on the first day: major disease category, acute physiology (17 variables), age, co-morbidity-points only assigned with AIDS, lymphoma, solid tumour with metastasis, leukaemia, myeloma, hepatic failure and cirrhosis, origin and timing of patient selection.

Other scoring systems have been used, including SAPS and SAPS II (simplified acute physiology score).

2.13   a) False   b) True   c) True   d) False   e) True

EXPLANATION
Routine chest X-rays are not necessary on every patient and no longer justified because of cost. Preoperative chest X-rays should be done on the following patients:

1. Those with acute respiratory disease
2. Those with possible metastasis
3. Those with suspected or established cardiorespiratory disease who have not had an X-ray in the previous 12 months
4. Recent immigrants from countries where tuberculosis is endemic who have not had an X-ray within the previous 12 months.

Table 2.4   Glasgow coma scale

Eye opening		Best verbal response		Best motor response	
Spontaneous	4	Orientated	5	Obeys commands	6
To speech	3	Confused	4	Localized pain	5
To pain	2	Inappropriate words	3	Normal flexion to pain	3
None	1	Incomprehensible sounds	2	Abnormal flexion to pain	3
		None	1	Extension to pain	2
				None	1

A score of 14–15 indicates minor injury; 9–13 moderate injury; and 3–8 severe injury.

Chest X-rays are not useful in assessing lung function, but can be extremely beneficial in diagnosis of lung disease and may influence anaesthetic management (e.g. presence of pneumothorax, effusion, etc.). It is important to allow for effects of patient position, over- and underexposure, the effect of rotational distortion (i.e. mediastinal widening) and phase of breath holding. Hypoinflation results in mediastinal widening, enlargement of heart and hilar areas, and increased opacity of lung fields which can mimic heart failure or pneumonia. A normal chest X-ray should show a central trachea with no deformity of the rib cage. The right lobe of the diaphragm should lie at the 6th rib anteriorly and be approximately 1-2 cm higher than the left. Vascular markings in the lung fields should be symmetrical, but larger in the lower zones. The transverse diameter of the heart on the posteroanterior projection should be less than 50% of the chest width.

2.14   a) False   b) False   c) True   d) True   e) True

EXPLANATION
Antihypertensives can be divided into six groups depending on their mode of action:

1. Sedatives. These act by decreasing anxiety. Methyldopa, apart from its antihypertensive action, has a marked sedative effect.
2. Drugs interfering with adrenergic transmission:
- Ganglion blockers, e.g. trimetaphan. These drugs block both sympathetic and parasympathetic activity.
- Adrenergic neuron blockers. These drugs block the uptake of noradrenaline (e.g. guanethidine, reserpine).
- Competitive antagonism at alpha or beta adrenoceptors:
  - Alpha receptor antagonists, e.g. phentolamine or phenoxybenzamine used for phaeochromocytoma.
  - Alpha-2 agonists, e.g. clonidine which acts both on the CNS and peripherally. CNS action causes inhibition of central sympathetic outflow.
  - Beta antagonists. Beta blockade leads to diminution of sympathetic activity and reduction in cardiac contractility and rate causing a drop in cardiac output (e.g. atenolol, metoprolol).
  - Alpha and beta blockers, e.g. labetolol.

3. Peripheral vasodilators, e.g. hydralazine, sodium nitroprusside.

4. Calcium channel blockers. Since calcium plays a part in activating cardiac muscle, calcium blockers cause negative inotropism and a decreased atrioventricular conduction as well as coronary vasodilatation. Some, like verapamil have strong antidysrhythmic properties, while nifedipine mainly dilates the systemic and coronary arteries. Diltiazem's actions are in between verapamil and nifedipine.

5. Angiotensis converting enzyme (ACE) inhibitors. Since renin is a precursor of angiotensin these drugs are especially useful when hypertension is associated with high renin levels (e.g. renal hypertension, malignant hypertension). They are not so effective if the renin levels are not elevated (e.g. captopril, enalapril).

6. Diuretics. The hypotensive action of diuretics is related to sodium diuresis and volume depletion (e.g. thiazides, spironolactone which being an aldosterone antagonist reduces the potassium loss which occurs with thiazides and frusemide).

2.15	a) True	b) False	c) False	d) True	e) False

EXPLANATION

MAC is defined as the minimum alveolar concentration of anaesthetic that prevents movement in 50% of subjects in response to a surgical incision. It is a reflection of potency and the MAC for different agents is as follows:

N_2O	105%	least potent
Desflurane	4.6–6%	
Sevoflurane	1.71%	
Enflurane	1.58%	
Isoflurane	1.28%	
Halothane	0.75%	most potent

A number of factors influence MAC:

1. *Age.* MAC is higher in the first year, then steadily decreases with age until by age 80 it is reduced by 40%.

2. *Pregnancy.* This reduces MAC by about 40%.

3. *Temperature.* Hypothermia decreases MAC (about 5% for every degree centigrade fall in temperature).

4. *Drugs.* CNS stimulants (e.g. amphetamines) increase MAC, while depressants (e.g. alcohol, sedative premedication) reduce it. The addition of other drugs to inhalational agents reduces MAC (e.g. narcotics, sedatives, etc.).

5. *Physiological factors.* Hypercarbia, hypoxia, acidosis reduce MAC because the CNS does not function properly under these conditions.

NB: Obesity, sex and general health do not affect MAC. 'MAC awake' is the alveolar concentration when emergence occurs; for halothane this is 59% of MAC, for isoflurane it is 29% of MAC.

2.16	a) False	b) True	c) False	d) False	e) True

EXPLANATION

In treating metabolic acidosis it is most important to treat the cause of the acidosis. When the underlying cause is treated, the excess acid will be metabolized and excreted. The use of sodium bicarbonate is controversial. Even in a cardiac arrest situation, the most important treatment for lactic acidosis is improving cardiac output with mechanical cardiopulmonary resuscitation and adrenergic agonists. Bicarbonate is indicated in prolonged periods of cardiac arrest, in patients where metabolic acidosis contributed to the arrest, and where cardiac arrest is caused by hyperkalaemia. Even so, it should be administered carefully, i.e. 1 mg/kg initial dose and half that amount if required every 10 minutes. When bicarbonate is administered, the blood is alkalized more quickly than the cerebrospinal fluid (CSF) because of the blood-brain barrier, and the persistent CSF acidosis sustains the hyperventilatory response. Complications of sodium bicarbonate include hypocalcaemia, hypokalaemia, hypernatraemia, fluid overload, increased production of organic acids, intracranial haemorrhage in the neonate, and shift of the haemoglobin oxydissociation curve to the left increasing the affinity of oxygen for haemoglobin, thus reducing oxygen release to tissues and undermining tissue oxygenation. Therefore the current recommendation is for judicious use of sodium bicarbonate.

2.17	a) True	b) False	c) True	d) False	e) False

EXPLANATION

Diabetic ketoacidosis usually presents with thirst, polyuria and also abdominal pain, nausea and vomiting. Therefore, it is important to check the blood sugar before taking an acute abdominal emergency to theatre. The ketoacidosis must be differentiated from diabetic hyperosmolar crisis. In both cases there is severe hyperglycaemia and dehydration, but there is little or no ketosis or acidosis with hyperosmolar crisis.

Treatment. The principles of treating ketoacidosis are: (a) insulin; (b) i.v. fluids; (c) potassium and insulin are given by continuous i.v. infusion with dosage adjusted according to hourly blood sugars.

Intravenous fluids. These should be almost entirely isotonic saline as the average deficit is about 6 litres. Bicarbonate should not be given as metabolic acidosis improves with insulin and saline. Bicarbonate can cause hypernatraemia and further falls in potassium and possible metabolic alkalosis. When the blood sugar falls, an addition may be indicated (1 litre of 5% dextrose contains 50 g dextrose: 1% solution = 10 mg/ml; thus 1 litre contains 50 g).

Potassium. Insulin causes potassium to migrate out of cells; therefore diabetic acidosis is associated with considerable hypokalaemia which is a common cause of death. Therefore potassium is required with the saline infusions.

Table 2.5   Properties of vitamins

Vitamin	Clinical signs of deficiency	Cause of deficiency	Comments
Vitamin A (retinal)	Night blindness; permanent blindness; skin degeneration and respiratory tract degeneration causing respiratory infections; also kidney stones	Malabsorption; malnutrition	High levels during pregnancy can cause teratogenic anomalies
Vitamin B₁ (thiamine)	Beriberi: wet – high output heart failure dry – muscle wasting; polyneuropathy infantile – cardiac failure; spasticity; gastrointestinal symptoms	Nutritional, especially when there is excessive intake of polished rice which provides little energy	
Vitamin B₂ (riboflavin)	Anorexia; weakness; scaly and greasy skin and mucosa especially tongue, nose, eyes; normochromic anaemia	Malnutrition; malabsorption; diarrhoea	
Vitamin B₆ (pyridoxine)	Normoblastic anaemia	Malabsorption; drugs – isoniazid, hydralazine	
Vitamin B₁₂ (cyanocobalamin)	Pernicious (megaloblastic) anaemia; peripheral neuropathy; subacute degeneration of the cord affecting lateral and posterior columns	Malnutrition; failure of production of intrinsic factor, e.g. blind loop syndrome; malabsorption	Required for RBC maturation; neurological features of pernicious anaemia aggravated by folic acid
Folic acid	Megaloblastic anaemia	Pregnancy; premature infants; malabsorption; drugs, e.g. phenytoin	Required for RBC maturation

Table 2.5 (*Cont'd*)

Nicotinic acid	Pellagra – diarrhoea, dementia, debility dermatitis (especially glossitis and stomatitis) – 4Ds	Nutritional	
Vitamin C	Scurvy – bleeding of gums and into skin, anaemia	Nutritional lack of oranges, lemons	
Vitamin D	Hypocalcaemia causing rickets and osteomalacia in adults (soft brittle bones); tetany	Lack of vitamin D (cold winters); lack of calcium in foods especially milk	Produced in skin in presence of sunlight; required for calcium absorption
Vitamin E	Haemolytic anaemia in premature infants		
Vitamin K	Hypoprothrombinaemia causing bleeding	Failure of fat absorption, e.g. malabsorption; diseases causing lack of intestinal fatty bile salts, e.g. biliary obstruction, liver disease	Vitamin K (as well as A, D and E) is fat soluble, the rest water soluble. Vitamin K is required for production of clotting factors and bone calcification

2.18 a) True b) False c) True d) True e) False

EXPLANATION
See Table 2.5.

2.19 a) False b) False c) False d) False e) False

EXPLANATION
In the lateral position with both lungs ventilated the dependent lung receives more perfusion because of gravitational effects, but less ventilation because anaesthesia reduces functional residual capacity (FRC) of the dependent lung. When the non-dependent lung is deflated, PaO_2 drops and one should increase the FiO_2 to compensate for this. However, the fall in PaO_2 is not dramatic because of hypoxic pulmonary vasoconstriction which reduces the blood flow and shunting in the deflated lung. Vasodilators such as volatile agents (nitrates, nitroprusside) cause pulmonary vasodilatation and increase shunting, causing a fall in PaO_2. The application of high airway pressures or PEEP to the dependent lung will divert blood

47

flow to the deflated lung again reducing PaO_2 and this is more relevant than the positive effect of PEEP on increasing FRC and oxygenation. If PaO_2 is too low, the addition of continuous positive airway pressure (CPAP) or oxygen insufflation to the non-dependent lung may improve oxygenation.

$PaCO_2$ is not usually a problem as blood in the ventilated lung can eliminate enough CO_2 to compensate for the non-ventilated lung.

2.20   a) False   b) True   c) True   d) False   e) True

EXPLANATION
Tacrine hydrochloride acts as an anticholinesterase and was used in the past to prolong and potentiate suxamethonium.

Factors which potentiate non-depolarizing muscle relaxants include:

- Metabolic acidosis often accompanied by hypoventilation and tracheal tug.
- Myasthenia gravis/myasthenic syndrome. With myasthenia gravis there is usually resistance to suxamethonium and increased sensitivity to non-depolarizing relaxants. Myasthenic syndrome is a muscular weakness occasionally seen in patients with bronchial carcinoma, thyroid disease and connective tissue disorders like systemic lupus erythematosus and dermatomyositis. These patients are sensitive to both suxamethonium and non-depolarizers.
- Electrolytic disturbances – hyponatraemia, hypo- or hyperkalaemia, hypocalcaemia.
- Antibiotics, e.g. neomycin, gentamicin, polymyxin and other aminoglycosides.
- Renal failure especially with relaxants which have significant renal excretion, e.g. gallamine, pancuronium, curare.
- Hypothermia.

3.1 **In regard to maternal deaths, the current situation is that:**

a) Maternal deaths primarily due to anaesthesia have not diminished in the last 10 years
b) The administration of H_2 receptor blocking drugs and antacids to maternal patients who require anaesthesia reduces considerably the incidence of anaesthetic deaths
c) The latest maternal mortality rate is 10 per 100 000 maternities
d) Anaesthetic complications account for a higher proportion of maternal deaths than do obstetric complications
e) The most common cause of maternal death is related to hypertensive disease

3.2 **With regard to anaesthetic molecules:**

a) Iodinated hydrocarbons are often useful anaesthetic agents
b) The substitution of some hydrogen atoms in hydrocarbons and ethers with fluoride or chloride increases narcotic potency
c) The substitution of hydrogen atoms in hydrocarbons and ethers by halogens makes the compounds more flammable
d) Substitution of some hydrogen atoms in hydrocarbons and ethers with halogens causes convulsant properties
e) Halogenated hydrocarbons are more prone to produce cardiac arrhythmias and hepatotoxic effects than halogenated ethers

3.3 **Causes of raised intracranial pressure include:**

a) Polycythaemia
b) Meningitis
c) Acidosis
d) Water intoxication
e) Uraemia

3.4 **Acute pancreatitis:**

a) Is more common in alcoholics
b) Always causes a rise in serum amylase – a high serum amylase is diagnostic
c) Has features which may include hypocalcaemia and hyperglycaemia
d) May be treated with Trasylol
e) Has higher mortality in the haemorrhagic type

3.5 **To avoid accidental oesophageal intubation, one should be aware that:**

a) With preoxygenation, pulse oximetry is still a reliable method of determining correct tracheal intubation
b) The presence of condensation in the lumen of a clear endotracheal tube is a sure sign of tracheal placement
c) The negative pressure test is more reliable than chest auscultation in determining tracheal intubation
d) Flexion and extension of the neck during surgery can cause a tracheal tube to move by up to 5 cm with possible oesophageal displacement
e) If accidental oesophageal intubation is preceded by positive pressure mask ventilation, no expired CO_2 is detected on a capnograph

3.6 **In the supine position:**

a) Abduction of the arm to 90° with the hand supinated (palm upwards) and the head turned away from the abducted arm is a safe posture against brachial plexus traction injuries
b) The cornea can be left exposed if the operation is less than 20 minutes
c) Crossing of legs is safe
d) Oxygen absorption is reduced
e) Cardiac workload is reduced

3.7 **With regard to bleeding disorders:**

a) Massive blood transfusions cause bleeding because the blood is deficient in factor VIII and platelets
b) Disseminated intravascular coagulation is characteristically associated with excessive fibrinolysis and a low fibrinogen level
c) Heparin is a prime indication in disseminated intravascular coagulation because of the underlying thrombosis
d) Bleeding in Von Willebrand's disease is due to low factor VIII
e) Thrombin time reflects the amount of circulating heparin

3.8 **Drug interactions are such that:**

a) A patient on ecothiopate for glaucoma requires more suxamethonium
b) Buprenorphine is a suitable analgesic for postoperative pain relief in a patient who is a known heroin addict
c) A patient on lithium carbonate for depression requires larger doses of non-depolarizing relaxants
d) A parkinsonian patient with a history of anaesthetic vomiting can be treated with droperidol
e) Patients on spironolactone are likely to have a prolonged action of non-depolarizing relaxants

3.9 **In drug poisoning:**

a) Cyanide poisoning due to sodium nitroprusside can be treated with amyl nitrite
b) Cysteamine to treat paracetamol overdose can be administered successfully up to 1 week following ingestion
c) Alkaline diuresis is of no value in salicylate overdose
d) Digoxin overdose typically produces cardiac arrhythmias and hyperkalaemia
e) Chelating agents are of value in treating iron and lead poisoning

3.10 **Effects of hypercapnia include:**

a) Retention of bicarbonate and sodium
b) Reduction in thiopentone requirements
c) Cerebral vasodilatation and rise in intracranial pressure
d) Shift of the haemoglobin dissociation curve to the left
e) Dysrhythmias

3.11 **When using endotracheal tubes and masks:**

a) Endotracheal tube sizes refer to the external diameter of the tube
b) When a laryngeal mask is used for intermittent positive-pressure ventilation (IPPV) it is recommended that a pressure of 20 cm water should not be exceeded
c) In a child who is 3–12 months old an appropriate tracheal tube length is 12 cm for oral intubation and 15 cm for nasal intubation
d) Endotracheal tubes with floppy cuffs are of the high-volume, low-pressure type
e) Modern breathing connections use a 22-mm diameter taper while adult tracheal tube connectors have a 15-mm diameter taper

3.12 **In Guillain-Barré syndrome:**

a) Autonomic dysfunction and arrhythmias are a common feature
b) Cerebrospinal fluid protein is unaltered in most cases
c) Typically motor loss initially occurs distally and then ascends
d) Plasma exchange is valuable in treatment
e) Suxamethonium is the relaxant of choice if intubation is required urgently

3.13 **Cardiovascular effects of muscle relaxants include:**

a) Suxamethonium causes bradycardia by stimulating muscarinic receptors
b) Rocuronium reduces blood pressure by histamine release
c) Curare causes hypotension by histamine release and ganglion blockade
d) Pancuronium blocks muscarinic receptors and predisposes to arrhythmias
e) Atracurium causes bradycardia by vagal nerve stimulation

3.14 **Rocuronium:**

a) Is a bisquaternary benzyl isoquinoline agent
b) Is mainly metabolized in liver
c) Has few cardiovascular actions
d) Causes histamine release
e) Has a quicker onset of action than atracurium

3.15 **Non-depolarizing block is potentiated by:**

a) Desflurane
b) Motor neuron disease
c) Burns and massive trauma
d) Calcium blockers
e) Muscular dystrophy

3.16 **With regard to inhalational anaesthetics:**

a) Isoflurane and enflurane are isomers
b) Metabolism of sevoflurane is minimal
c) Isoflurane causes a fall in cardiac output and blood pressure due to myocardial depression
d) Desflurane boils at room temperature
e) The addition of an ether link tends to reduce myocardial sensitization to catecholamines

3.17 Of the inhalational anaesthetics:

a) Desflurane causes 'coronary steal syndrome'
b) Halothane increases cerebral blood flow more than isoflurane or desflurane
c) Desflurane is more suitable as an induction agent than sevoflurane
d) Sevoflurane cannot be used in closed circuits
e) Renal blood flow is reduced more with isoflurane than with halothane

3.18 Nitrous oxide:

a) Is a poor analgesic
b) Has little effect on cerebral blood flow
c) Undergoes considerable liver metabolism
d) Inhibits vitamin B_{12} metabolism
e) Is more soluble than nitrogen in blood

3.19 Lignocaine:

a) Is one of the constituents of EMLA cream
b) Has systemic analgesic effects
c) Is broken down by cholinesterase
d) Is effective in the treatment of supraventricular tachycardia
e) Is more protein bound than bupivacaine

3.20 With regard to the non-steroidal anti-inflammatory drugs (NSAIDs):

a) They are very effective analgesics even in the absence of inflammation
b) They inhibit cyclo-oxygenase
c) Ibuprofen causes less gastric bleeding than most NSAIDs
d) Ketorolac has marked anti-inflammatory actions
e) 50% of asthmatic patients are allergic to aspirin

3.1   a) False   b) False   c) True   d) False   e) True

EXPLANATION

The number of maternal deaths between 1988 and 1990 (3 years) was 238 compared to 223 in the previous 3 years and 390 in 1973–1975. The maternal mortality rate is 10 per 100 000 compared to 20 in 1973–1975. The deaths directly due to anaesthesia were 4 in 1988–1990, 6 in 1985–1987 and 27 in 1973–1975. The incidence of death directly related to anaesthesia is therefore diminishing, especially when one considers that the number of caesarean sections and abortions has increased dramatically. There is no conclusive evidence that antacid and H_2 blocker prophylaxis in women in labour has resulted in lower morbidity. However, many obstetric units adopt this practice routinely. The causes of maternal deaths (238) in 1988–1990 are as follows:

Hypertensive disease	18.6%
Other obstetric causes	16.6%
Pulmonary embolism	16.6%
Haemorrhage	15.2% (a considerable increase over previous years)
Ectopic	10.3%
Amniotic fluid embolism	7.6%
Abortion	6.2%
Sepsis	4.8%
Anaesthesia	2.8%
Ruptured uterus	1.4%

In about 50% of cases there was substandard care especially in the postoperative period, and the use of appropriate monitoring (pulse oximetry and capnography) both intraoperatively and postoperatively is recommended.

3.2   a) False   b) True   c) False   d) True   e) True

EXPLANATION

Volatile anaesthetic agents in common use today are usually halogenated hydrocarbons (e.g. halothane) or halogenated ethers (e.g. enflurane, isoflurane which is an isomer of enflurane, sevoflurane, desflurane). The addition or substitution of bromo- or iodohalogens to hydrocarbons and ethers does not make useful anaesthetics as these compounds are hydrolysed into the corresponding alcohol or into the parent hydrocarbon. Therefore halogenation is usually achieved by chlorination and more commonly by fluorination. As the hydrogen atoms in hydrocarbons and ethers are increasingly replaced by chlorine or fluorine, the agents become more potent narcotic anaesthetics and become more stable and less flammable, but also acquire convulsant properties up to a point where all the hydrogens are completely replaced by halogens in which case the compounds become pharmacologically inert. On the whole, halogenated ethers are more useful than halogenated hydrocarbons because the latter produce more cardiac effects and liver damage.

3.3   a) True   b) True   c) True   d) True   e) True

EXPLANATION

The classical signs of raised intracranial pressure are headache, vomiting papilloedema. Other symptoms include drowsiness, giddiness, blurred vision. The symptoms are usually worse in the morning because of CO_2 retention during sleep. Acute rises in intracranial pressures cause a rise in blood pressure, bradycardia and possibly coma and convulsions.

Causes of raised intracranial pressure are:

1. Space-occupying lesions, e.g. tumour, haematoma, abscess (meningitis may be complicated by a cerebral abscess).
2. Increase in cerebrospinal fluid volume, e.g. hydrocephalus.
3. Increase in brain water. Cerebral oedema may be due to a number of causes, e.g. hypoxia, water intoxication, excessive intake of hypotonic fluids, falls in plasma osmolarity which encourage movement of water into brain cells (e.g. uraemia, hyperglycaemic diabetic coma).
4. Increase in intracranial blood volume. Thus any factor which causes cerebral vasodilatation will increase intracranial pressure (e.g. hypoxia, hypercapnia, acidosis, polycythaemia where the increased viscosity causes a compensatory cerebral vasodilatation to maintain normal cerebrovascular resistance). Low cortisol levels and a number of drugs such as volatile anaesthetic agents increase intracranial pressure, as also does ketamine.

3.4   a) True   b) False   c) True   d) False   e) True

EXPLANATION

Predisposing factors. Alcoholism, biliary tract pathology (e.g. cholecystitis, biliary surgery), viral infections (e.g. mumps), following abdominal trauma and investigations (e.g. endoscopic retrograde cholangiopancreatography – ERCP) or translumbar aortography, drugs (e.g. phenformin, thiazides).

Clinical features. Severe epigastric pain radiating to back with nausea and vomiting and can be confused with other causes of acute abdomen (e.g. perforated ulcer, leaking aneurysm, myocardial infarction, cholecystitis, etc.). Paralytic ileus is common. The patient is usually shocked and cyanosed. Haemorrhage and coagulation disorders can also occur. Other features include jaundice, renal failure and respiratory failure. 50% of patients develop pseudocysts while 5% develop a pancreatic abscess with haemorrhage and septicaemia.

Diagnosis. Biochemical: hypocalcaemia, hyperglycaemia (impaired insulin production) hyperlipidaemia. Serum amylase is elevated in 75% of cases and an elevated serum amylase is not specific to acute pancreatitis.

Ultrasound or CT scan usually confirms the diagnosis.

Treatment. Symptomatic and supportive, i.e. nasogastric suction, analgesia, parenteral fluid replacement, possibly insulin, antibiotics, coagulation factors, ventilatory support, haemodialysis, surgery to drain a cyst or abscess. Trasylol used in the past is no longer thought to be of any value.

Prognosis. Mortality is 10%; 90% in the severe haemorrhagic type.

3.5　　a) False　　b) False　　c) True　　d) True　　e) False

EXPLANATION

Oesophageal intubation is still a major cause of anaesthetic mortality and morbidity and it is thus very important to detect correct tracheal placement. The clinical signs of tracheal intubation include:

1. Visualization of tube passing through cords.
2. Auscultation over trachea, apices, bases and epigastrium.
3. Observation of chest movement.
4. Lack of abdominal distension.
5. Lack of cyanosis.
6. Presence of water vapour condensing in the breathing system during expiration. This is unreliable as condensation can arise from the stomach.
7. Capnography to detect expired CO_2. One great advantage of a capnograph is that it gives a continuous end-tidal CO_2 readout and therefore if accidental extubation occurs during surgery this will be detected on the capnograph (*NB* flexion/extension of neck can move a tube by up to 5 cm). If one applies positive pressure mask ventilation prior to accidental oesophageal intubation, the CO_2 inflated into the stomach may for a few minutes give a CO_2 readout on a capnograph. This 'oesophageal' capnograph is characterized by a stepwise decrease in CO_2.
8. Negative pressure test. Because the trachea is more rigid than the oesophagus a negative pressure (i.e. aspirating on a syringe attached to the endotracheal tube) applied to the oesophagus will cause the oesophageal wall to wrap round the tube making aspiration difficult, while air within the trachea is freely aspirated.
9. Oxygen saturation. With preoxygenation becoming a common practice it can take many minutes for desaturation to occur.

3.6　　a) False　　b) False　　c) False　　d) True　　e) True

EXPLANATION

Positional hazards include:

1. *Facial damage:* supraorbital nerve or facial nerve damage with connectors; masks; eye pressure with a mask; corneal damage (10 minutes' exposure without eyelid movement causes corneal drying).
2. *Upper limb damage:* brachial plexus traction injury. If the arm is abducted to 90° the hand should be pronated (palm downwards) and the head turned to the abducted arm; both radial nerve and ulnar nerves can be compressed by screens or mattress.
3. *Lower limb:* deep vein thrombosis and pulmonary embolism due to pressure on calf muscles; skin on posterior ankles can also be damaged; therefore, the Achilles tendons should be supported with foam rubber or, preferably, external pneumatic compression applied to the legs. If the legs are crossed, the underlying long saphenous vein and dorsalis pedis can be compressed.
4. *Respiratory system:* functional residual capacity is reduced because the abdominal contents especially in the obese patient push the diaphragm upwards. The distribution of inspired gases is altered as well as the distribution of blood

55

(perfusion greatest in the dependent areas because of gravitational effects). There is therefore ventilation/perfusion imbalance and less oxygen is absorbed.

5. *Cardiovascular:* gravity no longer impedes venous return from the lower body and there is therefore increased venous return to the heart, with consequent increase in cardiac output though this may be slightly offset by intermittent positive-pressure ventilation (IPPV).

Conclusion. The supine posture is the one least likely to upset the normal physiology.

3.7   a) True   b) True   c) False   d) False   e) True

EXPLANATION
When a bleeding disorder is suspected a number of tests are required:

- prothrombin time (PT) – reflects the extrinsic coagulation system
- partial thromboplastin time (PTT) – reflects the intrinsic system
- thrombin time – reflects circulating heparin
- fibrinogen level – dangerous if less than 100 mg/100 ml
- platelet level – dangerous if less than 100 000/ml
- bleeding time – detects abnormal platelet function.

A coagulopathy is usually multifactorial and is in most cases treated with fresh frozen plasma (FFP) and platelets.

1. Massive transfusion causes bleeding because of the dilutional effect and deficiency of platelets and factor VIII if blood is over 48 hours old.
2. Disseminated intravascular coagulation (DIC) is a manifestation of severe underlying disease. It is initially a thrombotic problem and secondarily a bleeding disorder due to excess fibrinolysis. Platelets, fibrinogen and factor VIII are low. One must treat the cause and FFP, fibrinogen and platelets are indicated. Heparin is not indicated, neither should agents to reverse fibrinolysis be given.
3. Liver disease. Treat with FFP, platelets and vitamin K.
4. Congenital disorders. The most common disorder is haemophilia where there is factor VIII deficiency. PTT is prolonged but bleeding time is normal. In Von Willebrand's disease there is impaired (but not low) factor VIII activity plus platelet disorder. FFP or factor VIII is indicated. Factor VIII activity must be above 60%.

3.8   a) False   b) False   c) False   d) False   e) False

EXPLANATION
Ecothiopate is an organophosphate which is a pseudocholinesterase inhibitor and therefore prolongs the action of suxamethonium.

Being an agonist-antagonist-type analgesic, buprenorphine may produce a withdrawal syndrome because of its antagonistic actions. The perioperative period is not the time for withdrawal and the addict should be maintained with adequate narcotics. A regional technique should be chosen for postoperative pain relief.

Lithium carbonate causes hypokalaemia and decreases acetylcholine release and therefore prolongs non-depolarizing muscle relaxants.

Droperidol can cause extrapyramidal symptoms because of block of dopaminergic receptors and should therefore not be used in Parkinson's disease.

Hypokalaemia potentiates non-depolarizing relaxants. Being an aldosterone antagonist, spironolactone does not cause hypokalaemia (as other diuretics do) and therefore should not potentiate the effects of muscle relaxants.

3.9   a) True   b) False   c) False   d) True   e) True

EXPLANATION

Excessive nitroprusside administration produces cyanide poisoning which causes tissue hypoxia due to inactivation of the cytochrome oxidase system. The cyanide can be neutralized with:

1. Amyl nitrite. Inhalation of amyl nitrite converts haemoglobin into methaemoglobin which combines with cyanide to form cyanmethaemoglobin.
2. Sodium thiosulphate intravenously converts cyanide into the non-toxic thiocyanate.
3. Cobalt edentate intravenously chelates cyanide.

Paracetamol overdosage causes hepatic failure due to overloading of the glutathione conjugation pathway which normally neutralizes a highly hepatotoxic metabolite. Treatment with cysteamine or methionine must be given within 10 hours of ingestion to be effective.

Forced diuresis is an attempt to alter the urinary pH to trap the filtered drug within the renal tubule by increasing the ionized fraction. This is achieved in salicylate and barbiturate overdose by alkaline diuresis and in amphetamine overdose by acid diuresis.

Digoxin overdose causes cardiac dysrhythmias and hyperkalaemia. Bradycardia is treated with atropine/pacing; dysrhythmias with lignocaine, beta blockers, etc. Hyperkalaemia is treated with dextrose and insulin. Toxicity of digoxin is enhanced by hypokalaemia.

Chelating agents are of value mainly in heavy metal poisoning. Desferrioxamine is the chelating agent of choice in iron overdose, calcium edentate in lead poisoning.

3.10   a) True   b) False   c) True   d) False   e) True

EXPLANATION
See Table 3.1.

Table 3.1 Effects of hypercapnia and hypocapnia

	Hypercapnia	Hypocapnia
Central nervous system	Progressive narcosis; increased cerebral blood flow and increased intracranial pressure	Progressive clouding of consciousness. Reduced cerebral blood flow and fall in intracranial pressure. If CO_2 below 30 mmHg (4 kPa) the cerebral vasoconstriction can impair cerebral oxygenation
Autonomic system	Sympathetic system stimulated causing tachycardia; hypertension dilated pupils and sweating	
Respiration	Stimulated, Bohr effect – Hb dissociation curve shifted to the right; thus more oxygen is liberated to the tissues	Depressed, Hb dissociation curve shifted to left. Less available oxygen to tissues
Cardiovascular system	Tachycardia; increase in blood pressure and cardiac output due to sympathetic stimulation. Dysrhythmias. Sympathetic stimulation causes vasoconstriction but peripheral effect of CO_2 is vasodilatation.	Fall in blood pressure and cardiac output, vasoconstriction. Maternal hyperventilation not recommended as the vasoconstriction can lead to diminished fetal oxygenation
Biochemical	Respiratory acidosis, fall in pH leading to compensatory metabolic alkalosis with secretion of acid urine and retention of sodium and bicarbonate. Rise of potassium	Respiratory alkalosis. Rise in pH and fall in sodium
Effects on drug action	pH changes affect ionization of many drugs and the amount of protein binding. Requirements of thiopentone increased	

3.11   a) False   b) True   c) True   d) True   e) True

EXPLANATION

Endotracheal tube sizes refer to the internal diameter of the tube. All modern adult

Table 3.2   Tracheal tube sizes and lengths

Age	Size	Oral length (cm)	Nasal length (cm)
0–3 months	3.0	10	
3–12 months	3.5	12	15
3 years	4	13	16
4 years	4.5	14	17
5 years	5	14	17
5–6 years	5.5	15	18
6–8 years	6.0	16	19

tube connectors have a 15-mm diameter taper while the British Standard connections with a 22-mm diameter taper are used in breathing systems. Modern tubes are of two types – low-volume high-pressure cuff where a high pressure may be exerted on the tracheal mucosa if overinflated especially if nitrous oxide is used, because it can diffuse through the plastic. The second type is the floppy high-volume low-pressure cuff which exerts less tracheal pressure, but may cause more trauma during insertion.

Tracheal tube size and lengths in children

Table 3.2 lists tube sizes and lengths according to the age of the child. Below age 10 non-cuffed tubes should be used because in a child the narrowest part of the airway is in the trachea at the level of the cricoid cartilage.

Laryngeal masks are best suited for spontaneous respiration. If used with IPPV it is recommended that a pressure of 20 cm water should not be exceeded. They should not be used with IPPV in patients who are at risk from regurgitation.

3.12   a) True   b) False   c) True   d) True   e) False

EXPLANATION

Guillain–Barré syndrome is thought to be caused by immunologically mediated nerve injury.

The patient often has a minor respiratory or gastrointestinal illness prior to development of the neurological symptoms. The initial symptoms are usually paraesthesia in hands and feet, muscle pains, followed by motor weakness and reduced reflexes distally, which typically spreads upwards and may involve the intercostal muscles, so that respiration may be compromised. Sensory loss is usually mild. Cranial nerve involvement occurs in about 50% of cases, especially facial, glossopharyngeal and vagus. Autonomic dysfunction is common, and can be precipitated by changes in position – sweating, tachycardia, hypertension and tachyarrhythmias are all possible. The disease is self-limiting and recovery starts 2–4 weeks after halt of progression of neurological signs.

Cerebrospinal fluid protein is increased in most cases. White cell count is normal.

Treatment. Prognosis is usually good. Mortality is about 8%. The mainstay of treatment is supportive, i.e.:

- Respiratory support, physiotherapy and possibly intermittent positive-pressure ventilation.
- Cardiovascular support. Treatment of accompanying hypotension and arrhythmias. If tachycardia compromises cardiac output, beta blockers may be required.
- Fluids, electrolytes and nutrition.
- Plasma exchange may be of value, and may accelerate recovery. Steroids are of no benefit.
- Anaesthesia. If a general anaesthetic is required, suxamethonium should be avoided, because it may be associated with transient severe hyperkalaemia, and rhabdomyolysis, which can cause acute renal failure.

3.13   a) True   b) False   c) True   d) True   e) False

EXPLANATION
See Table 3.3.

3.14   a) False   b) False   c) True   d) False   e) True

EXPLANATION
See Table 3.3.

3.15   a) True   b) False   c) False   d) True   e) True

EXPLANATION
Sensitivity to non-depolarizers is associated with:
- Neonates
- Neuromuscular disease: myasthenia; muscular dystrophy
- Drugs: volatile anaesthetics – desflurane more so than isoflurane; local anaesthetics; aminoglycoside antibiotics, e.g. neomycin, polymyxin; calcium blockers; steroids; diuretics; cytotoxics and immunosuppressants
- Electrolyte abnormalities; acidosis (respiratory or metabolic), hypokalaemia; hypocalcaemia; hypernatraemia; hyponatraemia; hypermagnesaemia
- Renal/hepatic failure due to delayed metabolism/excretion
- Hypothermia.
Resistance to non-depolarizers is associated with:
- Burns and massive trauma
- Motor neuron disease
- Drugs: aminophylline; phenytoin.

3.16   **a) True**   **b) False**   **c) False**   **d) True**   **e) True**

EXPLANATION
See Table 3.4.

3.17   **a) False**   **b) True**   **c) False**   **d) False**   **e) False**

EXPLANATION
See Table 3.4.

3.18   **a) False**   **b) False**   **c) False**   **d) True**   **e) True**

EXPLANATION
See Table 3.4.

3.19   **a) True**   **b) True**   **c) False**   **d) False**   **e) False**

EXPLANATION
EMLA cream is a local anaesthetic cream containing 25 mg lignocaine and 25 mg prilocaine in a eutectic mixture as an oil/water emulsion. It has to have been applied for at least 1 hour for anaesthetic action and lasts about 5 hours. EMLA causes blanching of skin and vasoconstriction which can make venepuncture more difficult. Amethocaine gel does not cause this and it has a quicker onset of action. Apart from local anaesthetic action, lignocaine and other local anaesthetics provide systemic analgesia when administered intravenously. The mode of action is unclear – it may be related to local anaesthetic effects on damaged nerve fibres; to partial sympathetic blockade which counteracts the vasoconstriction from the pain; or to the abolition of nerve response to the pain transmitter bradykinin. Intravenous local anaesthetics (especially lignocaine because of its relatively low toxicity) have been used in chronic pain when other treatments fail, e.g. neuralgias especially post-herpetic, deafferentation syndrome, peripheral neuropathies and also chronic back pain. Repeated infusions are often required.

The ester-type local anaesthetics (e.g. procaine) are hydrolyzed by cholinesterase, the amide local anaesthetics (e.g. lignocaine, bupivacaine) are primarily metabolized in the liver. The duration of action of local anaesthetics is related primarily to the degree of protein binding. Lignocaine is 55% protein bound, while bupivacaine is 95% bound explaining its longer duration of action. Of the local anaesthetics, procaine has a short duration, lignocaine and prilocaine moderate, while bupivacaine has a long duration. The addition of adrenaline causes vasoconstriction and prolongs the action but not with bupivacaine because it is so highly protein bound.

61

Table 3.3 Actions of muscle relaxants

	Physical	Metabolism	Liver/renal
Curare	Bisquaternary benzyl isoquinoline agent. Non-depolarizer	Two methods of elimination: 50% renally in unchanged form; rest in bile in glucuronidated form	Prolonged action in liver and renal disease
Pancuronium	Synthetic steroid molecule. Non-depolarizer	75% renally excreted and has long action in renal disease. Rest metabolized in liver – metabolites excreted renally	Prolonged action in liver and renal disease
Vecuronium	Monoquaternary analogue of pancuronium. Non-depolarizer	Eliminated unchanged in bile and action prolonged in liver disease. Also metabolized in liver – metabolites eliminated renally	Prolonged action in liver disease. Can be used in renal disease except in prolonged operations
Atracurium	Bisquaternary nitrogen benzyl isoquinoline diester compound. Non-depolarizer	Spontaneous Hofmann degeneration to laudanosine and a monoacrylate agent. Breakdown is pH and temperature dependent. Laudanosine stimulates CNS and can cause fits, but not in doses usually employed	Best relaxant for liver/ renal disease. Elimination not organ dependent
Rocuronium	Aminosteroid. Non-depolarizer	Less than 25% excreted renally	? prolonged action in liver disease, but not in renal disease
Mivacurium	Bisquaternary benzyl isoquinoline choline-like diester. Non-depolarizer	By plasma cholinesterase and other esterases in liver. Action prolonged when cholinesterase level low (liver disease, congenitally)	Not dependent on organ elimination
Suxamethonium	Molecules of linked acetylcholine. Depolarizing but repeated doses/infusions lead to initial depolarizing (phase 1 block), then to non-depolarizing (phase 2 block)	By cholinesterase into succinyl monocholine and then into succinic acid and choline. 96% of patients are homozygous for cholinesterase gene (dibucaine number (DN) > 70); 4% heterozygous (1 normal, 1 atypical gene) (DN 30–70); 0.04% homozygous for atypical gene causing prolonged apnoea (DN < 30). Some have cholinesterase which is resistant to fluoride but not dibucaine. With fluoride-resistant homozygotes apnoea lasts about 1 h; with heterozygotes it lasts about 10 min	In cholinesterase absence, drug eliminated by redistribution and slow renal excretion
Specific problems with suxamethonium	High potassium – suxamethonium increases K by 0.5–1 mEq/l and more with damaged muscles or nerves: massive trauma; burns – first 6 weeks. Neuromuscular disorders; Guillain–Barré syndrome; Friedreich's ataxia; spinal cord trauma – lasts 6–12 months; cerebrovascular accidents. Bradycardia due to vagal stimulation especially with repeated doses. Very rarely, suxamethonium can cause cardiac arrest in children with undiagnosed myopathy which may not be apparent until age 6–8. Increase in intraocular pressure – open eye injuries; increase in intracranial pressure, i.e. intracranial pathology. Malignant hyperpyrexia		

Dose/onset/duration	Histamine	Cardiovascular
ED_{95}: 5 mg/kg Onset: 3–5 min Duration to 95% recovery: 120–140 min	Moderate	Histamine release causes low BP and tachycardia. Ganglion block also causes fall in BP
ED_{95}: 0.07 mg/kg Onset: 3–5 min Duration to 95% recovery: 120–140 min	None	Blocks muscarinic receptors and stimulates sympathetic system leading to tachycardia, high BP and dysrhythmias
ED_{95}: 0.05 mg/kg Onset: 1.5–3.5 min Duration to 95% recovery: 80–120 min	None	No significant cardiovascular effects
Ed_{95}: 0.2 mg/kg Onset: 3–5 min Duration to 95% recovery: 60–80 min depending on dose	Slight	Histamine release can cause tachycardia and hypotension
Dose: 0.1 mg/kg Onset: 45 s–2 min Duration to 75% recovery: 33–117 min	None	No significant cardiovascular effects
ED_{95}: 0.07 mg/kg Onset: 1–2 min Total recovery in 25 min; partial recovery in 14 min and can then be reversed with neostigmine	Slight	No significant cardiovascular actions
ED95: 0.25 mg/kg Onset: 24–84 s duration to 95% recovery: 12–15 min	Slight	Effects similar to acetylcholine, i.e. stimulation of muscarinic receptors causes bradycardia and nodal rhythm especially after second dose. Arrhythmias in sensitive patients due to K release

Table 3.4   Actions of anaesthetic vapours

	Nitrous oxide N_2O	Isoflurane $CF_3CHCl–O–CF_2H$	Enflurane $CHFClCF_2–O–CF_2H$
MAC			
In O_2	105	1.28	1.28
In 70% N_2O	–	0.56	0.57
Awake	0.7	–	–
Physical		Ethane with ether link to reduce myocardial sensitization to catecholamines. Substitution of fluorine for chlorine to increase stability and reduce potency and solubility	Isomer of isoflurane
Cardiovascular	Sympathetic stimulation causing increase in BP and CO	Fall in BP due to fall in SVR. CO maintained. ? coronary steal – blood flow diverted from collaterals to normal vessels causing ischaemia in collateral dependent area	Fall in BP and CO due to myocardial depression and low SVR. Tachycardia. Dysrhythmias uncommon
Respiration and bronchi	Little respiratory depression	Respiration depressed – fall in PaO_2 and rise in $PaCO_2$. Bronchodilatation	Respiratory depression and bronchodilatation
Central nervous system and cerebral blood flow	Mild increase in CBF	No seizure activity in EEG. 60% increase in CBF but less than with halothane and reduced with hypocarbia	Seizure activity on EEG. Increase in CBF more than isoflurane but less than halothane
Renal and hepatic blood flow	Little effect	Fall in renal flow due to decreased perfusion pressure. Fall in hepatic flow but less than with halothane/enflurane	25% fall in renal flow. Fall in hepatic flow
Metabolism	Eliminated by pulmonary ventilation	0.2% metabolism into fluorine and trichloroacetic acid – not enough to cause liver damage	Most eliminated by ventilation 2% by liver metabolism to fluorine and difluoromethoxy-difluoroacetic acid. Dangerous in severe renal failure
Induction/ emergence	Insoluble gas; thus rapid uptake and rapid elimination leads to rapid recovery	Rapid recovery. Nausea, vomiting and shivering similar to other agents	Rapid emergence
Complications and problems	Possible pneumothorax as gas expands in a cavity as the more soluble N_2O exchanges with N_2 in blood. Bone marrow depression after long use owing to inhibition of methionine synthetase (required for vitamin B_{12} synthesis)	Possible coronary steal in patients with coronary disease	Seizure activity on EEG. Fits, however, very rare and usually without any sequence

Inhalational agent		
Halothane CF$_3$CHClBr	**Desflurane** CF$_3$.CHF.O.CHF$_2$	**Sevoflurane** C$_3$HF$_4$.OF$_2$.CH$_2$F
0.75 0.29 0.52	4.6–6.0 – 0.53	1.71 0.66 –
Halogen substituted ethane	Fluorinated methyl ethyl ether. Further substitution of fluorine for chlorine decreases potency and solubility causing rapid induction and recovery	Fluorinated methyl isopropyl ether similar to desflurane
Fall in BP and CO due to myocardial depression. Bradycardia. Reduction in coronary flow. Dysrhythmias possible	Similar to isoflurane. Fall in BP due to fall in SVR. No coronary steal	Similar to isoflurane. Fall in BP due to reduced SVR
Respiratory depression and bronchodilatation	Respiratory depression and bronchodilatation	Respiratory depression and bronchodilatation
Marked increase in CBF and vasodilatation even with fall in cardiac output. Not recommended in neurosurgery	No seizure activity on EEG. Increase in CBF	No seizure activity on EEG
35% fall in renal flow due to fall in perfusion pressure. Marked fall in hepatic flow	No significant effects on renal or hepatic perfusion	No significant effects on renal or hepatic perfusion
20% liver metabolism to bromine, chlorine, trifluoroacetic acid. Liver damage and cirrhosis probably due to liver metabolites	Minimal biotransformation; less than isoflurane	Metabolism into fluorine which can cause renal damage over long time
Non-pungent and best for inhalational induction. Fairly rapid emergence. Nausea, vomiting, shivering similar to other agents	Pungent and can cause coughing, laryngospasm in inhalational induction. Prompt emergence is main advantage (day cases)	Rapid induction and emergence
Hepatic dysfunction after repeated exposure. 1 in 10 000 adults, less in children. Arrhythmias. Uterine relaxation can cause increased bleeding after delivery	Boils at room temperature. Thus very volatile and has to be diluted from a heated pressurized vaporizer. Should be used in closed-circuit systems because of cost	

Table 3.4 (*Cont'd*)

	Nitrous oxide N_2O	Isoflurane $CF_3CHCl-O-CF_2H$	Enflurane $CHFClCF_2-O-CF_2H$
Strengths/ weaknesses	Analgesia; little cardiac respiratory depression; rapid induction/recovery. Sympathetic stimulation; expansion of closed air spaces; needs high concentration	Stable heart rate; good muscle relaxation. Strong vasodilator. Pungent, not ideal for inhalational induction	Stable heart rate; good muscle relaxation. Pungent, not ideal for inhalational induction. Seizure activity on EEG

Key: BP = blood pressure; CBF = cerebral blood flow; CO = cardiac output; EEG = electroencephalogram; MAC = minimum alveolar concentration; SVR = Systemic vascular resistance

Lignocaine is the drug of choice in the treatment of ventricular dysrhythmias. It has been shown to be effective in the prevention of ventricular fibrillation after acute myocardial infarction. It decreases the slope of phase 4 of the action potential of Purkinje fibres. Lignocaine has no effect on atrial tissue and is ineffective in supraventricular tachycardias.

3.20   a) False   b) True   c) True   d) False   e) False

EXPLANATION

Mode of action
Prostaglandins are released by tissue trauma, and, in conjunction with other chemical mediators – histamine, bradykinins and serotonin, sensitize peripheral nociceptors to cause pain. NSAIDs exert their analgesic action by blocking the synthesis of prostaglandins by inhibiting the enzyme cyclo-oxygenase (prostaglandin synthetase). There are two types of cyclo-oxygenase, type I and type II. Type I is associated with gastric acid and mucus production and maintaining blood flow. Type II is associated with inflammatory response. At present, meloxicam is the only available NSAID which is a specific Type II inhibitor but others are being developed. NSAIDs that act on type II (e.g. ibuprofen) are less toxic. Cyclo-oxygenase catalyzes the conversion of the prostaglandin precursor arachidonic acid to prostaglandins. Prostaglandins are responsible for many effects of the inflammatory response, i.e. fever, pain, vasodilatation. NSAIDs also inhibit neutrophil and lymphocyte activity, which contributes to their analgesic and anti-inflammatory properties.

NSAIDs are rapidly absorbed in the gut and metabolized in the liver into inactive metabolites, which are excreted in the urine. NSAIDs are highly protein bound in the blood.

Major common problems
Gastrointestinal problems. A number of prostaglandins (PGE_1, PGE_2 and prostacyclin – PGI_2) protect the gastric mucosa by reducing gastric acid secretion,

Inhalational agent		
Halothane $CF_3CHClBr$	Desflurane $CF_3.CHF.O.CHF_2$	Sevoflurane $C_3HF_4.OF_2.CH_2F$
Cheap; effective in low concentration; not irritant to airway, thus good as inhalation agent. Uterine relaxation. Fairly slow uptake and elimination; arrhythmias; cardiac depression; biodegradable – hepatic damage	Rapid uptake and elimination. Low boiling point – special vaporizer; potent vasodilator; expensive	Rapid uptake and elimination. Potent vasodilator; expensive

and increasing gastric bicarbonate secretion, blood flow and mucus production. Prostaglandin inhibition by NSAIDs reduces this protection, and predisposes to peptic ulcerations. Apart from gastric ulcers, NSAIDs can cause dyspepsia, epigastric pain, anorexia, oesophagitis, constipation and diarrhoea. Risks are increased with prolonged NSAID use, alcohol abuse and advanced age. The NSAID most likely to cause gastric bleeding is azapropazone (Rheumox); the least likely is ibuprofen, while piroxicam, ketoprofen, indomethacin, naproxen and diclofenac are associated with intermediate risks. The incidence of peptic ulceration and bleeding can be reduced by:

- H_2 antagonists, e.g. cimetidine, ranitidine, which reduce histamine and therefore gastric acid secretion.
- Proton inhibitors, e.g. omeprazole, which inhibit gastric acid secretion by blocking the hydrogen/potassium adenosine triphosphatase enzyme system of the gastric parietal cell.
- Synthetic prostaglandins, e.g. misoprostol which reduces gastric acid secretion, and protects the gastric mucosa.

Coagulation problems. NSAIDs inhibit the prostaglandin thromboxane A_2 present in platelets. Thromboxane A_2 is a potent vasoconstrictor and stimulates platelet aggregation, leading to clot formation. Thus bleeding time is prolonged by NSAIDs. Aspirin inhibits platelet cyclo-oxygenase irreversibly and, when stopped, coagulation is affected until the platelet is regenerated within 6–10 days. Conversely, when other NSAID medication is terminated, the bleeding time is only prolonged until the drugs are excreted, because platelet cyclo-oxygenase is reversibly inhibited. One must also remember that since NSAIDs are highly protein bound, they displace other drugs (including coumarin anticoagulants) from their binding sites, causing further coagulation problems in patients on concurrent anticoagulant therapy.

Renal problems. In healthy patients, renal blood flow and glomerular filtration rate are not dependent on prostaglandins. However, patients with renal or hepatic damage, congestive heart failure, or who are volume depleted have high renin-angiotensin levels which promote the release of renal prostaglandins, causing renal vasodilatation and inhibition of tubular reabsorption of water and sodium. In these situations, NSAIDs can lead to decreased renal blood flow and decreased glomerular filtration rate, as well as water retention and hyperkalaemia.

Table 3.5   Properties of common non-steroidal anti-inflammatory analgesics

Drug	Half-life	Daily dose	Routes
Carboxylic acids			
Salicylic acids			
Acetylsalicylic acid (aspirin)	4–15 h	1000–6000 mg	Oral
Diffusinal (Dolobid)	7–15 h	500–1500 mg	Oral
Acetic acids			
Indomethacin (Indocin)	3–11 h	50–200 mg	Oral rectal
Ketorolac (Toradol)	3–8 h	75–150 mg	i.m., i.v.
Diclofenac (Voltarol)	2 h	100–200 mg	Oral, i.m., rectal
Tolmetin (Tolecitin)	1–2 h	600–2000 mg	Oral
Propionic acid			
Ibuprofen	2 h	1200–3200 mg	Oral
Ketoprofen (Orudis)	2 h	10–400 mg	Oral, i.m., rectal
Naproxen (Naprosyn)	13 h	250–1500 mg	Oral, rectal

Comments	Side-effects
Used widely for prophylaxis against cerebrovascular and myocardial ischaemia	Nausea; peptic ulceration with bleeding; tinnitus, rarely deafness; vertigo; allergy – rashes, oedema, bronchospasm; coagulation disorders – especially thrombocytopenia; rarely renal damage due to reduced blood flow; Reye's syndrome, thus should be avoided in children under age 12
Effects more similar to ibuprofen than aspirin	Similar to aspirin
Potent anti-inflammatory	Similar to aspirin Specific problems: CNS: headache, dizziness, mood swings, light-headedness, blurred vision; peripheral neuropathy
Can be used i.v.; non irritant; potent analgesic; weak anti-inflammatory	
Irritant. i.m. injection painful and tissue necrosis possible; rectal can cause proctitis	Similar to aspirin Specific problem: hepatitis
	Like aspirin Specific problem: aseptic meningitis
Fewer side-effects but weak anti-inflammatory and not indicated for acute rheumatic conditions	Gastrointestinal – nausea, diarrhoea; occasionally peptic erosions and bleeding; tinnitus, dizziness, vertigo; allergy – rashes, oedema, bronchospasm; rarely acute reversible renal failure; hepatic damage Specific problem: aseptic meningitis – headache, stiff neck, photophobia, fever
i.m. – pain, rarely tissue necrosis Suppositories – rectal irritation	Similar to aspirin and ibuprofen
Suppositories may cause rectal irritation	Similar to aspirin and ibuprofen Specific problem: bilateral pulmonary infiltrates causing dyspnoea and cough

Table 3.5 (*Cont'd*)

Drug	Half-life	Daily dose	Routes
Pyrazoles			
Phenylbutazone (Butazolidine)	40–80 h	200–800 mg	Oral
Oxicams			
Piroxicam (Feldene)	30–80 h	20 mg	Oral, rectal

Anaphylactic problems. These vary from mild skin rashes or urticaria to severe bronchospasm. 5–10% of asthmatic patients are allergic to NSAIDs; therefore one should be very careful in administering NSAIDs to asthma patients, and to patients who have a history of allergic reactions, and a history of allergic nasal polyps.

Properties of common non-steroidal anti-inflammatory analgesics are listed in Table 3.5.

Other non-opioid analgesics

Apart from opioids, agonist-antagonists and NSAIDs there are a number of other analgesics which may be of use in mild to moderate pain.

Paracetamol. Paracetamol is as analgesic as aspirin, but has no anti-inflammatory action. It is less irritant to the stomach, but an overdose can cause liver and more rarely renal damage. Rashes, blood disorders and acute pancreatitis are also possible.

Dextropropoxyphene. This is a mild opioid analgesic, which is less potent than codeine. It is not very effective on its own.

Nefopam. This may be useful for moderate pain. It does not cause any respiratory depression but may have sympathomimetic side-effects – tachycardia, sweating; and atropine-like actions – dry mouth, blurred vision, urinary retention. Other side-effects include nausea and CNS symptoms – headache, confusion, drowsiness, insomnia, hallucinations. It is available as oral or intramuscular preparations.

Tramadol. Tramadol is a potent analgesic, which has a dual action; it acts on opioid receptors and also increases noradrenaline and 5-HT levels. It does not cause respiratory depression or sedation, and causes less constipation and addiction than opioids, but nausea and vomiting are common. Other side-effects include hypotension, hypertension, allergic reactions, confusion, hallucinations. It is available as oral, intramuscular and intravenous preparations.

Analgesic combinations. Analgesic combinations are popular. They include: aspirin-paracetomal combinations, e.g. benorylate; aspirin-codeine preparations, e.g. co-codaprin; paracetamol-codeine combinations (i.e. tablets usually containing 500 mg paracetamol with varying amounts (8–30 mg) of codeine), e.g. co-codamol, co-dydramol, dihydrocodeine, Tylex, Kapake, Solpadol, Remedeine, etc.; paracetamol-dextropropoxyphene preparations, e.g. co-proxamol (32.5 mg dextropropoxyphene and 325 mg paracetamol).

Comments	Side-effects
Potent anti-inflammatory	Similar to aspirin and ibuprofen Specific problem: bone marrow toxicity – aplastic anaemia, leucopenia, thrombocytopenia; parotitis; stomatitis; hepatitis
Painful i.m. injections	Similar to aspirin and ibuprofen

4.1 Nitric oxide:

a) Is a pulmonary vasodilator
b) Is inactivated by soda lime
c) In increased levels, is associated with general anaesthesia
d) Is released by nitroprusside and nitroglycerine
e) Is an impurity in nitrous oxide synthesis

4.2 Delayed recovery from general anaesthesia may be due to:

a) Potassium imbalance
b) Sodium imbalance
c) Parathyroid surgery
d) Hypercapnia
e) Steroid overdose

4.3 Of the local anaesthetics:

a) Like all other ester local anaesthetics, cocaine is metabolized by cholinesterase
b) Compared to 'EMLA' gel amethocaine gel used for surface analgesia has a quicker onset of action and causes less vasoconstriction
c) One must wait at least 15 minutes before starting a bronchoscopy under local anaesthesia with lignocaine
d) Allergic reactions are more likely with lignocaine than with procaine
e) Bupivacaine is the best agent to use in intravenous regional analgesia because it provides prolonged analgesia

4.4 With regard to peripheral neuropathies:

a) Diabetic neuropathy is confined to severe diabetics and is very unlikely in mild cases
b) Neuropathy due to a lumbar intervertebral disc prolapse is most common at S1 and lower lumbar root levels
c) Alcoholic neuropathy is associated with vitamin B_{12} deficiency
d) Both diabetic and porphyria neuropathy can be associated with autonomic nerve involvement
e) Nerve conduction velocity is reduced in all types of neuropathies

4.5 In anaesthetic practice, allergic reactions:

a) Are more likely with etomidate than thiopentone
b) May occur as a result of cross-sensitivity when a carbapenem antibiotic is given to a patient with a known history of penicillin allergy
c) Are unlikely to include bronchospasm in patients with a history of aspirin-induced reaction
d) Are more likely with bupivacaine than with amethocaine
e) To non-steroidal anti-inflammatory drugs and aspirin analgesics are likely to be more severe than to opioids

4.6 Of the sympathomimetic drugs:

a) Alpha-2 adrenergic drugs stimulate noradrenaline release
b) Beta-2 adrenergic drugs stimulate glycogenolysis and gluconeogenesis
c) Alpha-1 agonists decrease intracellular calcium
d) Adrenaline has alpha-1 and -2 actions and beta-1 and -2 actions
e) Beta-2 agonists cause uterine relaxation

4.7 Of the antiemetic drugs:

a) Those which act as antidopaminergic agents can cause extrapyramidal symptoms
b) Domperidone reduces vomiting by an antiserotonin action
c) Extrapyramidal symptoms after administration of droperidol are unlikely 6 hours after administration
d) Phenothiazines reduce nausea and vomiting by antidopaminergic, antihistamine and antimuscarinic actions
e) Domperidone exerts its action by its sedative effect on the central nervous system

4.8 With regard to pulmonary aspiration:

a) The incidence of regurgitation and aspiration is higher in patients undergoing 'mask' anaesthesia compared to endotracheal anaesthesia
b) In the supine position aspiration is more likely in the right lung
c) Patients especially at risk are those with gastric pH less than 2.5 and gastric volumes greater than 25 ml
d) Metoclopramide is more effective at reducing gastric volume and increasing gastric pH than ranitidine
e) It can cause pulmonary and cardiovascular pathology

4.9 Ropivacaine:

a) Is an aminoamide-type local anaesthetic
b) Is more cardiotoxic than bupivacaine
c) Produces a motor block of more pronounced degree and duration than bupivacaine
d) Gives rise to a sensory block that is similar to bupivacaine
e) Is more lipid soluble than bupivacaine

4.10 Pleural effusion:

a) Is transudate when the protein level is above 30 g/litre; and exudate when it is below 30 g/litre
b) When small, is more likely to be detected clinically than with chest X-ray
c) Can be due to hypoproteinaemia
d) If malignant, is often bloodstained
e) Of chyle (chylothorax) is likely in penetrating wounds in the right chest because of thoracic duct trauma

4.11 Compared to atracurium, cisatracurium:

a) Is a mixture of 10 stereoisomers
b) Produce higher levels of laudanosine
c) Causes less histamine release
d) Is less potent
e) Has a slower onset and shorter duration of action

4.12 With regard to the use of antibiotics during surgery:

a) Antibiotic prophylaxis given immediately after surgery is just as effective as when administered prior to surgery
b) Patients with ventricular septal defect have a higher risk of endocarditis than patients with atrial septal defect
c) Antibiotic prophylaxis is necessary in dirty cases but of no benefit in clean cases
d) Aminoglycosides can potentiate both depolarizing and non-depolarizing relaxants
e) In view of their sterile nature, prosthetic devices do not require prophylactic antibiotic cover

4.13 Bowel motility is increased with:

a) Vagal stimulation
b) Anticholinesterase drugs
c) High spinal/epidural with local anaesthetics
d) Intrathecal/epidural opiates
e) Diazepam

4.14 With regard to the kidney and anaesthesia:

a) Renal autoregulation is abolished during general anaesthesia
b) Fluoride levels from volatile anaesthetics less then 50 µm/litre are unlikely to be associated with renal failure
c) Hypotension accompanied by vasoconstriction is less likely to be harmful than hypotension with vasodilatation
d) Diuretics are indicated to treat oliguria in shocked patients
e) PGE_1 prostaglandins cause renal vasodilatation and increase salt excretion

4.15 Problems with closed circle systems include:

a) Cranial nerve damage with methoxyflurane/soda lime
b) Potential nephrotoxic ethers with sevoflurane/soda lime
c) Higher carbon monoxide production when the soda lime has a high water content
d) Increased resistance to breathing
e) Carbon monoxide production is higher with halothane than with desflurane

4.16 These anaesthetic agents increase sympathetic tone:

a) Pancuronium
b) High concentrations of desflurane
c) Nitrous oxide
d) Ketamine
e) Curare

4.17 In neuroleptic malignant syndrome:

a) The condition is congenital and familial
b) Rigidity is not relieved with non-depolarizing relaxants
c) Dantrolene is ineffective in treatment
d) Suxamethonium often triggers off the syndrome
e) Temperature is never elevated

4.18 In HELLP syndrome:

a) Characteristic features include haemolytic anaemia and elevation of liver enzymes
b) Occurrence can be pre- and postpartum
c) There is always an association with hypertension
d) Epidural anaesthesia is the preferred method of delivery
e) Steroids are contraindicated

4.19 Pulmonary complications are increased with:

a) Operations lasting over 4 hours
b) Thoracotomy done through a median sternotomy rather than a lateral approach
c) Prolonged antibiotic therapy
d) Inadequate control of postoperative pain
e) Patients with low functional residual capacity

4.20 Of the antiplatelet drugs:

a) Aspirin exerts its antiplatelet action by increasing the synthesis of thromboxane A_2
b) Dipyridamole can be of great benefit in venous thromboembolism
c) All prostaglandins encourage platelet aggregation
d) None should ever be administered in conjunction with oral anticoagulants
e) Low molecular weight dextrans reduce platelet aggregation

4.1   a) True   b) True   c) False   d) True   e) True

EXPLANATION

Nitric oxide (NO) reacts with ozone to produce nitrogen dioxide and photons, and this photo-emission property is used in the detection and measurement of nitric oxide.

Nitric oxide is produced from L-arginine in a number of cells including vascular endothelium. The enzyme nitric oxide synthetase (NOS) is required for its production. The main function of NO is regulation of vascular tone. It is produced by the endothelium and diffuses into the vascular smooth muscle where it activates soluble guanylate cyclase which in turn increases levels of the vasodilator, cyclic GMP. Increased NO synthesis may be responsible for vasodilatation in septic shock. Nitrate vasodilators such as nitroglycerine and nitroprusside act by releasing nitric oxide. Inhaled NO has been used to produce pulmonary vasodilatation in pulmonary disease, but is not so effective as a systemic vasodilator because NO is rapidly inactivated by haemoglobin. (NO combines with haemoglobin much more so than carbon monoxide.) Adult respiratory distress syndrome (ARDS) is associated with hypoxaemia and pulmonary hypertension, and inhaled NO (5–20 parts per million) has been used for this condition and for other pulmonary diseases where pulmonary vasodilatation is required. NO itself is not toxic but its metabolites (such as nitrogen dioxide – NO_2) can cause pulmonary toxicity (pneumonitis). (Both nitric oxide and nitrogen dioxide are impurities in the synthesis of N_2O.) NO_2 is absorbed by soda lime and this property may be useful when NO inhalation therapy is employed. However, NO is also absorbed by soda lime, and the inspired levels must therefore be measured at a point distal to the soda lime.

It is likely that nitric oxide interacts with analgesics and general anaesthetics, both intravenous and inhalational. Nitric oxide synthetase is reduced by all anaesthetic agents and it is likely that inhibition of nitric oxide production augments anaesthesia and this may play a role in producing anaesthesia in humans. Nitric oxide is thought to act as a neurotransmitter involved in consciousness, learning and memory.

4.2   a) False   b) True   c) True   d) True   e) False

EXPLANATION

The three major causes of prolonged awakening following general anaesthesia are:

1. prolonged action of anaesthetic agents
2. metabolic causes
3. neurological causes.

Prolonged action of anaesthetic agents. This may be due to drug overdose, drug interaction, decreased protein binding or increased sensitivity (advanced age, hypothermia, hypothyroidism, liver and renal disease which slows metabolism/excretion).

Metabolic causes:

● Hypoxia – often presents with agitation or delirium.
● Hypercapnia causes acidosis which depresses the central nervous system; the acidosis also prolongs the action of neuromuscular agents. Hypocapnia can cause cerebral vasoconstriction and prolong awakening.

- Endocrine: renal failure; liver failure; hypothyroidism; adrenal insufficiency.
- Glucose imbalance: hypoglycaemia; hyperosmolar non-ketotic hyperglycaemia; diabetic ketoacidosis.
- Electrolyte imbalance: hyponatraemia (e.g. TURP syndrome causing water intoxication); hypernatraemia (dehydration, hypercalcaemia (malignancy) or hypocalcaemia (e.g. parathyroid surgery)); hypermagnesaemia due to magnesium sulphate therapy.

Neurological causes. These include cerebral ischaemia, intracranial haemorrhage, cerebral embolus, cerebral fits; etc.

In order to make a diagnosis, one needs to review the history of pre-existing disease and drug administration; make a detailed neurological examination and possibly take blood gases and measure electrolyte and biochemical levels (e.g. Na, glucose, etc.). A CT scan of the head may also be required.

4.3   a) False   b) True   c) False   d) False   e) False

EXPLANATION
See Table 4.1.

4.4   a) False   b) True   c) False   d) True   e) False

EXPLANATION
Causes of peripheral neuropathies. Peripheral neuropathy usually starts in the distal areas with loss of vibration, followed by tendon loss, motor weakness and muscle wasting. It can be associated with autonomic neuropathy (e.g. diabetes) which is characterized by loss of sweating, hypotension, pupil abnormalities, bladder sphincter disturbances and impotence. Nerve conduction times are not altered in ascending types of neuropathy, but are reduced when it is due to nerve demyelination.

1. Acute neuropathy (i.e. Guillain–Barré – ascending polyneuritis). Usually follows a viral infection, often glandular fever but also mumps, herpes, hepatitis. Porphyria can also cause an acute neuropathy.
2. Chronic neuropathy:
- Ischaemia and pressure, e.g. prolapsed intervertebral disc especially at S1 and lower lumbar levels or C5–C6 in the neck. Other examples include nerve entrapment syndrome, carpal tunnel syndrome, Volkmann's ischaemic contracture.
- Myopathic, e.g. Bell's facial palsy – usually primary, but may follow leukaemia, multiple sclerosis, sarcoid, parotid tumour. Steroids may be helpful.
- Nutritional, e.g. thiamine deficiency in alcoholics may be associated with Wernicke's encephalopathy, vitamin B_{12} deficiency in pernicious anaemia causing subacute degeneration of the spinal cord.
- Metabolic – most commonly in diabetics, even mild or undetected diabetics, and often associated with autonomic neuropathy. Also possible in renal failure,

hepatic failure, myxoedema, acromegaly, porphyria (again often associated with autonomic neuropathy).
- Carcinomas, especially carcinoma of the bronchus; also after Hodgkin's disease and other reticuloses.
- Collagen diseases, e.g. polyarteritis nodosa, dematomyositis, systemic lupus erythematosus.
- Drugs, e.g. heavy metals (environmental pollution), phenytoin, vincristine.

4.5   a) False   b) True   c) False   d) False   e) True

EXPLANATION
Agents likely to induce allergic reaction in anaesthetic practice are numerous:

1. *Antibiotics.* The incidence of penicillin fatal anaphylaxis is about 1 in 75 000. About 15% of patients have a history of penicillin allergy. Like penicillins, cephalosporins and carbapenems (e.g. imipenem) have a betalactam ring, and allergy to these antibiotics is possible in patients with a history of penicillin allergy. Vancomycin and the sulphonamides have also been associated with anaphylactic reactions.

2. *Muscle relaxants.* Allergic reactions are possible with relaxants that release histamine, e.g. curare, suxamethonium, atracurium and mivacurium.

3. *Induction agents.* Etomidate is the induction agent least likely to cause allergic reactions; thiopentone is probably most likely, though reactions to the latter are still rare.

4. *Local anaesthetics.* True allergic reactions to local anaesthetics are very rare. If they occur they are to agents in the ester group (i.e. procaine, tetracaine, etc.) rather than the amide group (lignocaine and bupivacaine).

5. Analgesics.

- Aspirin and non-steroidal anti-inflammatory drugs (NSAIDs): reactions to aspirin and NSAIDs are usually skin reactions (urticaria, oedema) or respiratory system (bronchospasm, rhinitis, sinusitis). Aspirin-induced bronchospasm is rare in non-asthmatics but occurs in 10% of asthmatics, 35% of asthmatics with a history of nasal polyps and allergic rhinitis, and 75% in asthmatics who give a history of aspirin-induced reactions. All NSAIDs should be avoided in asthmatics and in patients with a history of nasal polyps.
- Narcotics (e.g. morphine, pethidine, codeine): cause histamine release from skin mast cells and opiate-induced reactions are usually cutaneous.
- *Contrast media.* Incidence of reactions is about 7%—nausea, vomiting, flushing, urticaria, wheezing, hypotension.

6. Others:

- Protamine/insulin preparations: both protamine and insulin can cause allergic reactions. Insulin usually causes local skin reactions which often disappear with repeated treatment because of antibody production. Severe reactions to insulin are very rare. Reactions to protamine are more severe and include bronchospasm and hypotension. Moreover, diabetics on protamine/insulin preparations have a 50-fold increased risk of severe reactions if protamine is administered.

Table 4.1 Properties of local anaesthetics

	Cocaine	Procaine	Amethocaine
Ester/amide	Ester	Ester	Ester
Onset/duration	Rapid onset Duration: 20–30 min	Slow onset Short duration: 45–90 min with adrenaline	Slow onset Long duration: 1.5–3 h
Potency/protein binding		Potency: 1 6% protein bound	Potency: 8
Metabolism	Liver. 10% excreted unchanged via kidney	By cholinesterase into p-aminobenzoic acid which can cause allergy	Hydrolysed by cholinesterase; allergic reactions possible
Specific uses	Topical use in nasal surgery in concentrations of 4–20%	Infiltration; spinals; not much used now. Used in treatment of malignant hyperpyrexia	Topical (amethocaine lozenge – 65 mg for analgesia in mouth and pharynx). Gel 4%: onset 30–40 min and causes vasodilatation, viz EMLA
Dose NB: 1% solution equals 10 mg/ml	1.5 mg/kg of 10% solution		Maximum dose for 70-kg adult: 100 mg without adrenaline
Specific problems/ comments	Sympathomimetic: addition; high pulse rate and BP; vasoconstriction and dilated pupils	Allergy possible due to p-aminobenzoic acid	Highly toxic

Local anaesthetic

Lignocaine	Prilocaine	Bupivacaine	Ropivacaine
Amide	Amide	Amide	Amide
Fast onset Moderate duration: 1 h without adrenaline; 1.5–2 h with adrenaline	Fast onset Moderate duration	Moderate onset Long duration: 3–10 h	Onset and duration same as bupivacaine
Potency: 2 55% protein bound	Potency: 2	Potency: 8 95% protein bound	Potency: 8
Metabolized in liver	Liver metabolism	Liver metabolism	Liver metabolism
Infiltration; spinal/ epidural; topical nerve blocks; Bier's; EMLA; systemic analgesia – used in chest pain; ventricular arrhythmias 1 mg/kg	Infiltration; peripheral, nerve blocks; Bier's	Infiltration; peripheral nerve blocks, epidurals/spinals	Obstetrics/ postoperative analgesia
3 mg/kg without adrenaline; 7 mg/kg with adrenaline Corneal analgesia 4%; urethra 2% Maximum dose for 70-kg adult: 200 mg plain; 500 mg with adrenaline	6 mg/kg without adrenaline; 9 mg/kg with adrenaline Maximum dose: 400 mg plain; 600 mg with adrenaline	2 mg/kg without adrenaline – addition of adrenaline does not prolong action Maximum dose: 150 mg plain; 150 mg with adrenaline	Used as 1% solution Maximum dose plain: 250 mg
Low toxicity; metabolism can cause methaemoglobinaemia – rarely a problem; vasodilatation	Least toxic; less vasodilatation than lignocaine. Methaemo-globinaemia – neonate cyanosis after epidurals	Highly toxic; not suitable for Bier's block because i.v. injection can cause CVS collapse	As highly protein bound as bupivacaine but less lipid soluble; less cardiotoxic; less CNS toxicity; degree and duration of motor block less than bupivacaine

Table 4.1   (Cont'd)

	Cocaine	Procaine	Amethocaine
General problems	CNS: tinnitus; confusion; numbness around mouth; convulsions; co		
	CVS: initial hypertension; tachycardia; myocardial depression; hypo		
	Allergy: with procaine-type ester, due to formation of *p*-aminobenzo		
Factors increasing activity	Dosage; addition of vasoconstrictor		
	Site of administration: shortest onset spinal, subcutaneous, bronchi		
	Carbonation: more rapid onset and increased block; alkalinization:		
	Pregnancy: increased spread and depth of spinals/epidurals owing		

- Mannitol: dextrans and other hyperosmotic agents cause histamine release from mast cells.
- Streptokinase: about 10% of patients show allergic reactions.
- Latex: latex is a component of Foley catheters, surgical gloves, rubber tips of syringes, some adhesives, some electrodes and oximeter probes, etc. Latex is associated with type 4 and type 1 anaphylactic reactions. Type 4 are cell mediated, i.e. when exposed to the offending rubber material, the T cells become sensitized to these haptens (allergens); when re-exposure occurs, the T lymphocytes multiply and cause a delayed hypersensitivity reaction—skin rashes and dermatitis, which are irritating but not life threatening. The more serious reaction is type 1 hypersensitivity, where the rubber antigen promotes the production of an antibody of the immunoglobulin E class (IgE); at re-exposure, even to a tiny amount of antigen, histamine, prostaglandins, etc. are released to cause an anaphylactic picture which can vary from itching, oedema and mild hypotension to severe shock. Latex allergy is present in about 1% of the general public, 10% of health workers, and as high as 67% of patients with spina bifida (owing to repeated catheterizations).

4.6   a) False   b) True   c) False   d) True   e) True

EXPLANATION
See Table 4.2.

4.7   a) True   b) False   c) False   d) True   e) False

EXPLANATION
See Table 4.3.

Local anaesthetic

Lignocaine	Prilocaine	Bupivacaine	Ropivacaine

)ression

tion; bradycardia; arrhythmias; CVS collapse

onset major nerve blocks

Table 4.2 Actions of sympathomimetics

	Example	Antagonist	Mechanism	Actions
Alpha-1 agonist	Adrenaline, ephedrine, noradrenaline, metaraminol, methoxamine – pure alpha	Phentolamine, phenoxybenzamine	Increase in intracellular calcium causing smooth muscle contraction. Present mainly in smooth muscle	Vasoconstriction; contraction of smooth muscles of iris, ureter and sphincters. Relaxation of gut smooth muscle; increased salivary and sweat gland secretions
Alpha-2 agonist	Clonidine, adrenaline, noradrenaline	Yohimbine	Decreased cyclic AMP and increase in intracellular calcium. Present in peripheral vasculature and coronary arteries	Peripheral vasoconstriction; dilatation of coronary arteries; bradycardia; platelet aggregation; inhibition of lipolysis in adipose tissue
Beta-1 agonist	Adrenaline, ephedrine, noradrenaline, dobutamine	Atenolol, propranolol	Mainly present in the heart. Activation of calcium channels	Increased rate and contractility of heart
Beta-2 agonist	Adrenaline, ephedrine, isoprenaline, salbutamol	Propranolol	Present in smooth muscle of peripheral vessels, bronchi and uterus. Also in adipose tissue, liver, skeletal muscle, endocrine and salivary glands	Vasodilatation and bronchodilatation; lipolysis, glycogenolysis and gluconeogenesis

4.8   a) False   b) True   c) True   d) False   e) True

EXPLANATION

Incidence. Silent regurgitation is common and often unnoticed (about 9%), while the incidence of aspiration is about 0.8%.

Table 4.3 Properties of antiemetics

Drugs	Antidopaminergic	Muscarinic antagonists
Anticholinergics Hyoscine Atropine Glycopyrolate		Strong
Antihistamines e.g. cyclizine	Mild	Moderate
Phenothiazines e.g. prochlorperazine, chlorperazine	Strong	Strong
Butyrophenones e.g. droperidol	Strong	
Others Metoclopramide	Strong	
Domperidone	Strong	
Ondansetron (granisetron similar)	Nil	

Predisposing factors. Obesity, hiatus hernia, oesophageal carcinoma, peptic ulcers, gastro-oesophageal reflux, pregnancy, swallowing disorders secondary to neurological or anatomical abnormalities, postoperative period before full return of laryngeal reflexes. There is no evidence to suggest that endotracheal intubation reduces the risk; in fact in some studies mask anaesthesia was associated with a lower risk of regurgitation. It has been shown that patients mostly at risk are those with gastric pH less than 2.5 and gastric volumes greater than 25 ml.

Clinical. Aspiration of liquid material produces a pneumonia in the affected areas of the lung. In the supine position bronchial anatomy favours right-sided aspiration, though both lungs are often involved. An hour or two after aspiration there is cyanosis, tachycardia and tachypnoea. Auscultation reveals rhonchi and crepitations. Because significant fluid can be absorbed into the circulation, there may be pulmonary oedema and circulatory collapse (pulmonary oedema may also be due to chemical pneumonitis from aspiration of acid material). Chest X-ray reveals areas of lung collapse and/or patchy areas of pulmonary oedema. In some cases minor

Antihistamines	Antiserotonin	Comments
		Reduced sweating and secretion; tachycardia; muscle relaxation
Strong		CNS depression: sedation; vestibular sedative (therefore useful in vertigo and tinnitus – cinnarizine); possible extrapyramidal
Strong		symptoms; atropine-like actions: drying of secretions; smooth muscle relaxation; tachycardia
Mild		Sedation; extrapyramidal symptoms even 24 h after administration. Alpha-adrenergic action: hypotension; hypothalamic depression reducing shivering; alpha-blocking action: hypotension and antihistaminic action
Mild	Moderate	Reduces oesophageal and gastric tone; sedation; restlessness; extrapyramidal symptoms possible
Nil	Nil	Useful for cytotoxic-induced vomiting; sedation; extrapyramidal symptoms less likely because it does not cross blood-brain barrier
Nil	Strong	Especially useful for cytotoxic emesis but not more effective than droperidol for anaesthetic vomiting and the latter is much cheaper; headaches; transient liver impairment; sedation; constipation

degrees of aspiration can cause massive pneumonitis. In others, significant aspiration can lead to hardly any pulmonary pathology.

Prevention:

1. Cricoid pressure and crash inductions in patients at risk. Patients at risk, indeed all patients, should be extubated only on full recovery and in the lateral position with suction readily available.

2. Aim to keep gastric pH above 2.5 and gastric volumes below 25 ml.

- Antacids alone increase pH but may increase gastric volume.
- Metoclopramide alone reduces gastric volume and increases pH.
- H_2 antagonists, e.g. ranitidine, are the most effective measures available to significantly reduce gastric volume and increase pH. Therefore ranitidine (150 mg 2–4 h preoperatively) should probably be administered to all patients having a general anaesthetic.

4.9   a) True   b) False   c) False   d) True   e) False

EXPLANATION

Ropivacaine has been evaluated in recent years as an alternative to bupivacaine in an effort to find a local anaesthetic which is less cardiotoxic than bupivacaine. Although the high lipid solubility of bupivacaine is beneficial in reducing absorption, this protection is lost when bupivacaine is directly injected into a vein and there is a high concentration of free drug which is likely to cause cardiac and CNS toxicity. Ropivacaine is very similar to bupivacaine in many respects. It is a long-acting aminoamide (duration similar to bupivacaine), as highly protein bound as bupivacaine but less lipid soluble. Its molecular weight is also similar: 274 – ropivacaine; 288 – bupivacaine. The advantages of ropivacaine over bupivacaine are that it is less cardiotoxic (thus injections are less likely to cause cardiovascular depression) and also has less CNS toxicity. Moreover, the degree and duration of motor blockade are significantly less than those of bupivacaine and this property is very useful in obstetric and postoperative analgesia. Sensory block is similar to bupivacaine. It can be used for surgical anaesthesia in concentration up to 1%. The maximal dose plain is 250 mg.

4.10   a) False   b) False   c) True   d) True   e) False

EXPLANATION

Types and causes of pleural effusions include:

1. Transudate (protein less than 30 g/litre):
   - Heart failure: left ventricular failure is the most common cause, constricture pericarditis
   - Hypoproteinaemia: due to hepatic or renal failure
   - Meigs' syndrome: effusion associated with ovarian fibroid.
2. Exudate (protein more than 30 g/litre):
   - Malignancy: usually bloodstained
   - Infections: pneumonia, tuberculosis
   - Connective tissue disorders: e.g. rheumatoid arthritis, systemic lupus erythematosus
   - Pulmonary infarction: following pulmonary embolism (usually small and bloodstained)
   - Pancreatitis
   - Drugs: e.g. some beta blockers (practolol, oxprenolol), methysergide.
3. Haemothorax: trauma; malignancy; pulmonary infarction.
4. Empyema, i.e. pus in pleural cavity: pneumonia; tuberculosis; subphrenic abscess; ruptured oesophagus; chest trauma.
5. Chylothorax: usually due to thoracic duct involvement in the left chest either following trauma or because of malignancies (carcinoma of bronchus or lymphoma).

   Clinical. In the early stages there is pleuritic pain, then breathlessness depending on the size of the effusion. On the side of the effusion there is reduced movement; absent breath sounds; dull percussion and bronchial breathing. There must be at least 500 ml of effusion to be detected clinically and 300 ml to be visible on a chest

X-ray. Ultrasound and CT scans may be useful in the differential diagnosis, especially with mediastinal lesions.

If the effusion is due to hypoproteinaemia, this must be treated. In other cases pleural aspiration relieves breathlessness and helps to establish the diagnosis by protein estimation in the fluid (i.e. transudate or exudate), differential cell counts, cytology for neoplastic cells, bacteriology, detection of rheumatoid factor, detection of carcinoembryonic antigen (CEA).

Recurrent effusions (especially in malignant disease) require pleural ablation either by talc pleurodesis or pleurectomy.

4.11   a) False   b) False   c) True   d) False   e) False

EXPLANATION
Atracurium is a mixture of 10 stereoisomers which are distributed into three main groups depending upon whether the arrangement is 'cis' or 'trans' at each end of the molecule. There are three isomers in the 'cis-cis' group, three in the 'trans-trans' group and four in the 'cis-trans' group. One isomer in the cis-cis group (cisatracurium) has now been released.

Cisatracurium is very similar to atracurium in action with some minor differences (see Table 4.4).

4.12   a) False   b) True   c) False   d) True   e) False

EXPLANATION

Prophylactic antibiotics during surgery
Antibiotics are important to anaesthetists during surgery because they may interact with anaesthetic drugs and because anaesthetists often have to administer them for prophylaxis against wound infection and endocarditis.

Prevention of wound infection. Sepsis is common postoperatively even when surgery is carried out with strict aseptic technique. This is probably because even in uncomplicated procedures there is depression of the immune response. This depression occurs early in the perioperative period. It is obviously important to administer antibiotics in 'dirty' cases; however, there is increasing evidence that even in 'clean' cases prophylactic antibiotics reduce the incidence of postoperative infection. Antibiotic cover started before wound contamination renders bacteria inactive; thus prophylaxis should be started before the incision (ideally 30 min parenterally), which would ensure adequate tissue levels at least until the wound is closed. It is probable that coverage beyond 24 hours is unnecessary.

Prevention of endocarditis. Prophylaxis against endocarditis is recommended in patients and procedures with a high incidence of bacteraemia. Patient conditions with a risk of endocarditis are:

1. High risk – artificial valve, patent ductus arteriosus, ventricular septal defect (VSD), mitral valve disease
2. Medium risk – mitral valve prolapse, pulmonary/tricuspid valve disease, idiopathic hypertrophic subaortic stenosis
3. Low risk – atrial septal defect (ASD), previous coronary grafts, pacemakers.

Table 4.4   Atracurium and cisatracurium

	Atracurium	Cisatracurium
Potency	ED$_{95}$ 0.23 mg/kg	ED$_{95}$ 0.05 mg/kg; thus more potent
Onset/duration/dose	Maximum block 3 min after injection. Duration about 35 min. Dose 0.5 mg/kg	Slower onset; maximum block after 5 min. Duration about 45 min. Easily reversed with anticholinesterase drugs, supposedly more so than with with atracurium. Dose 0.1–0.15 mg/kg
Pharmacokinetics	Hofmann degradation pH and temperature dependent, organ independent. Metabolites: laudanosine and monoquaternary acrylate which are eliminated by liver and kidneys, but have no neuromuscular activity. Ideal in liver or renal failure	Hofmann degradation; because it is more potent, the concentration of metabolites is much less than with atracurium (laudanosine 1/10 level of atracurium). Ideal in liver/renal failure
Histamine	Histamine release	Much less histamine release, again because of its potency and thus reduced mass of drug
Cardiovascular system	Possible hypotension and tachycardia due to histamine	No cardiovascular effects because of lack of histamine release

Procedures most likely to cause bacteraemia are dental operations, operations on the respiratory tract (e.g. tonsillectomy, nasal operations, intubations; head and neck surgery, thoracic surgery), operations on the gut (e.g. cholecystectomy, colorectal surgery, hysterectomy, etc.), operations on the urinary tract (e.g. prostatic surgery, nephrectomy, etc.), cardiac surgery.

Antibiotic prophylaxis as recommended by the British Society of Antibiotic Chemotherapy
Prophylaxis against endocarditis. In patients having dental operations or operations on the respiratory tract, genitourinary procedures, obstetric, gynaecological or gut operations:
Low risk, e.g. ASD, coronary grafts:

1. Parenteral:
   - Adults: amoxycillin i.m. or i.v. at induction followed by oral amoxycillin 6 hours later
   - Children: age 5-10, half adult dose; below 5, one-quarter adult dose.

2. Oral:
  - Adults: 3 g amoxycillin 4 hours preoperatively
  - Children: age 5-10, half adult dose; below 5, one-quarter adult dose.

High risk, e.g. VSD, prosthetic valve:

- Adults: 1 g amoxycillin i.m./i.v. plus 120 mg gentamicin i.m./i.v. at induction followed by oral amoxycillin 500 mg 6 hours later
- Children: age 5–10, amoxycillin, half adult dose plus gentamicin, 2 mg/kg; below 5: amoxycillin, one-quarter adult dose plus gentamicin, 2 mg/kg.

If a patient is sensitive to penicillin:

- Adult: vancomycin, 1 g i.v. given over 1 hour followed by gentamicin, both given 2 hours preoperatively
- Child: vancomycin, 20 mg/kg; gentamicin, 2 mg/kg.

Prophylaxis in abdominal surgery:

  - Upper gastrointestinal surgery (e.g. carcinoma of the oesophagus or stomach, gall bladder operations): single dose of gentamicin or cephalosporin 2 hours preoperatively. ˙
  - Lower gastrointestinal surgery (e.g. colon resections): single dose of gentamicin plus metronidazole or cephalosporin plus metronidazole 2 hours preoperatively.
  - Major gynaecological surgery (e.g. hysterectomy): metronidazole as suppository or single intravenous dose.

Complications associated with antibiotic administration
Penicillin: allergic reactions.
Cephalosporins: allergic cross-sensitivity with penicillin (5–10%); renal toxicity, bleeding abnormalities.
Aminoglycosides: renal toxicity, ototoxicity, potentiation of neuromuscular block especially with non-depolarizing relaxants.
Vancomycin: hypotension due to histamine release, venous thrombosis, renal and ototoxicity.
Metronidazole: neuropathy, encephalopathy (fits), potentiation of vitamin K antagonists (e.g. warfarin).
Erythromycin: phlebitis.

4.13   a) True   b) True   c) True   d) False   e) False

EXPLANATION
Parasympathetic drugs (e.g. anticholinesterases – neostigmine) increase intestinal activity especially in the colon. When the colon is diseased (e.g. ulcerative colitis, diverticulitis) this effect seems to be more pronounced. Conversely, parasympatholytic agents (e.g. atropine, glycopyrolate) reduce intestinal peristalsis. Sympathetic block with high spinals/epidurals promotes intestinal motility because of unopposed parasympathetic activity. Intrathecal/epidural narcotics do not block the sympathetic system and intestinal motility is actively reduced because of the action of opiates on intestinal tone. Apart from opiates, diazepam has also been shown to reduce intestinal activity, while thiopentone has been shown to increase it.

4.14   a) False   b) True   c) False   d) False   e) True

EXPLANATION

Renal blood flow and glomerular filtration rate remain constant between a systolic pressure of 80–180 mmHg. This autoregulation is not usually abolished during anaesthesia. However, hypotension results in oliguria even if renal blood flow (RBF) and glomerular filtration rate (GFR) are maintained by autoregulation.

The kidney's functions include homeostasis of blood pressure, volume and tonicity. The sympathetic system, antidiuretic hormone, and renin-angiotensin-aldosterone system protect against hypotension and hypovolaemia by promoting vasoconstriction and salt retention, while prostaglandins, bradykinins and other peptides protect against hypertension and hypervolaemia by promoting vasodilatation and salt excretion.

Factors causing vasoconstriction and salt retention:

1. *Sympathetic system.* Circulating adrenaline or release of noradrenaline from sympathetic system T12–L4 provides the sympathetic effects on the kidney. Alpha stimulation causes renal vasoconstriction and decreases RBF and GFR. Beta stimulation increases cardiac output and RBF, but also releases renin from the juxtaglomerular apparatus increasing secretion of angiotensin and aldosterone.

2. *Renin-angiotensin.* Renin controls the formation of the vasoconstrictor angiotensin II which decreases RBF and GFR. Renin release is increased by decreased renal perfusion pressure. Renin also stimulates aldosterone release by the adrenal cortex.

3. *Aldosterone.* Aldosterone is secreted by the adrenal cortex in response to hypokalaemia, angiotensin II and adrenocorticotrophic hormone (ACTH). It increases absorption of sodium and water causing hypervolaemia.

4. *Antidiuretic hormone* (ADH). ADH (vasopressin) is secreted in the anterior hypothalamus. Its secretion is dependent on osmoreceptors so that an increased osmolarity increases the secretion of ADH to cause water retention and prevent dehydration. Stress response to surgery causes profound release of ADH for 2–3 days postoperatively.

Factors causing vasodilatation and salt excretion. Prostaglandins, kinins and other peptides cause renal vasodilatation; thus prostaglandin inhibitors (NSAIDs) can lead to renal vasoconstriction and renal impairment in predisposed patients.

Effects of anaesthesia and surgery on renal function

Epidurals/spinals decrease renal blood flow if accompanied by vasodilatation and hypotension, but this hardly causes any problems because hypotension associated with vasodilatation is rarely harmful, as opposed to hypotension accompanied by vasoconstriction (e.g. shock).

General anaesthesia. All anaesthetic agents decrease GFR and urine flow and may decrease RBF especially if cardiac output is reduced. However, this is rarely a problem. Renal toxicity is more likely to be caused by nephrotoxins especially inorganic fluoride which is a metabolite of methoxyflurane and to a lesser extent enflurane and sevoflurane. Fluoride levels of less than 50 μm/litre are not usually associated with renal failure; and with enflurane, levels above 25 μm/litre are seldom achieved. Methoxyflurane can cause high levels leading to polyuric renal failure. Intravenous induction agents reduce GFR and RBF by about 10–15%.

Intermittent positive-pressure ventilation decreases RBF, GFR, sodium excretion and urine flow because of the reduced venous return and reduced cardiac output caused by positive intrathoracic pressure.

Risk factors:

1. Pre-existing disease: advanced age; pre-existing renal dysfunction; obstructive jaundice; shock (cardiogenic, septic or hypovolaemic); massive blood transfusion; myoglobinaemia.

2. Surgical/anaesthetic risk procedures: cardiac surgery; aortic cross-clamping; biliary surgery; urology surgery; major trauma; complicated obstetrics (eclampsia, haemorrhage, amniotic fluid embolism).

3. Nephrotoxins:

- Endogenous, e.g. myoglobins, haemolysed haemoglobin, conjugated bilirubin in obstructive jaundice, uric acid (e.g. myelomas, leukaemia)
- Exogenous – volatile anaesthetic agents (fluoride metabolite of methoxyflurane), cytotoxics and immunosuppressants, iodine contrast dyes, low molecular weight dextrans.

Management

1. Maintain adequate renal blood flow by maintaining an adequate cardiac output, i.e. keep normal cardiac rate and rhythm; keep normal blood volume.

2. Pharmacological renal protection:

- Low-dose dopamine or dopexamine acting on dopaminergic receptors in renal beds to cause vasodilatation
- Mannitol – beneficial actions include increased in intravascular volume and RBF, osmotic diuresis, and possible free radical scavenging
- Diuretics, e.g. frusemide, induce excretion of sodium and potassium and increases urine flow, but they should not be used until hypovolaemia has been corrected
- Vasodilators, e.g. nitroglycerine, nitroprusside, PGE1 prostaglandins, calcium blockers.

4.15   a) False   b) True   c) False   d) True   e) False

EXPLANATION

The principle of a closed circuit is that at equilibrium there is no net exchange of anaesthetic between the patient and the circuit. Theoretically if the carbon dioxide is absorbed completely by soda lime and the basal oxygen requirement is supplied (i.e. 250–400 ml/min), the mixture of gases can be used repeatedly as it is exhaled unchanged. Unfortunately even with very insoluble agents it takes a long time to reach full equilibrium. Moreover, CO_2 is not completely absorbed by the soda lime. Furthermore, any change in respiratory rate will alter anaesthetic uptake, while if basal flows are to be employed, the circuit must be denitrogenated before use by filling it with oxygen. For all these reasons a basal flow of 250 ml/minute is not sufficient. Flows above basal flow should be used and then the circuit is semi-closed rather than closed. Even in a semi-closed system some economy is achieved. Apart from economy in consumption of anaesthetic vapours, other advantages of closed circuits include less pollution, bacteriostatic properties and conservation of heat and moisture. Soda lime is a mixture of calcium hydroxide, with sodium hydroxide and about 15% water. The hydroxide combines with CO_2 to form carbonates, water and heat (more so with baralyme than soda lime). Baralyme is 80% calcium hydroxide and 20% barium hydroxides; it produces more heat than soda lime. Anaesthetics containing a CHF_2 group can break down in dry soda lime or baralyme to form carbon monoxide. Carbon monoxide is only formed if the absorbent mixture is allowed to dry out completely (i.e. water content less than 3%). Therefore, if dried out, the soda lime should be changed. Of the inhaled anaesthetic agents, desflurane produces the most carbon monoxide, followed by enflurane, isoflurane, sevoflurane and halothane in that order. Apart from carbon monoxide production, some volatile agents have specific interactions with CO_2 absorbents. Trichloroethylene is degraded by soda lime into toxic products which can paralyse all cranial nerves except I, II and IX, but usually the fifth nerve is affected. The motor part of the trigeminal nerve is not involved and recovery usually occurs within 14 days. Sevoflurane is also absorbed and degraded by soda lime and baralyme. The breakdown products are designated as A, B, C, D and E and compound A has been found to cause renal toxicity in rats when levels reach 25–50 parts per million. These levels are routinely achieved during sevoflurane anaesthesia, yet renal damage is very unlikely in humans. The probable reason for this is that rats have a very high level of the enzyme B-lyase, which catalyses the conversion of compound A into a toxic thiol. The level of this enzyme in humans is 30 times lower. The degradation into compound A is temperature dependent and because heat production is greater with baralyme than with soda lime the concentration of compound A is higher with baralyme. The production of compound A is reduced in the presence of water (another reason for not allowing soda lime to dry out) and by increasing fresh gas flows. There is still a controversy over whether sevoflurane causes renal damage in humans. There are no changes in urea and creatinine levels following sevoflurane anaesthesia, but more sensitive parameters of renal impairment, such as urine albumin and glucose levels, are increased with prolonged, low-flow sevoflurane anaesthesia. Therefore if surgery is going to last many hours, sevoflurane should probably be avoided and, moreover, fresh gas flow should not fall below 2 litres/minute.

Resistance to breathing is increased in circle systems and this may be important in the very young and old.

4.16   a) True   b) True   c) True   d) False   e) False

EXPLANATION

Diethyl ether increases sympathetic tone so that pulse rate and blood pressure are maintained or increased. Arrhythmias do not occur and there is no increased sensitivity to catecholamines.

If the inspired concentration of desflurane is increased above 6%, the sympathetic system is stimulated causing tachycardia and increased blood pressure.

There is increasing evidence suggesting that nitrous oxide increases sympathetic tone, elevating blood pressure and cardiac output. However, some cardiac anaesthetists avoid nitrous oxide because it limits the inspired oxygen concentration and may expand any gas bubbles that enter the circulation.

Ketamine causes increase in pulse rate and hypertension; these effects are due to direct action on neuronal pathways in the CNS and increased catecholamine levels; the sympathetic tone is not actually increased.

Curare causes histamine release leading to hypotension and tachycardia. Blood pressure also falls from ganglion blockade.

4.17   a) False   b) False   c) False   d) False   e) False

EXPLANATION
Causes. Neuroleptic-type drugs: butyrophenones, e.g. droperidol, haloperidol; phenothiazines, e.g. chlorpromazine, trifluoperazine, etc.; and psychedelic drugs. Suxamethonium is not thought to cause this syndrome.
Incidence. Rare but potentially fatal. Not familial or congenital.
Symptoms. Symptoms may occur on the day of therapy or may start after several months of treatment. As with malignant hyperpyrexia, there is muscular rigidity and inhibition of central dopaminergic activity leading to disturbed regulation and elevated temperature. Apart from rigidity and pyrexia there is muscle breakdown causing myoglobinaemia, autonomic dysfunction (hypo- or hypertension, tachycardia and cardiovascular collapse), renal failure and CNS changes leading to delirium and permanent damage—dementia, parkinsonism. Serum creatine kinase is often elevated.
Treatment. Supportive therapy and dantrolene – relieves pyrexia and muscle breakdown. L-dopa and bromocriptine (a dopamine agonist) relieve rigidity and tremor.
 Neuroleptic malignant syndrome can easily be confused with malignant hyperpyrexia and differential diagnosis is therefore important (Table 4.5).

4.18   a) True   b) True   c) False   d) False   e) False

EXPLANATION
HELLP syndrome equates to haemolysis, elevated liver enzymes and low platelet count. It is a variant of pre-eclampsia and the main features are (a) microangiopathic haemolytic anaemia; (b) abnormal elevation of liver enzymes; (c) low platelet count. There is reduction of prostacyclin levels and EDRF (endothelium-derived relaxing

Table 4.5 Differences between neuroleptic malignant syndrome and malignant hyperpyrexia

	Neuroleptic malignant syndrome	Malignant hyperpyrexia
Triggering agents	Phenothiazines, butyrophenones. Suxamethonium and inhalational agents should be avoided if possible	Usually halothane or suxamethonium
Clinical	Rigidity relieved with non-depolarizing relaxants. CNS symptoms not as fulminant and development of complications less rapid. Pyrexia not so marked	Rigidity not relieved with non-depolarizing drugs. CNS symptoms less evident, fulminant symptoms

factor) and increase in the prostaglandin thromboxane all of which lead to platelet aggregation.

Clinical features. The syndrome can occur before 36 weeks, or after delivery (up to 6 days postpartum). Initially there may be minimal changes in platelet count, liver function tests and blood pressure. 90% present with right-sided abdominal/epigastric pain due to blood flow obstruction in the liver sinuses. There is often malaise and nausea and vomiting. There is usually weight gain due to oedema, but hypertension is not always present. Neurological manifestations include headache, fits, retinal detachment and vitreous haemorrhage. Acute renal failure, disseminated intravascular coagulation (DIC) and haematomas of liver can follow.

Laboratory findings include haemolysis, increased bilirubin and increased SGOT (serum glutamic oxaloacetic transaminase) and lactic dehydrogenase. There is also a low platelet count (below 100 000/ml).

Management:

1. Plasma volume expansion: bed rest, crystalloids.
2. Antithrombolytic agents: low-dose aspirin, dipyridamole, heparin, prostacyclin infusions, thromboxane synthetase, e.g. dazoxiben.
3. Immunosuppressants: steroids to increase fetal maturity.
4. Others: fresh frozen plasma, dialysis, plasmapheresis if thrombocytopenia or haemolysis do not resolve.
5. Treatment of major problems: i.e. hypertension control, control of fits, renal support.

Labour induction is indicated if there is fetal distress, worsening thrombocytopenia, worsening hypertension, worsening neurological status, worsening renal or liver function or if gestation has reached 34 weeks or more. Delayed delivery is associated with high perinatal mortality.

Epidural anaesthesia is not recommended because of thrombocytopenia and coagulopathy. Platelet infusions are not very successful in treating the low platelet count, because consumption of platelets occurs rapidly. These patients often require caesarean section and general anaesthesia is usually employed for this. The danger here is exacerbation of hypertension (tracheal intubation, surgical excision) which carries the risk of intracranial haemorrhage. Short-acting hypotensive agents (e.g. nitroprusside) may be required to reduce blood pressure.

4.19   a) True   b) False   c) True   d) True   e) True

EXPLANATION

The incidence of pulmonary complications for all surgery is 6%. The rate increases to 35% for abdominal and thoracic surgery, and 12% in lower abdominal operations. Incidence is also increased with obesity, smoking and pre-existing pulmonary diseases (e.g. asthma and chronic obstructive airways disease (COAD)) and cardiac disease.

Causes of pulmonary complications

Anaesthesia. Length: operations over 3–4 hours, possibly because of impaired mucociliary clearance.

Inhalational anaesthetics inhibit hypoxic pulmonary vasoconstriction which could cause hypoxia in patients with preoperative ventilation/perfusion abnormalities.

Absorption atelectasis can be caused if 100% oxygen is used during anaesthesia. Pulmonary function is also altered during general anaesthesia. The diaphragm is shifted upwards, especially in the dependent portions of the diaphragm, reducing lung volumes and functional residual capacity (FRC). There is also airway closure in the dependent portions of the lungs so that the non-dependent portions have increased ventilation leading to ventilation-perfusion mismatch, causing hypoxaemia. The decrease in FRC during anaesthesia means that the closing volume of some alveoli encroaches upon the tidal volume leading to collapse of alveoli.

Surgery. Anaesthetic causes of postoperative pulmonary dysfunction are of little significance after 2 hours. As stated above, thoracic and upper abdominal surgery cause most postoperative problems because of reduced vital capacity and FRC. Moreover, pain, abdominal distension and immobilization impair breathing and coughing and lead to further reduced FRC, increased airway closure and atelectasis.

Decreased respiratory drive. By drugs (opiates, barbiturates, inhalational anaesthetics), CNS abnormalities (infarction, neoplasm, infection), myxoedema, metabolic alkalosis, sleep apnoea.

Decreased respiratory muscle function. Inadequate reversal from muscle relaxants, metabolic causes (hypokalaemia, hypo- and hypermagnesaemia), myasthenia gravis and myasthenic syndrome, muscle diseases.

Pulmonary disease:

1. *Collapse*: most common cause of postoperative dysfunction and often related to the pulmonary problems of surgery and anaesthesia mentioned above. Specific causes include bronchial carcinoma, aspiration, excess mucus, endobronchial intubation.

2. *Pulmonary oedema*: either due to fluid overload or myocardial dysfunction or increased permeability, e.g. adult respiratory distress syndrome (ARDS), or secondary to upper airway obstruction. With cardiogenic pulmonary oedema and fluid overload the central venous pressure (CVP) and wedge pressures are elevated; with ARDS there are diffuse lung infiltrates and the CVP and wedge pressures are usually low.

3. *Aspiration pneumonia*: i.e. pulmonary inflammation caused by aspiration of gastric or nasopharyngeal secretions, especially if the pH of gastric secretions is less than 2.5. Antibiotics and corticosteroids are of doubtful value.

4. *Pulmonary infection*: The incidence of postoperative pulmonary infection is about 20%. Predisposing causes include prolonged intubation (Gram-negative rods infect the upper airway); prolonged antibiotic therapy leading to infection with antibiotic-resistant strains of Gram-negative bacteria especially in patients with reduced resistance.

5. *Exacerbation of COAD*: i.e. asthma and bronchitis. Patients with pre-existing COAD not uncommonly have exacerbations postoperatively and the patients should be improved as much as possible before elective surgery. A number of factors can trigger off bronchitis or asthma perioperatively – infections, heart failure, airway irritation by endotracheal tube irritants, allergic reactions, pulmonary emboli.

6. *Pulmonary embolism*: usually presents with dyspnoea but may be silent. With larger emboli there may be chest pain, bronchospasm, pulmonary opacities and atelectasis, and possibly cardiac failure. If ventilation/perfusion lung scanning is normal, a significant pulmonary embolus is unlikely; if ventilation/perfusion is abnormal, pulmonary angiography is required for diagnosis.

4.20   a) False   b) False   c) False   d) False   e) True

EXPLANATION

Platelets encourage the production of arterial thrombi in patients with atheromatous vascular disease; thus antiplatelet drugs have been found to be of use in the prevention and treatment of thromboembolic arterial disease, e.g. following cardiac/arterial surgery, in the prevention and treatment of cerebral ischaemia/myocardial ischaemia and in the prevention of thrombus formation in haemodialysis machines and in pump oxygenators. Antiplatelet drugs are thought to have little effect on venous thromboembolism.

Antiplatelet drugs

Aspirin and NSAIDs. Aspirin inhibits platelet cyclo-oxygenase. Cyclo-oxygenase is required for the synthesis of thromboxane A_2 which is a vasoconstrictor and induces platelet aggregation by releasing ADP. The antiplatelet action of aspirin occurs even with single doses and may last for up to 1 week because aspirin irreversibly inhibits cyclo-oxygenase and new platelets must be produced for normal function to return.

Dipyridamole. This is similar to papaverine and a coronary vasodilator, but since it does not alter peripheral resistance is not of much benefit in myocardial ischaemia. Its main use is its ability to reduce platelet aggregation by reducing ADP levels and by sequestrating calcium ions. It has been used with oral anticoagulants to prevent thrombus formation on artificial valves and in the prevention of ischaemic episodes. Side-effects: headaches, hypotension.

Low molecular weight dextrans. These are primarily used as plasma expanders but dextran 40 and dextran 70, apart from maintaining blood volume, reduce plasma viscosity and reduce platelet function thus prolonging bleeding time. Other colloids (e.g. Haemaccel) may also diminish platelet aggregation. Dextrans are sometimes used for the prevention of thromboembolic episodes following surgery. Side-effects: overloading and allergic reactions (bronchospasm, skin reactions, hypotension).

Epoprostenol (prostacylin). Some prostaglandins are potent vasodilators and inhibit platelet aggregation. Epoprostenol is an example of one and has been used as an alternative to heparin in renal dialysis. Because it has a very short half-life (3 min) it has to be given by infusion. Side-effects: headache, hypotension.

Others. Sulphinpyrazone inhibits cyclo-oxygenase; dazoxiben is a thromboxane inhibitor. Other drugs which have antiplatelet action include biguanides, some anabolic steroids and the antimalarial drug chloroquine.

5.1 **When considering plasma substitutes:**

a) Allergic reaction to gelatins are more common than to albumins
b) Gelatins (e.g. Gelofusine) and starches (e.g. Hespan) are excreted via the kidney
c) The volume required for resuscitation with crystalloid is two to four times the volume of colloid required
d) Gelatins (Gelofusine/Haemaccel) stay in the circulation longer than hetastarch
e) Dextran 40 is preferable to dextran 70 when renal function is compromised

5.2 **With regard to suxamethonium:**

a) In a patient with no plasma cholinesterase/pseudocholinesterase, the suxamethonium is eventually totally excreted unchanged by the kidney
b) A patient recovering from a prolonged suxamethonium block due to abnormal pseudocholinesterase is likely to demonstrate equal train of four responses 60 minutes after the suxamethonium was administered
c) A patient with a dibucaine number of 50 is likely to be heterozygous for cholinesterase/pseudocholinesterase
d) The rise in intragastric pressure due to suxamethonium is related to the intensity of muscle fasciculation
e) Postoperative myalgia following use of suxamethonium is related to the intensity of muscle fasciculation

5.3 **In gas analysis:**

a) Gas chromatography can be used for the analysis of volatile agents in blood
b) A mass spectrometer can be used for the simultaneous analysis of a number of gases
c) Oxygen concentration in a gas mixture can be measured with a paramagnetic analyser
d) A halothane meter depends upon the absorption of ultraviolet light by vapour
e) A capnograph for CO_2 measurement uses infrared spectroscopy

5.4 **Of the inherited disorders:**

a) When two heterozygous individuals mate, 25% of their offspring will exhibit the recessive characteristic
b) A patient with full-blown sickle cell anaemia has the homozygous form of the disease
c) Malignant hyperpyrexia is transmitted as an autosomal recessive gene
d) Hereditary porphyria is transmitted as an autosomal dominant gene
e) A suxamethonium-sensitive patient with a fluoride number of 25 is homozygous

5.5 A lumbar (L3–L4) epidural is performed on a 63-year-old woman. After a negative aspiration test 14 ml of 0.25% plain bupivacaine are administered. 6 minutes later the patient complains of numbness and weakness in arms and neck, slight difficulty in breathing and numbness in face. However, the lower limbs are not affected by any motor or sensory loss until 30 minutes after the injection. Blood pressure falls to 80 mmHg systolic. The term which best describes this series of events is:

a) Subarachnoid block
b) Total spinal block
c) Inadvertent intravascular injection of bupivacaine
d) Massive extradural block
e) Subdural block

5.6 With regard to alternative opioid delivery systems:

a) Plasma concentrations with transdermal fentanyl are less constant than with intermittent intravenous or intramuscular injections
b) Incidence of side-effects is low with transdermal fentanyl compared to other routes of administration
c) Iontophoretic opioid delivery is more rapid than the transdermal route
d) Onset of action of an opioid delivered transnasally is likely to be faster than with the oral route
e) Morphine is more suitable than fentanyl when used by the oral transmucosal (buccal) route

5.7 End-tidal CO_2:

a) Falls with pulmonary embolus
b) Falls with methaemoglobinaemia
c) Increases with hyperthermia
d) Falls when fresh gas flow in a Mapleson D circuit is less than alveolar ventilation
e) Rises when oxygen tissue delivery is reduced

5.8 Drug interactions are such that:

a) Erythromycin prolongs the action of alfentanil
b) Epidural chlorprocaine decreases analgesia of the subsequently administered epidural morphine
c) Intrathecal clonidine reduces the minimum alveolar concentration (MAC) of volatile anaesthetics
d) Barbiturates used for induction and non-depolarizing relaxants can be mixed in the same syringe
e) Trimetaphan enhances the action of suxamethonium

5.9 In cardiopulmonary resuscitation:

a) Dobutamine is just as effective as adrenaline in maintaining cardiovascular support
b) End-tidal CO_2 is useful in predicting effectiveness
c) Because acidosis lowers fibrillation threshold and impairs response to sympathomimetics, sodium bicarbonate should be given without delay
d) Calcium administration improves outcome
e) Cardiac output during effective resuscitation is primarily directed to the organs above the diaphragm

5.10 Cancer patients on cytotoxic drugs presenting for general anaesthesia may have the following problems:

a) Chronic pneumonitis and fibrosis
b) Cardiomyopathy
c) Anaemia if cytotoxics have been administered for longer than 1 week
d) Meningeal irritation after intrathecal administration
e) Hepatic and renal dysfunction

5.11 With regard to the diaphragm:

a) It is the principal muscle of respiration
b) Its motor innervation is primarily via the lower six intercostal nerves
c) Unilateral paralysis maintains normal tidal exchange
d) Total paralysis normally requires intermittent positive-pressure ventilation (IPPV)
e) The nerves passing through it are vagal, phrenic, and sympathetic chain

5.12 Tramadol:

a) Produces analgesia by acting on opiate receptors and inhibition of noradrenaline re-uptake
b) Is eliminated by hepatic metabolism and renal excretion
c) Results in more pronounced sedation and constipation than morphine
d) Has an analgesic effect that is potentiated by carbamazepine
e) Causes respiratory depression that is reversed with naloxone

5.13 With regard to perioperative arrhythmias:

a) A preoperative patient, found to have a prolapsing mitral valve and symptomless runs of ventricular tachycardia but no evidence of cardiac problems, requires urgent treatment
b) A patient presenting for operation with ventricular arrhythmias after a myocardial infarction has increased morbidity and mortality if arrhythmias are left untreated
c) Most patients presenting for surgery with atrial fibrillation or flutter have underlying heart disease
d) Hypomagnesaemia predisposes to arrhythmias by reducing intracellular K^+ concentrations
e) Mexiletine reduces arrhythmias by its calcium-blocking action

5.14 **Physiological changes during pregnancy mean that:**

a) Hypoxaemia and hypercarbia are more likely
b) More local anaesthetic is required in epidurals or spinals
c) There is a reduced likelihood of thrombosis
d) pH rises because of increased alveolar ventilation
e) There is a rise in blood pressure because of increased cardiac output

5.15 **With regard to local anaesthetics:**

a) Prilocaine is ideal for epidural anaesthesia because of its very low toxicity
b) In general, amide agents cause vasodilatation at low concentrations and vasoconstriction at higher concentrations
c) Allergic reactions to amide agents are due to the metabolite *p*-aminobenzoic acid
d) Duration of action is related to degree of protein binding
e) An ankle block involves blocking the posterior tibial nerve, sural nerve, saphenous nerve, deep and superficial peroneal nerves

5.16 **Problems during a laparoscopic cholecystectomy include:**

a) Fall in cardiac output with an intra-abdominal pressure of above 15 mmHg
b) Acidosis and hypercarbia in patients with cardiovascular disease after CO_2 insufflation
c) Stress response significantly less than with open cholecystectomy
d) Increased incidence of regurgitation
e) Pneumothorax

5.17 **The following agents are metabolized by plasma cholinesterase:**

a) Mivacurium
b) Lignocaine
c) Amethocaine
d) Propanidid
e) Rocuronium

5.18 **A patient with polycythaemia:**

a) May have a history of chronic hypoxaemia
b) Will have abnormal platelet function if the polycythaemia is secondary to chronic hypoxaemia
c) Is more likely to develop venous thrombosis
d) Has a reduced oxygen saturation
e) May have low erythropoietin levels

5.19 In a patient who presents for general anaesthesia for relief of bowel obstruction due to a carcinoid tumour, and in whom urinary 5-hydroxyindoleacetic acid levels are high preoperatively:

a) Hypertension, hypotension and tachycardia could be due to serotonin release
b) Liver metastasis is likely
c) There may be symptoms of left heart failure
d) Atracurium is the relaxant of choice
e) Cardiovascular collapse should be treated with catecholamines

5.20 Intraocular pressure is increased by:

a) Trabeculectomy
b) Extrinsic compression of the globe with an anaesthetic mask
c) Suxamethonium
d) Intubation
e) Deep inhalational and thiopentone anaesthesia

EXPLANATION

Fluids with a similar osmotic pressure to plasma can be used to replace plasma or blood within certain limits. Human albumin is probably the best available product for this purpose but is very expensive. Similarly, human plasma protein fraction (PPF), which is prepared from donor plasma and contains albumin in saline has fewer side-effects then the gelatins and starches used for volume expansion, but PPF is also expensive and in short supply. Therefore in most cases artificial volume expanders are now being used which are much less expensive and have a very long shelf life (up to 5 years). These are usually high molecular weight gelatins (Haemaccel/Gelofusine) or starches (Hetastarch/Hespan) or dextrans (40 or 70). The characteristics of volume expanders are shown in Table 5.1.

EXPLANATION

The greatest advantage of suxamethonium is its short duration of action. This is due to enzymatic hydrolysis with plasma cholinesterase and plasma pseudocholinesterase. Breakdown occurs in two stages:

1. Suxamethonium (succinyldicholine) in the presence of cholinesterase gives rise to succinylmonocholine plus choline. This stage is very rapid.
2. Succinylmonocholine is broken down by a specific liver enzyme to produce succinic acid and choline. This stage is slow.

Normal adults convert at least 80 mg succinyldicholine into succinylmonocholine per minute and succinylmonocholine only has about 1/50th of the potency of succinyldicholine. When pseudocholinesterase/cholinesterase is deficient or abnormal, suxamethonium is eliminated by alkaline hydrolysis (5% per hour), renal elimination (2% per hour) and by redistribution. The dibucaine number refers to the percentage inhibition of pseudocholinesterase by dibucaine. The dibucaine test separates patients into three groups:

1. dibucaine number above 70 would be a homozygote with two normal genes and normal enzyme
2. dibucaine number below 30 would be a homozygote with two abnormal genes and only abnormal enzyme
3. dibucaine number 40–70 would be a heterozygote with one normal and one abnormal gene and a mixture of normal and abnormal enzyme.

Patients who have a prolonged action to suxamethonium go initially through a phase I depolarizing block: i.e. sustained response to single stimuli; sustained tetanus; absence of post-tetanic potentiation; equal train of four responses; and block potentiated by anticholinergic drugs. Eventually the block changes to a phase II non-depolarizing block: i.e. tetanic fade; post-tetanic potentiation; train of four fade; and reversal with anticholinesterases. Therefore, the patient recovering from a suxamethonium apnoea would have a phase II block with typical train of four fade.

Suxamethonium can raise intragastric pressure by as high as 85 cmH$_2$O and the degree of rise is related to the intensity of muscle fasciculation.

Postoperative myalgia following suxamethonium occurs mostly in ambulatory patients having minor surgery. It is more common in females and less common in children and the elderly. There is no correlation between the intensity of fasciculation and myalgia.

5.3   a) True   b) True   c) True   d) True   e) True

EXPLANATION

Gas chromatography can be used for the analysis of volatile agents in blood and also for simultaneous analysis of various gases, but changes in a single breath cannot be measured because the estimation takes several minutes. The principle relies on the separation of the gases by a partition column. The column is a metal or glass tube packed with a solid support material which is impregnated with a liquid (e.g. a high boiling point wax or silicone) which has a high affinity for the gases to be separated. The liquid is kept stationary by the support material in the tube. This liquid is the stationary phase. An inert carrier gas passes through the tube at a constant rate. The mixture to be separated and analysed is introduced at the proximal end of the tube, and if all its components are insoluble in the stationary liquid phase, they will all come out at the distal end of the tube at the same rate as the inert carrier gas. However, if the components are soluble in the stationary phase, they will be held up, and the delay in passing through the column is directly proportional to the partition coefficient between the stationary liquid and the component gas.

When the gases are separated, each gas has to be identified by a detector and its amount calculated. There are various types of detectors: the katharometer, a heated thermistor which is sensitive to vapours of different thermal conductivity; the flame ionization detector in which a carrier gas (hydrogen) is ignited by organic compounds resulting in ionized particles which travel to alter voltages on electrically charged plates; electron capture devices (for halogenated compounds) where the agent to be identified is bombarded by γ-rays and the electrons emitted from the halogen collected.

A mass spectrometer can be used for the simultaneous analysis of various gases. The molecules are ionized, accelerated by an electric field and deflected by a magnetic field. The angle of deflection is related to molecular weight. Therefore gases (e.g. N$_2$O and CO$_2$) with similar molecular weights have to be differentiated by special electronic circuits.

Oxygen (as well as nitric oxide) is a paramagnetic gas, i.e. it seeks the area of strongest flux in a magnetic field, and this characteristic can be used to identify it. Fuel cells are more commonly used today.

Halothane can be detected with a halothane meter because of its ability to absorb ultraviolet light. The meter is used for monitoring the halothane concentration in closed-circuit anaesthesia and in checking the calibration of vaporizers.

The infrared analyser (Fig. 5.1) is used mainly for the detection of carbon dioxide, but it can be used for any gas or vapour which, like CO$_2$, absorbs infrared radiation. In the CO$_2$ analyser, infrared radiation is generated by an incandescent filament, and split by mirrors into two parallel beams. The reference beam passes through a

Table 5.1   Colloid properties

Agent	Composition	Molecular weight	Osmolarity	Electrolytes mEq/l	Plasma volume expansion
Albumin 5%	5 g/100 ml > 85% albumin	66 500	300	Na: 130–160	100%
Albumin 20%	20 g/100 ml > 85% albumin	66 500	1500	Na: 130–160	250%
Gelatins					
Haemaccel	Polypeptide of bovine collagen	35 000	300	NaCl: 145 K: 5.1 Ca: 6.25	80% in 2 h
Gelofusine	Polypeptide of bovine collagen	30 000	279	Na: 154 Cl: 125	80% in 2 h
Starches					
Hespan: 6%	Hydroxyethyl substituted amyloprotein	450 000	310	Na: 154 Cl: 154	100% in 2 h
Pentaspan: 10%	Hydroxyethyl substituted amyloprotein	250 000	320	Na: 154 Cl: 154	145% in 2 h 100% in 4 h
Haessteril: 6%	Hydroxyethyl substituted amyloprotein	20 000	308	Na: 154 Cl: 154	100% in 4 h
Haessteril: 10%	Hydroxyethyl substituted amyloprotein	20 000	308	Na: 154 Cl: 154	145% in 2 h 100% in 4 h
Elo-haessteril: 6%	Hydroxyethyl substituted amyloprotein	20 000	308	Na: 154 Cl: 154	100% in 8–12 h
Dextrans					
Dextran 40 in 6% saline or 5% dextrose	Plasma substrate produced by bacterial action on sugars	40 000	Slightly hyperoncotic	Na: 77	180% in 2 h 100% in 4 h
Dextran 70 in 6% saline or 5% dextrose		70 000	Iso-osmotic	Na: 77	100% in 2 h 80% in 4 h

Duration of PVE	Metabolism	Excretion	Allergy	Comments
About 24 h	Interstitial translocation	Gut, renal	Very low incidence	PPF: plasma with added saline and albumin. Albumin and PPF: expensive
About 24 h	Interstitial translocation	Gut, renal	Very low incidence	
4 h	Proteolytic enzymes	Renal	1 in 6000	
4 h	Proteolytic enzymes	Renal	1 in 6000	NB: 500 ml of all these expand the blood volume by about 500 ml, as compared to Hartmann's which expands it by 175 ml. The volume required for resuscitation if crystalloids are used is two to four times that of colloid because crystalloids are shifted quickly into interstitial fluid
24–36 h	Intravascular hydrolysis by serum amylase	Renal	1 in 46 000	
16–18 h	Intravascular hydrolysis by serum amylase	Renal	1 in 46 000	
16–18 h	Intravascular hydrolysis by serum amylase	Renal	1 in 46 000	
16–18 h	Intravascular hydrolysis by serum amylase	Renal	1 in 46 000	
18–24 h	Intravascular hydrolysis by serum amylase	Renal	1 in 46 000	
4–6 h		Renal. High concentrations can cause renal failure	1 in 2000. Serious reactions 1 in 12 000	Both prevent platelet aggregation and have been used for DVT prophylaxis; but may increase surgical bleeding
24 h		Renal	1 in 2000. Serious reactions 1 in 12 000	

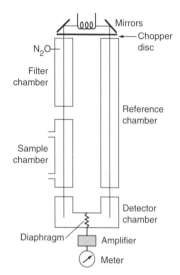

Fig 5.1 *The infrared gas analyser.*

reference chamber filled with an inert gas such as nitrogen; the sample beam passes through a filter chamber, then the sample chamber. The beams then end up in the detector chamber, which is divided into two by a flexible metal diaphragm. If the radiation beams are equal in intensity, the pressures are the same in the two detector chambers and the diaphragm does not move; however, if they are unequal because, for example, the CO_2 in the filter chamber absorbed infrared radiation; then the pressures in the chambers will be unequal and the diaphragm is pushed over towards the sample half of the detector where the pressure is lower. The diaphragmatic movement is amplified and correlated with the CO_2 concentration. Since nitrous oxide also absorbs infrared radiation, and may be present in the sample gas, it would be detected as CO_2 by the analyser. Therefore, to prevent this false interpretation, the filter chamber is filled with 100% nitrous oxide.

5.4   **a) True**   **b) True**   **c) False**   **d) True**   **e) True**

EXPLANATION

Mendel identified characteristics which were dominant or recessive. A dominant characteristic is apparent when only one dominant gene is present on both chromosomes; while with a recessive character the recessive genes have to be present on both chromosomes for the disease to be overt. Thus when two heterozygous individuals mate, 25% of the offspring will exhibit the recessive characteristic but 75% will exhibit a dominant one.

    Sickle cell disease is a hereditary autosomal recessive haemolytic anaemia where haemoglobin A is replaced by haemoglobin S. There are two forms; sickle cell trait

Hom o 8y   wter—-.
(heterozygous – S$ form) and sickle cell disease (homozygous – SA). It is found in individuals of tropical African or West Indian descent, and also in parts of India and some Mediterranean areas. Sickling is precipitated by acidosis, stasis, hypoxia, hypothermia; pyrexia; tourniquets, etc., which increase blood viscosity and cause stasis, sludging, thrombosis, reduced oxygen availability and thus infarctions. A patient with sickle cell trait usually presents no problems; on the other hand, sickle cell disease is associated with small vessel occlusion causing infarctions in affected organs and bone (osteomyelitis); bone marrow (aplastic anaemia); spleen; brain; lung (chest pain, fever, pulmonary infiltrates); kidney (papillary necrosis, haematuria). Gall bladder disease is also common in these patients. Sickle cell anaemia is diagnosed by the Sickledex test which tests for insoluble deoxygenated Hb S. A positive test does not differentiate between trait or disease; haemoglobin electrophoresis is required for this. During anaesthesia, one must avoid all the factors which predispose to sickling, i.e. hypoxia, acidosis, hypothermia, local stasis (e.g. vasopressors), dehydration, tourniquets.

Malignant hyperpyrexia is transmitted as a dominant disorder and the incidence varies between 1 in 15 000 and 1 in 200 000.

Suxamethonium is normally broken down by plasma cholinesterase. Plasma cholinesterase is inhibited by cinchocaine (nupercaine, dibucaine) (normally 80% inhibition) and fluoride (60–65% inhibition); therefore dibucaine numbers of less than 80 or fluoride numbers less than 60 are abnormal and signify a low plasma cholinesterase. A dibucaine number of below 60 (fluoride number below 30) indicates marked sensitivity to suxamethonium.

Porphyria is a group of diseases where there is an inherited defect in the   Dauin
metabolism of porphyrins. Porphyrins are essential for the production of respiratory   'aculin
pigments which form compounds with various metals, e.g. magnesium to form chlorophyll, and iron to synthesize the haem of haemoglobin. Haem normally inhibits D-aminolaevulinic acid (ALA) synthase. In porphyria haem levels are low, and therefore ALA synthase levels are high. Since ALA synthase is one of the enzymes responsible for porphyrin synthesis, accumulation of porphyrins is the result. Acute attacks of porphyria can be precipitated by barbiturates, sulphonamides, anticonvulsants, alcohol, oral contraceptives. Ketamine and propofol are safe induction agents; there is, however, some doubt about the safety of etomidate. Clinical features include:

- abdominal symptoms – nausea, vomiting, abdominal pain
- neurological symptoms – motor and sensory peripheral neuropathies, epilepsy
- psychiatric symptoms
- cardiovascular symptoms – tachycardia, raised blood pressure
- urine may be red or brown because of the presence of porphobilinogen which can be detected by spectroscopy.   As phobilinogon,

---

5.5   a) False   b) False   c) False   d) False   e) True

EXPLANATION

The subdural space is a narrow interval between the dura and subarachnoid mater and extends upwards into the cranium and around the cranial nerves and downwards to S1–S2 level. It is widest in the cervical area. The incidence of an accidental subdural block is approximately 0.1%. The clinical effects of a subdural block are intermediate between a subarachnoid and an epidural block; the block is usually widespread, presumably because the space has a limited capacity, and the fluid cannot escape. Features of subdural block are: after a negative aspiration test, onset of block is quicker than epidural, but slower than spinal; there is widespread cephalad sensory and motor blockade and possibly cranial nerve block causing pupil dilatation, trigeminal nerve block and possible progressive respiratory depression. The block affects upper dermatomes with sparing of lower dermatomes. Sympathetic block is variable and can be absent; thus hypotension is less than would be expected from spinal anaesthesia. Occasionally, a predominantly unilateral block occurs. Recovery is usually within 2 hours. An accidental subdural block should be suspected if abnormal symptoms follow epidural analgesia, especially if the block is widespread. It can be confirmed by injecting contrast media into the catheter; it will show a characteristic 'string of beads' appearance dorsally and laterally around the nerve roots, and a 'rail road track' appearance on the anteroposterior view.

It is very unlikely that a massive lumbar epidural is not associated with lumbar dermatomal block.

The symptoms of a total spinal (subarachnoid) block would occur within 3 minutes and are more catastrophic than in the patient described above. A total spinal block would cause marked hypotension, apnoea coma and dilated pupils. Intubation, fluid resuscitation and sympathomimetics are required. Breathing recommences within 1–2 hours.

Inadvertent intravenous administration is usually recognized by symptoms of acute intoxication with local anaesthetics, i.e. nausea, confusion, fits, irregular respiration, and possibly cardiovascular collapse. Antiepileptic drugs and resuscitation may be required.

5.6   a) False   b) False   c) True   d) True   e) False

EXPLANATION

Transdermal fentanyl is a relatively new method of fentanyl delivery. The advantages of transdermal fentanyl are mainly twofold:

1. Sustained release. This provides constant plasma concentrations of the drug, unlike intermittent intravenous, intramuscular or oral dosage.

2. Prolonged analgesia. The fentanyl from the transdermal patch accumulates in the skin to become available to the blood circulation. The fentanyl concentration gradually increases to reach a constant value within 12–24 hours and remains approximately at this value for 72 hours, thus providing prolonged analgesia.

The disadvantages of transdermal fentanyl are:

1. Prolonged onset of action and prolonged duration. There is a delay to a steady state of about 15 hours, and once the patch is removed the half-life is about 21 hours, as it continues to be absorbed from the skin depot. This may be an advantage for sustained analgesia; however, it can be a distinct drawback if the medication has to be discontinued because of overdosage or side-effects.

2. High incidence of side-effects. Compared to conventional opiate administration, the incidence of nausea, vomiting, urinary retention, pruritus and respiratory depression are significantly higher.

Transdermal fentanyl is available in four sizes, i.e. 25, 50, 75 and 100 µg/hour, containing 2.5, 5, 7.5 and 10 mg of fentanyl respectively.

There are obviously difficulties with the passive delivery of drugs through the skin, and only a few medications are available as skin patches – scopolamine for nausea, especially that caused by intrathecal/epidural opioids; nitroglycerine for angina; clonidine for hypertension; fentanyl for pain; oestrogen therapy during the menopause. Because of difficulties with passive delivery, active methods of transdermal drug delivery are being looked at. Iontophoresis is one such method where the electrically charged components of ionizable drugs are propelled through the skin by an external electrical charge. Unfortunately, this method is usually limited to drug delivery times of 15–30 minutes, as longer times can cause skin burns. Newer electrodes are being developed to increase delivery time.

Another new approach to administering fentanyl is via the transmucosal route (i.e. fentanyl lozenge). This route has the advantage over the oral route of avoiding the first pass hepatic metabolism. Moreover, because the oral cavity has a rich blood supply, drug absorption and onset of action are rapid. The preparation is available in 200, 300 and 400 mg sizes and the recommended dose is 5–15 µg/kg. The lozenge is sucked as a sucrose-based lozenge on a stick over a 10-minute period. Good analgesia and sedation occur within 20–30 minutes and last 4–6 hours. Respiratory depression is much less common than with the transdermal route. Buccal morphine has also been tried, but because it is so poorly lipid soluble, transmucosal absorption of this agent is not very effective.

A final promising alternative drug delivery system is the intranasal transmucosal route. The nose has a large blood supply; therefore absorption should be rapid, and will avoid the extensive inactivation of drugs that occurs in the gut following the oral route. The delivery of the drug is dependent upon a number of factors, i.e. temperature of nasal mucosa, airway resistance, pH, pK_a and lipid solubility of agent, and droplet size. Some drugs are already available via this route, e.g. vasopressin (antidiuretic hormone) for diabetes insipidus, oxytocin. Intranasal sufentanil has been tried as a premedicant, and has been found to provide rapid satisfactory sedation with few side-effects. Intranasal midazolam and ketamine have also been used for premedication.

5.7 a) False   b) True   c) True   d) False   e) False

EXPLANATION

End-tidal CO_2 ($P_{ET}CO_2$)/alveolar CO_2 (P_ACO_2) is altered by increase/decrease in CO_2 production, increases in inspired CO_2, and increase/decrease in alveolar ventilation.

1. Increase in CO_2 production (high P_ECO_2): hyperthermia, malignant hyperpyrexia, post-anaesthetic shivering, fighting the ventilator, endocrine disease (e.g. thyrotoxicosis).

2. Decrease in CO_2 production (low P_ECO_2): this is either due to (a) reduced oxygen delivery (e.g. reduced cardiac output, fall in haemoglobin, CO poisoning, methaemoglobinaemia, aortic cross-clamping) or (b) reduced tissue oxygen uptake (hypothermia, myxoedema, cyanide poisoning, leg tourniquet).

3. Decreased alveolar ventilation (high P_ECO_2): there are numerous causes for this, i.e. increased depth of anaesthesia with a spontaneously breathing patient; anaesthetic machine problems, e.g. reduced fresh gas flow, leak; disconnection;

ventilator problems, e.g. ventilator malfunction or not enough minute volume; breathing circuit problems, e.g. obstructed circuits, fresh gas flow too low causing rebreathing, CO_2 absorption due to exhaustion of soda lime; pulmonary problems; upper airway obstruction (mask, soft tissue, endotracheal tube); bronchial intubation; secretions or blood in airway; asthma; aspiration; pneumothorax; haemothorax; congestive heart failure; extrathoracic problems, e.g. increased abdominal muscle tone; excessive retraction causing reduced lung compliance; dead space problems due to increased anatomical or alveolar dead space, e.g. pulmonary embolus; reduced cardiac output.

4. Increased alveolar ventilation (low $P_E CO_2$): by increasing tidal volume or respiratory rate.

5.8   a) False   b) True   c) True   d) False   e) True

EXPLANATION

Interactions can occur by four mechanisms:

1. Physical or chemical interaction, e.g. barbiturates and non-depolarizing relaxants form a precipitate when mixed together.
2. Pharmacokinetic, when one drug alters the absorption, distribution, metabolism or excretion of another:
   - absorption, e.g. N_2O enhances uptake of halothane (second gas effect)
   - distribution, e.g. contrast media displace barbiturates from proteins
   - metabolism, e.g. barbiturate and antiepileptic therapy increase metabolism of other drugs by liver enzyme induction, echothiophate reduces suxamethonium metabolism
   - excretion: bicarbonate enhances barbiturate excretion by pH alteration, erythromycin inhibits alfentanil clearance
3. Pharmacokinetic, owing to interactions at effector sites having enhancing effects (additive, agonistic, synergistic) or inhibitory effects (antagonistic, competitive), e.g. antagonism of opiates with naloxone.
4. Unknown mechanisms, e.g. pancuronium reduces halothane MAC.

Specific interactions

1. Antihypertensives affecting noradrenaline storage/release: reserpine and methyldopa reduce the MAC of volatile anaesthetics because they deplete catecholamine stores in the CNS.

2. Ganglion blocks: trimetaphan enhances the action of suxamethonium by inhibiting pseudocholinesterase.

3. Alpha-adrenergic receptor drugs: alpha blockers such as phenoxybenzamine decrease the ability to vasoconstrict and respond to hypovolaemia. Clonidine is an alpha-2 agonist with inhibitory and analgesic effects on the CNS and thus reduces the MAC of volatile anaesthetics.

4. Beta-adrenergic receptor drugs: beta agonists can cause hypertension and dysrhythmias during anaesthesia; beta agonist drugs may exacerbate the myocardial depressant effects of anaesthetics or other cardiac depressant drugs such as calcium antagonists. On the other hand, they may prevent dangerous rises in blood pressure and heart rate and any patient on beta blocker therapy should carry on the medication before surgery.

5. ACE inhibitors: renin is released from the kidney and converted in the liver to angiotensin which is a vasoconstrictor and increases aldosterone secretion. ACE inhibitors (e.g. captopril) lower blood pressure and decrease aldosterone secretion with possible hyperkalaemia.

6. Vasodilating drugs: e.g. hydralazine, diazoxide, are peripheral vasodilators and thus may potentiate hypotensive effects of anaesthetics. Nitroglycerine and nitroprusside prolong neuromuscular block.

7. Calcium antagonists: can enhance the cardiovascular effects of anaesthetics but on the whole are of more benefit than risk.

8. Diuretics: many diuretics can cause hypokalaemia which increases the incidence of arrhythmias, increases toxicity of digoxin and enhances neuromuscular block.

9. Monoamine oxidase inhibitors (MAOI): e.g. phenelzine, administration of a sympathetic stimulant to a patient on MAOI may, during anaesthesia, cause hypertension and hyperpyrexia and subarachnoid haemorrhage. Hypotension and respiratory depression are also possible. MAOI should therefore be discontinued at least 2 weeks before surgery.

10. Tricyclic antidepressants: block noradrenaline uptake and when administered acutely can cause myocardial depression and arrhythmias but when administered chronically do not appear to cause any problems and need not be discontinued.

11. Cocaine: also blocks noradrenaline uptake – myocardial depression and arrhythmias. Avoid drugs that cause arrhythmias (e.g. halothane) and sympathomimetics.

12. Chlorprocaine and epidural opioids: prior administration of chlorprocaine decreases the duration and intensity of analgesia from subsequent epidural opiates, probably owing to a local effect at spinal receptors.

13. Anti-arrhythmic drugs: quinidine potentiates depolarizing and non-depolarizing relaxants. Amiodarone and bretylium can cause bradycardia and low cardiac output during anaesthesia.

14. H_2 antagonists: acute administration of H_2 antagonists has no drug interaction effect, but prolonged use has been associated with reduced clearance of drugs metabolized in the liver, and actions of opiates, local anaesthetics and sedatives may be prolonged.

15. Cytotoxic drugs: cyclophosphomide inhibits pseudocholinesterase. Bleomycin can cause pneumonitis and pulmonary fibrosis. Adriamycin can cause a cardiomyopathy. Methotrexate and nitrous oxide may act together to increase the myelosuppression effects of the former.

16. Immunosuppressants: cyclosporin potentiates non-depolarizing muscle relaxants; azathioprine (Imuran) increases depolarizing block and antagonizes non-depolarizing block. The mechanism is unknown.

17. Muscle relaxants: potentiation of non-depolarizing muscle relaxants by 'mycin' antibiotics.

18. Alcohol: acute alcohol intoxication reduces anaesthetic requirements; chronic alcoholism increases requirements.

5.9   a) False   b) True   c) False   d) False   e) True

EXPLANATION
The outcome of cardiopulmonary resuscitation (CPR) is dependent on the length of   111

cardiac arrest; the length of ventricular fibrillation and the adequacy of coronary and cerebral circulation during massage. Cardiac output is improved during CPR either because the heart is compressed between the spine and sternum, or because chest compression raises intrathoracic pressure forcing blood out of the chest. Cardiac output is approximately 25% of normal during CPR and it is directed mainly to organs above the diaphragm with the lower extremity and abdominal viscera receiving less than 5% of the cardiac output. The only drugs that are useful in resuscitation are the vasopressors with alpha effects. Pure beta-adrenergic agonists (e.g. dobutamine) are not effective, but alpha agonists such as methoxamine and noradrenaline are just as successful as adrenaline. Calcium administration has not been shown to be of any value. As regards sodium bicarbonate, it is true that acidosis lowers fibrillation threshold and impairs response to sympathomimetics; however, it causes hypernatraemia, hyperosmolarity and metabolic alkalosis and shifts the oxygen dissociation curve to the left reducing oxygen delivery. It can also increase intracellular acidosis by raising levels of CO_2; therefore bicarbonate should be used very carefully, if at all. Carbon dioxide elimination during CPR is flow, and not ventilation, dependent. Therefore there is a very good correlation between cardiac output and end-tidal CO_2 which is thus a very useful parameter to measure.

5.10   a) True   b) True   c) False   d) True   e) True

EXPLANATION

The anaesthetist should be aware of the toxic actions of cytotoxic agents:

1. Pulmonary toxicity:
   - acute hypersensitivity reactions
   - non-cardiac pulmonary oedema
   - chronic pneumonitis and fibrosis.
2. Cardiac toxicity:
   - acute: ECG changes and ectopics
   - subacute: myocarditis and endocarditis
   - chronic: cardiomyopathy and congestive heart failure.
3. Central nervous toxicity: meningeal irritation and even temporary paraplegia following intrathecal administration. Also peripheral neuropathies: autonomic neuropathy, muscle weariness and paraplegia, cranial nerve damage.
4. Haematological toxicity: leucopenia 4–6 hours after administration; thrombocytopenia after 7 days and anaemia after 120 days (occurs late because of prolonged life span of red blood cells). Disseminated intravascular coagulation and platelet dysfunction are also possible.
5. Hepatic and renal toxicity: hepatic and renal dysfunction is also possible leading to diminished metabolism/excretion of anaesthetic drugs.

NB: Many of these patients may have had radiotherapy. This leads to adhesions and fibrosis, making a subsequent operation on the irradiated area a prolonged, difficult and bloody procedure.

5.11 a) True   b) False   c) True   d) False   e) True

EXPLANATION

The diaphragm is the principal muscle of respiration but other muscles, i.e. intercostal, abdominal, scalene and sternomastoid, also contribute. All these muscles are attached to the thoracic cage. The diaphragm moves downwards in a vertical plain increasing intra-abdominal pressure and this increased abdominal pressure expands the lower rib cage. A 1.5 cm vertical movement achieves a tidal exchange of about 500 ml with deep breathing. The movement can increase to 6–10 cm enhancing tidal volumes considerably. The motor nervous supply to the diaphragm is primarily from the phrenic nerves. The lower intercostal nerves provide a minor motor supply and sensory and autonomic innervation. Unilateral paralysis of the phrenic nerve causes the paralysed half of the diaphragm to rise in the chest during inspiration and fall during expiration. Unilateral phrenic paralysis causes a reduction in breathing capacity of about 15%, while bilateral paralysis severely impairs ventilation with only adequate tidal exchange at rest or during gentle activity. The structures which go through the diaphragm include: nerves – phrenic (right and left), vagal (right and left), sympathetic chain; vessels – aorta and inferior vena cava; and oesophagus.

5.12 a) True   b) True   c) False   d) False   e) True

EXPLANATION

Tramadol is a synthetic opiate which achieves its analgesic action by acting on opiate receptors and by inhibiting noradrenaline and 5-hydroxytryptamine (5-HT) uptake. It is available in oral, intravenous and intramuscular preparations. Peak concentration is reached within 2 hours after oral uptake and 45 minutes after intramuscular injection. Half-life is 6 hours. It is eliminated both by hepatic metabolism and renal excretion. Central nervous system (CNS) effects are enhanced when used with other CNS depressant drugs, but analgesic effect and duration are reduced when combined with carbamazepine. It should not be administered to patients on monoamine oxidase inhibitors (MAOI). Compared to morphine it has a lower incidence of constipation and sedation and addiction is not a problem as it does not produce euphoria. Respiratory depression is also uncommon and if it occurs can be reversed with naloxone. Nausea, vomiting, dizziness and dry mouth are similar in incidence to morphine, while sweating is another not uncommon side-effect. Because of lack of sedation, some anaesthetists would not use it for interoperative analgesia because of the risk of awareness. If used as an intravenous infusion or for patient-controlled analgesia the loading dose is 100 mg, with incremental doses of 20 mg and a lock-out time of 5 minutes. The maximum dose is 500 mg per 4 hours.

5.13   a) False   b) True   c) True   d) True   e) False

EXPLANATION
Arrhythmias are common in healthy people – 50% have premature atrial contractions or premature ventricular contractions, 2% have sustained ventricular tachycardia. During surgery and anaesthesia arrhythmias are very common, e.g. bradycardia, premature atrial or ventricular contractions especially with pre-existing heart disease and electrolytic abnormalities; but significant benign arrhythmias during surgery are very uncommon.

Ventricular arrhythmias
Ventricular arrhythmias (unless benign and harmless) are usually associated with either organic heart disease or electrolytic disturbances.
   Organic heart disease:

   1. Mitral valve prolapse: common and symptomless in 15% of adults; may have premature ventricular contractions or unsustained runs of ventricular tachycardia. These arrhythmias are associated with increased levels of catecholamines, and beta blockers are the best drugs to use to treat them.
   2. Aortic stenosis: there is a very high incidence of ventricular arrhythmias with aortic valve disease.
   3. Ischaemic heart disease: myocardial ischaemia predisposes to atrial or ventricular arrhythmias.
   4. Congestive heart failure: ventricular arrhythmias are common in patients with congestive heart failure and cardiomyopathy.

   Treatment of all the above conditions reduces the incidence of arrhythmias perioperatively.
   Electrolytic disturbance. Hyperkalaemia and hypokalaemia can cause ventricular arrhythmias; hypokalaemia is the more common cause, either because of diuretics or associated with metabolic alkalosis.
   Hypomagnesaemia also predisposes to ventricular arrhythmias. Magnesium is required in the Na^+/K^+ pump and in its absence intracellular potassium falls leading to arrhythmias.
   Which ventricular arrhythmias are dangerous? Chronic ventricular arrhythmias may be classified into the following risk categories.

   1. Benign ventricular arrhythmias: no organic heart disease, no symptoms, occasionally associated with symptomless prolapsed mitral valve – frequent premature ventricular contractions or non-sustained tachycardia. Treatment is not usually required, but if necessary, beta blockers are best to use.
   2. Malignant ventricular arrhythmias associated with cardiac disease or post-myocardial infarction have frequent premature ventricular contractions, and runs of ventricular tachycardia are associated with significant cardiac disease and increased morbidity and mortality.

Anti-arrhythmic drugs
These can be classified as:

Class I: Local anaesthetic or sodium channel blocking properties
   IA: Slow conduction and prolong repolarization, e.g. quinidine, procainamide
   IB: Slow conduction and shorten repolarization, e.g. lignocaine, mexiletine
   IC: Slow conduction and variable effects on repolarization, e.g. flecainide

Class II: Beta blockers, e.g. propranolol
Class III: Prolong duration of action potential and effective refractory period, e.g.
              amiodarone, bretylium
Class IV: Calcium blockers, e.g. verapamil, diltiazem.

Supraventricular arrhythmias

Atrial fibrillation. This is usually associated with significant heart disease – mitral
heart disease, ischaemic heart disease, hypertension, thyrotoxicosis,
cardiomyopathies and congenital heart disease. Emboli occur in 22% of these
patients. Treatment consists in either converting the arrhythmia to sinus rhythm (e.g.
procainamide) or slowing the ventricular rate (e.g. digoxin, beta blockers or calcium
blockers). Electric cardioversion is indicated in patients who do not respond to drug
therapy.

Atrial flutter. This has the same predisposing conditions but is more difficult to
treat.

5.14   a) True   b) False   c) False   d) False   e) False

EXPLANATION

Physiological changes of pregnancy affect a number of systems.

Respiratory system

The gravid uterus elevates the diaphragm, causing the chest wall to increase in
anteroposterior and tranverse diameters. This causes a fall in functional residual
capacity (FRC) (by 20%) and residual volume. Ventilation increases because of
increased metabolic rate and the effect of progesterone which alters the sensitivity of
the respiratory centre to CO_2. Thus alveolar ventilation increases, with increases in
both respiratory rate and tidal volume. Oxygen consumption increases by 20%
owing to increased metabolism, and the oxyhemoglobin dissociation curve shifts to
the right, so that oxygen availability to the fetus is improved. Airway resistance
decreases by 50% because of the effects of progesterone on smooth muscle.

Clinical implications. Intubation is more difficult (weight gain, enlarged breasts,
enlarged neck and chest). The larynx is possibly oedematous; therefore a smaller
tube may be required. The induction rate with inhalational agents is increased due to
the decreased FRC and increased alveolar ventilation (also reduced MAC).
Decreased oxygen reserve (due to reduced FRC) and increased oxygen uptake
increase the likelihood of hypoxia and hypercarbia. Preoxygenation before induction
is thus important. The increased alveolar ventilation decreases PCO_2, but pH
remains the same owing to renal compensation with decreased HCO_3.

Cardiovascular system

Blood volume and cardiac output (increased rate and stroke volume) increases from
8–12 weeks' gestation and especially in the second trimester (by about 35%).
Peripheral vascular resistance and pulmonary vascular resistance decrease
significantly causing vasodilatation and a fall in blood pressure (BP). Hypotension may
also occur in the supine posture because of aortocaval compression by the uterus.

Clinical implications. Dilutional anaemia: haemoglobin (Hb) down to 11 g/100 ml
and haematocrit to 35%; vena caval compression causes ankle oedema; the

115

average blood loss at delivery is well tolerated because of increased blood volume. BP drops because of vasodilatation. Venous compression by the gravid uterus diverts blood into epidural veins making epidural venous puncture more likely. Supine posture should be avoided during anaesthesia in second and third trimester.

Central nervous system

Progesterone increases neural sensitivity to local anaesthetics and reduces MAC by about 30%.

Clinical implications. Less local anaesthetic (about 30% less) is required for epidurals/spinals. Decreased concentrations of inhaled anaesthetics are required.

Gut

Gastric pressure is increased by the uterus; gastrin levels are increased causing increased acidity. Increased progesterone levels decrease the tone of the lower oesophageal sphincter. Gut motility and gastric emptying are slowed by labour.

Clinical implications. Gastric reflux is common during pregnancy. A patient in labour must be regarded as having a full stomach and airway management should assume this, i.e. rapid sequence induction, decrease gastric volume and increase gastric pH with antacids and H_2 blockers.

Renal

The ureters and renal pelves dilate owing to obstruction by the gravid uterus. Renal blood flow and glomerular filtration rate (GFR) increase by 60%. Tubular reabsorption of water and electrolytes occurs, while the renal threshold for glucose decreases causing glycosuria.

Liver

The plasma protein level decreases as also does the alumin/globulin ratio with greater decrease in albumin than globulin. Plasma cholinesterase levels fall. Plasma levels of fibrinogen, and factors VII, VIII, X and XII increase. Therefore there is an increased likelihood of thrombosis (also because of increased platelet levels).

5.15   a) False   b) False   c) False   d) True   e) True

EXPLANATION

The potency of a local anaesthetic is primarily dependent on lipid solubility. This is because the nerve membranes where the local anaesthetic works consist primarily of lipids. The duration of action of local anaesthetics is primarily related to the degree of protein binding. Local anaesthetics act by binding to a protein receptor in the sodium channel; therefore the greater the protein binding of a specific agent, the longer is the period of sodium channel blockade and the longer the duration of local anaesthesia.

Local anaesthetics are divided into two groups: amino esters and amino amides. The esters (e.g. procaine, tetracaine) are relatively unstable, and are hydrolyzed by cholinesterase enzymes. p-aminobenzoic acid is one of the metabolites and this is the cause of the allergic reactions to amino esters. The amides (e.g. lignocaine, bupivacaine) are more stable, are broken down in the liver, and allergic reactions are extremely rare. At low concentrations these agents cause vasoconstriction, whereas in clinically employed concentrations they cause vasodilatation.

Prilocaine is also an amide agent and is the least toxic of the amide agents; it is therefore particularly useful for i.v. regional anaesthesia. It can, however, cause methaemoglobinaemia and is unsuitable for epidurals because the newborn babies may become cyanotic.

An ankle block requires block of five nerves – posterior tibial and sural nerves at the back of the ankle, and saphenous, superficial and deep peroneal at the anterior region of the ankle. The posterior tibial (supplying sole of foot) can be blocked behind the medial malleolus just posterior to the posterior tibial artery. Local anaesthetic is injected between the artery, Achilles tendon and tibia. The sural nerve is blocked by an injection behind the lateral malleolus, between it and the calcaneus. The other three nerves are anterior. The saphenous nerve is blocked anterior to the medial malleolus around the saphenous vein. The deep peroneal nerve (supplying dorsum of foot) is blocked on the anterior midline surface of the ankle just lateral to the anterior tibial artery. The superficial peroneal nerve is blocked by a subcutaneous injection between the anterior tibial artery and the lateral malleolus.

5.16   a) True   b) True   c) False   d) True   e) True

EXPLANATION

Pneumoperitoneum for laparoscopic cholecystectomy is usually achieved with CO_2 insufflation. Nitrous oxide and room air have been used for diagnostic laparoscopies but are unsuitable when cautery is required.

Problems associated with pneumoperitoneum include:

1. Technical: subcutaneous misplacement of trocar followed by insufflation can cause extensive subcutaneous emphysema which can involve neck, chest, abdomen and groin. Trocar insertion into the chest can lead to pneumothorax including tension pneumothorax. Bleeding is also possible from blood vessel injury. Other surgical complications include bile duct injuries, gut perforations, hepatic and splenic trauma.

2. Cardiovascular problems: nowadays an electronic variable flow insufflator is used which stops flow once an intra-abdominal pressure of 12–15 mmHg is reached. At this pressure no significant cardiovascular changes occur but if the intra-abdominal pressure is increased further, the accompanying increase in intrathoracic pressure, central venous pressure and femoral venous pressure leads to hypertension tachycardia and decreased cardiac output. Increase in vagal tone due to peritoneal irritation is also possible.

3. Respiratory function: functional residual capacity and lung compliance decrease with upward displacement of the diaphragm. Fit patients do not get significant rises in end-tidal and arterial PCO_2 but patients with cardiovascular disease develop significant acidosis and hypercarbia (CO_2 absorption from peritoneal cavity). The increased $PaCO_2$ may predispose to arrhythmias, especially with spontaneous respiration. Therefore intermittent positive-pressure ventilation (IPPV) is always best for this procedure.

4. Hormonal changes: significant increase in plasma concentrations of dopamine, vasopressin, adrenaline, noradrenaline, renin and cortisol.

5. Specific problems: pneumomentum, subcutaneous or mediastinal emphysema, pneumothorax, hypoxaemia, hypotension, cardiovascular collapse, venous gas

embolism, arrhythmias, increased likelihood of regurgitation and aspiration due to steep head-down tilt, insufflation of intraperitoneal gas and mechanical pressure exerted on the abdomen by the surgical team.

6. Anaesthesia: general anaesthesia is recommended because of patient discomfort associated with creation of pneumoperitoneum and constant position changes. Intubation is recommended to reduce the incidence of aspiration, together with controlled ventilation because of possible hypercarbia and mechanical impairment of ventilation by the pneumoperitoneum and steep head-down tilt. Postoperative nausea and vomiting are common, even if opioids are avoided.

5.17   **a) True**   **b) False**   **c) True**   **d) True**   **e) False**

EXPLANATION

Plasma cholinesterase is formed in the liver and is responsible for breaking down suxamethonium. In practice, the action of suxamethonium is not prolonged until about 80% of the enzyme is absent. Cholinesterase hydrolyses other agents including ester-type local anaesthetics, e.g. procaine, amethocaine (but not amide local anaesthetics, e.g. lignocaine, bupivacaine), propanidid and benzoylcholine. Mivacurium is also hydrolyzed by cholinesterase and there have been a few reports of prolonged neuromuscular block with mivacurium when cholinesterase levels are low.

Plasma cholinesterase levels may be low in advanced liver disease and malnutrition and its level is depressed by cholinesterase inhibitors, e.g. ecothiopate eye drops, tacrine; some cytotoxics; and organophosphate poisons including insecticides and nerve gases.

5.18   **a) True**   **b) False**   **c) True**   **d) False**   **e) False**

EXPLANATION

Polycythaemia is associated with increased haemoglobin (over 17 g/100 ml in males and over 16 g/100 ml in females). It can be primary or secondary.

Primary polycythaemia (polycythaemia rubra vera) is a bone marrow neoplastic disorder usually in males over 50. Symptoms are due to hypervolaemia and hyperviscosity, i.e. headaches, plethora, dyspnoea, visual disturbances, reduced cardiac output, hypertension, thrombosis due to abnormal platelets, and haemorrhagic episodes. Hepatosplenomegaly may be present. Apart from increased red cell mass and packed cell volume (50–70%), there is often an increased white cell and platelet count.

Secondary polycythaemia is due to raised erythropoietin levels either in response to chronic hypoxaemia from high altitude, pulmonary or cyanotic heart disease or in response to inappropriate secretion of erythropoietin (e.g. renal or liver carcinoma). Platelet function is not abnormal in secondary polycythaemia; therefore haemostasis is not affected.

The anaesthetic problems associated with polycythaemia are due to the very high blood viscosity which leads to reduced blood velocity and high left ventricular afterload. These patients often have normal cardiac outputs and blood pressure (sometimes increased cardiac output and hypertension), but they are often breathless on exertion even though oxygen saturation is normal. Other problems include increased haemorrhage due to abnormal platelets and increased incidence of venous thrombosis and pulmonary embolism. The anaesthetic technique should aim at optimizing tissue perfusion, i.e. either regional anaesthesia or general anaesthesia with vasodilatation. For elective surgery, venesection may be recommended to reduce the haematocrit to 55%. For emergency surgery, colloids and crystalloids are administered to reduce blood viscosity and haematocrit.

5.19	**a) True**	**b) True**	**c) False**	**d) False**	**e) False**

EXPLANATION

Carcinoid tumours occur mainly in the appendix, small intestine, rectum and bronchus, and especially in the first two sites. Carcinoid syndrome is caused by the release into the circulation of a number of active amines and peptides. The main mediator is serotonin, but there are a number of others including bradykinins, prostaglandins, histamine and substance P. The syndrome is usually the result of liver metastasis. Serotonin is metabolized into 5-hydroxyindoleacetic acid (5-HIAA) and a patient with carcinoid syndrome will have high urinary levels of 5-HIAA. 90% of patients with carcinoid syndrome have episodes of flushing of the face and upper body, 75% have diarrhoea, 33% have right-sided heart disease (right endocardial fibrosis with possible tricuspid insufficiency and pulmonary stenosis), while 20% suffer from bronchospasm. All the symptoms are associated with serotonin release except flushing and bronchoconstriction, the cause of which is multifactorial.

A patient with carcinoid syndrome presenting for anaesthesia may be on a number of medications which should be maintained prior to anaesthesia. These include digitalis and diuretics for right-sided heart failure, bronchodilators, sedatives to avoid stress which can be precipitated by pain, anaesthesia and surgery especially when the tumour is handled. This usually presents with cardiovascular collapse or tachycardia and hypertension. Bronchoconstriction and right heart failure are also possible. Catecholamines should not be administered for cardiovascular collapse as they may precipitate mediator release. If a crisis occurs, one should administer antimediator drugs such as ketanserin, aprotonin and antihistamines, and especially somatostatin analogues, e.g. octreotide, which have been found to inhibit the release of the active mediators from the carcinoid tumours. Because of histamine release in carcinoid syndrome, histamine-releasing drugs (e.g. atracurium, curare) should be avoided. Vecuronium is probably the relaxant of choice.

5.20	**a) False**	**b) True**	**c) True**	**d) True**	**e) False**

EXPLANATION

The intraocular pressure (IOP) is primarily determined by the aqueous humour and choroidal blood volume. An increase in these leads to increase in IOP and impairment of the retina and optic nerve. Normal IOP is between 10 and 20 mmHg. Intraocular pressure is increased by a number of causes:

1. Mechanical: when there is impairment of aqueous outflow, e.g. glaucoma. Trabeculectomy is a procedure to decrease IOP. An eye squeeze raises IOP to about 50 mmHg. A poorly placed anaesthetic mask could increase the IOP to a point where blood flow approaches zero.

2. Drugs:
- Anaesthetic: suxamethonium causes an increase in IOP of about 6–12 mmHg and lasts about 10 minutes. This must be taken into consideration when a rise in IOP is undesirable in eye surgery or open eye injuries. Pre-administration of non-depolarizers, lignocaine or diazepam, partially reduces the response. Ketamine is thought to increase IOP, but lately it has been suggested that ketamine has little, if any, effect on IOP. Inhalational agents cause dose-related depressions in IOP, owing to depression of CNS control, reduction in aqueous humour production, enhancement of aqueous outflow, or relaxation of the extraocular muscles. All CNS depressants – barbiturates, neuroleptics, narcotics, tranquillizers and hypnotics – lower IOP in both normal and glaucomatous eyes.
- Non-anaesthetic: anticholinergic drugs such as atropine/scopolamine increase IOP; cholinergic drugs such as pilocarpine/acetylcholine, and anticholinesterases such as ecothiopate reduce it. Ganglion blockers produce a dramatic decrease in IOP, including trimetaphan, despite mydriasis. Timodol is a beta blocker used to decrease aqueous humour production in the treatment of glaucoma. Intravenous hypertonic solutions, such as dextran, urea and mannitol, elevate plasma osmotic pressure, thereby decreasing aqueous humour formation and reducing IOP. Acetazolamide reduces IOP by inactivating carbonic anhydrase and thus interferes with the sodium pump which is responsible for aqueous humour production. Other diuretics also reduce IOP.

3. Ventilation: hyperventilation decreases IOP; hypoventilation and administration of carbon dioxide increase it. Hypoxia also increases IOP.

4. Temperature: hypothermia reduces IOP.

5. Changes in choroidal blood volume: hypercapnia increases choroidal blood volume and IOP. Increases in venous pressure caused by coughing, straining and intubation increase IOP to 30–40 mmHg.

6.1 Features of transcutaneous electrical nerve stimulation (TENS) include:

a) It is almost always ineffective in chronic cancer pain
b) It is more effective for somatic than for visceral pain
c) It is often effective in neurological pain and usually ineffective in psychogenic pain
d) It should not be used on the anterior cervical region
e) Pain relief is almost entirely due to the 'placebo' effect

6.2 Suxamethonium:

a) May cause sudden cardiac arrest in children with undiagnosed muscular dystrophy
b) Should be avoided in the first 6 weeks after a patient has suffered severe burns
c) Sensitivity is greater in neonates than in adults
d) May cause muscle pains which are more common in pregnant women following its use
e) Duration of action is increased in the presence of severe liver damage

6.3 Features of TURP (transurethral resection of prostate) syndrome include:

a) Pulmonary oedema
b) Glycine toxicity if glycine is used as the irrigating solution
c) Reduced severity of hyponatraemia if isotonic dextrose rather than glycine is used as the irrigating solution
d) A close relationship between symptoms and the falls in serum sodium levels
e) Hyponatraemia that should be corrected with the rapid administration of concentrated (hypertonic) salt solution

6.4 With regard to analgesia in renal and hepatic impairment:

a) Fentanyl and alfentanil are relatively safe in renal failure
b) Pethidine is preferable to morphine in patients with renal failure
c) Buprenorphine is contraindicated in renal failure
d) Ketorolac can be used in normal dosage with a creatinine of 300 μmol/litre
e) Non-steroidal anti-inflammatory drugs (NSAIDs) can cause water retention and hyperkalaemia in patients with renal or hepatic impairment

6.5 In a patient with a chronic spinal injury:

a) Pulmonary function tests are affected in lesions at T7 or above
b) In the first 2–3 weeks following the injury hypertension and tachycardia are characteristic
c) In the first 2–3 weeks following the injury flaccid paralysis is characteristic
d) Pre-treatment with a non-depolarizing relaxant prevents the hyperkalaemia caused by suxamethonium
e) Hypothermia is more likely during anaesthesia

6.6 **A pulse oximeter:**

a) Detects light transmitted through the skin at 540 and 660 nm wavelengths
b) Saturation approximates arterial saturation in the presence of carboxyhaemoglobin
c) Reading is not affected by jaundice
d) Reading may be affected by methylene blue injection
e) Detects falls in arterial saturation almost immediately when arterial oxygen tensions are above 10 kPa (75 mmHg)

6.7 **Lower oesophageal sphincter tone:**

a) Is increased by sympathetic beta stimulation and alpha block
b) Is reduced by suxamethonium
c) Is increased with vagal stimulation
d) Is increased with opiates
e) Is reduced with ranitidine

6.8 **Changes in pupil size (miosis – contraction; mydriasis – dilatation) are caused by:**

a) A successful stellate ganglion block, producing contralateral miosis
b) Pontine lesions, classically causing mydriasis
c) Hypercapnia, causing mydriasis
d) Carbachol, causing miosis
e) Sympathomimetic drugs, causing mydriasis by beta-stimulating action

6.9 **With regard to cardiomyopathy:**

a) Thromboembolism may be a feature of three types – congestive, hypertrophic or restrictive cardiomyopathy
b) Vasodilators are contraindicated in congestive (dilated) cardiomyopathy
c) Beta-stimulating sympathomimetic drugs are indicated for low cardiac output in hypertrophic (obstructive) cardiomyopathy
d) Spinal anaesthesia is preferable to general anaesthesia in a patient with hypertrophic (obstructive) cardiomyopathy
e) Restrictive cardiomyopathy is an autosomal dominant inherited disorder

6.10 **With regard to myocardial ischaemia:**

a) A normal resting electrocardiography (ECG) is a reliable indicator of absent coronary artery disease
b) Most old myocardial infarctions can be detected on an ECG
c) Prognosis of patients with coronary artery disease is highly dependent on left ventricular function and ejection fractions
d) Right bundle branch block is of greater significance than left bundle block when diagnosing myocardial ischaemia
e) Induction agents least likely to cause cardiovascular depression are etomidate and ketamine; thiopentone is more likely to cause it, and propofol is most likely

6.11 **With regard to blood products:**

a) Fresh frozen plasma contains all coagulation factors except platelets
b) Cryoprecipitate contains fibrinogen, factor VIII plus platelets
c) All coagulation factors are stable in stored blood except factors V and VIII
d) Stored blood anticoagulated with acid citrate dextrose has a longer shelf life than with citrate phosphate dextrose
e) One unit of platelets will increase the platelet count by about 50 000 per ml

6.12 **With regard to arterial cannulation:**

a) There is a higher incidence of infectious complications with femoral artery cannulation, compared to cannulation of the radial or brachial artery
b) Dorsalis pedis cannulation has a higher incidence of thrombosis than radial artery cannulation
c) The median nerve can be damaged with both brachial and radial artery cannulations
d) It is more likely to develop ischaemic complications with proximal artery cannulation (e.g. femoral, brachial) than with distal cannulation (e.g. radial, dorsalis pedis)
e) The radial artery has a better collateral circulation than the brachial artery

6.13 **Factors increasing renal blood flow include:**

a) Beta-2 agonists
b) Prostaglandins
c) Systolic blood pressure of 50 mmHg
d) Alpha agonists
e) Antidiuretic hormone (vasopressin)

6.14 **With regard to laryngeal and tracheal anatomy:**

a) The adult trachea is normally 10–12 cm long
b) The vocal cords lie just below the notch of the thyroid cartilage
c) In bilateral partial recurrent laryngeal nerve paralysis there is loss of voice but no respiratory impairment
d) The right main bronchus lies more vertically, and is shorter than the left main bronchus
e) In the desperate situation of a patient with complete respiratory obstruction, cricothyroid puncture is one of the safest ways of providing an airway

6.15 **Tachycardia occurs with the following agents/events:**

a) Pancuronium
b) Sodium nitroprusside
c) Cocaine
d) Raised intracranial pressure
e) Oculocardiac reflex

6.16 When using local anaesthetic agents:

a) Analgesia occurs prior to sympathetic block
b) Anaesthesia spreads in a proximal to distal direction when a limb is blocked
c) Hypersensitivity reactions are more likely with an amide-linked agent
d) They act by preventing sodium access to the axon interior by occupying the transmembrane sodium channels
e) The Cm of lignocaine is less than that of bupivacaine

6.17 With regard to postoperative spinal/epidural neurological complications:

a) The development of sudden back pain in a patient who has had vascular surgery and an epidural injection should arouse the possibility of an epidural haemorrhage
b) Postoperative anterior spinal artery thrombosis is often associated with perioperative hypotension and usually causes a flaccid paralysis without back pain
c) A myelogram/CT scan is of little use in the differential diagnosis of epidural haemorrhage/anterior spinal artery syndrome
d) Chronic adhesive arachnoiditis after epidural/spinal injection can cause cauda equina syndrome
e) Trauma to the spinal cord can be avoided by performing the dural (epidural) puncture below L2

6.18 With regard to temperature control:

a) It is regulated in the hypothalamus
b) 30% of heat loss during general anaesthesia occurs via respiration
c) Forced air-convective warming is more effective at preventing heat loss than water blankets
d) Hypothermia during general anaesthesia is minimal initially but increases markedly after 2–3 hours
e) Apart from causing heat loss, postoperative shivering does not cause any other deleterious effects

6.19 Liver function tests show:

a) No abnormalities before at least 75% of the liver has been destroyed
b) A lack of urobilin in urine and stercobilin in faeces in severe obstructive jaundice
c) An unchanged albumin/globulin ratio in severe liver failure
d) Raised serum acid phosphatase in conditions which cause liver damage (e.g. viral hepatitis)
e) Raised serum glutamic pyruvic transaminase (SGPT) and serum glutamic oxaloacetic transaminase (SGOT) in viral hepatitis

6.20 Patients with severe liver failure have:

a) Increased bleeding tendencies
b) Increased cardiac output
c) Typically diminished PaO_2 and decreased $PaCO_2$
d) Increased tendency to retain sodium and water
e) Increased drug tolerance

6.1   a) False   b) True   c) True   d) True   e) False

EXPLANATION
Mode of action:

1. Gate theory, i.e. activity in the myelinated afferent fibres (A fibres) inhibits the transmission of activity in the unmyelinated afferent C fibres. Therefore A fibre activity inhibits C fibre activity (closing the gate).

2. TENS releases inhibitory neurotransmitters in spinal cord and brain (e.g. endorphins, enkephalins, gamma-aminobenzoic acid (GABA)).

3. TENS stimulates descending inhibitory pain pathways which are activated by release of endorphins and monoamines (5-hydroxytryptamine (serotonin), noradrenaline, dopamine).

Techniques of electroanalgesia:

1. TENS – using surface electrodes applied to the skin.
2. Peripheral nerve stimulation through subcutaneously implanted electrodes.
3. Peripheral nerve stimulation using electrodes implanted directly on the nerve.
4. Stimulation of the dorsal columns either directly or through the dura.

Forms of TENS:

1. Continuous – continuous impulses at preset frequency.
2. Pulsed – (acupuncture-like) intermittent pulses at preset frequency; thus usually more effective. Shape of pulse – square wave; duration – 0.1–0.5 ms; current – 0–50 mA; frequency – 0–150 Hz.

Electrodes. The aim of TENS is to deliver sufficient charge to a pair of electrodes to excite the afferent fibres in an adjacent nerve in a controllable manner.

The most widely used electrodes are silicone rubber impregnated with carbon. They are strong, flexible and inert, but require adhesive tape. Therefore, self-adhesive disposable electrodes have been introduced, but are expensive. Electrode/skin resistance is reduced by electrolyte gel.

In use. Place electrodes over painful site and stimulate. If initial placement ineffective, relocate electrodes over nerve supplying the painful area. For widespread pain, multiple electrodes may be required. Sensation should be comfortable and not produce muscle twitching. The following are typical directions to the patient: begin with 1 hour three times a day; adjust according to need; you may get a bonus of post-TENS analgesia, i.e. pain relief after the stimulator is turned off.

Indications:

Postoperative pain. Although some studies have shown postoperative pain relief, the benefits may be placebo related.

Chronic pain. TENS is most effective with superficial somatic, deep somatic and neurological pain; less effective for visceral pain; and least effective for psychogenic pain.

Chronic conditions successfully treated with TENS. Peripheral nerve disorders (e.g. causalgia, trigeminal neuralgia, post-herpetic), spinal disorders (e.g. brachial plexus injuries), neoplastic, joint pains, acute pain (obstetric, acute trauma). Other conditions: itch, Raynaud's disease.

Conditions not likely to respond to TENS. Metabolic neuropathies, thalamic pain, headaches, pain scars, coccydynia, visceral pain, ischaemic pain, psychogenic pain.

125

Complications:

1. Allergic reactions to electrode, jelly or tape. This can be remedied by replacing the allergenic item with an alternative, e.g. carbon electrodes replaced by self-adhesive ones; the conductive jelly supplied with the stimulator may be replaced with KY jelly or another alternative; the offending tape can be replaced with transpore or micropore.
2. Tolerance.
3. Equipment failure – leads, battery, etc.
4. Electrical skin burn (very rare) due either to drying out of the jelly, or the electrical current having been applied to a poorly innervated area of skin.

Contraindications:

1. The anterior cervical region should be avoided because stimulation of the carotid sinus produces hypotension and possible laryngeal spasm by stimulation of the laryngeal muscles.
2. The pregnant uterus except for labour pains.
3. Cardiac pacemakers – one should check with manufacturers of pacemaker and TENS machine.
4. Unsuitable patients – low IQ, senility, etc.

Conclusion. TENS has two great advantages over drugs. The first is low cost – after the initial outlay, running costs are very low and, unlike drugs, when the machine is returned it can be used on another patient. Secondly a TENS machine is simple to use, non-invasive, has very few problems, and can be combined freely with other forms of treatment, thus reducing medication requirements.

6.2   a) True   b) True   c) False   d) False   e) True

EXPLANATION

In recent years there have been a number of reports of sudden cardiac arrest in children who have received suxamethonium. In most cases they were found to have an undiagnosed myopathy, symptoms of which may not become apparent before the age of 6–8 years. These children are therefore at risk of suxamthonium-induced hyperkalaemia.

Suxamethonium causes an increase in serum potassium of 0.5–1 mEq/litre. This response is exaggerated in the presence of muscle damage following burns (first 6 weeks), massive trauma, spinal trauma, and neuromuscular disorders such as Guillain–Barré syndrome, motor neuron diseases and various myopathies.

Neonates are relatively (on a weight for weight basis) resistant to depolarizing agents and sensitive to non-depolarizing drugs.

Muscle pains following the use of suxamethonium occur especially in shoulders, trunk and back and may last for a few hours or a few days. They are more common in ambulant patients and less common in the young, aged and pregnant women. Pre-treatment with non-depolarizing agents only has a partial effect in reducing suxamethonium (scoline) pains. Patients should be warned about the possibility prior to suxamethonium administration.

Since pseudocholinesterase is formed in the liver, in the event of severe liver damage, cachexia or malnutrition, an increased duration of action of suxamethonium should be anticipated.

6.3   a) True   b) True   c) False   d) False   e) False

EXPLANATION

TURP syndrome

Cause. This syndrome occurs during transurethral resection of the prostate (or endometrial resection of the uterus), and is caused by absorption into the circulation of large volumes of the irrigating fluid, glycine 1.5%. Glycine is used because it is non-electrolytic and conducts electricity to allow the resection. It is hypotonic, and is absorbed through the open prostatic veins into the extracellular fluid, causing water intoxication and hyponatraemia. The amount of glycine absorbed will depend upon a number of factors: length of resection; extent of open prostatic veins; the amount of bladder distension; the hydrostatic pressure of the irrigating fluid. The amount absorbed varies from 10–50 ml/minute, and up to 2.5 litres can be absorbed. The incidence of TURP syndrome may be reduced by administering saline solutions during the resection, keeping the irrigating pressure to 60–70 cmH$_2$O and replacing the glycine irrigation with saline postoperatively. Some surgeons have used isotonic dextrose as the irrigating solution, but apart from the risk of hyperglycaemia, hyponatraemia is actually more marked than with glycine irrigation.

Features.

1. Pulmonary oedema due to the intravascular absorption of the irrigating fluid, causing respiratory distress and cyanosis.

2. Hyponatraemia, again due to the dilutional effect of the absorption of the irrigating fluid. The symptoms of hyponatraemia (cerebral oedema) usually appear when the serum sodium drops below 120 mEq/litre, and levels below 100 mEq/litre have been reported. On the other hand, sodium levels close to 100 mEq/litre are often asymptomatic. Symptoms include restlessness, headache, confusion, convulsions, coma. Treatment is controversial. In many cases the hyponatraemia corrects itself within 24 hours. Rapid correction of hyponatraemia may be dangerous, because it can cause osmotic gradients between the brain and vascular compartments, and may cause cerebral damage. If therapy is deemed to be necessary, normal saline with frusemide is usually sufficient. In severe cases, concentrated (hypertonic) salt solutions may be required, but if administered rapidly can cause central pontine myelinolysis; therefore hypertonic salt solutions are given at a rate not exceeding 100 ml/hour.

3. Glycine toxicity. Glycine is an inhibitory neurotransmitter in the brain, spinal cord and retina, and its metabolites, such as ammonia, oxalate and glycolate, may have similar actions. Symptoms of glycine toxicity include nausea, vomiting, malaise, confusion, coma and transient blindness.

6.4   a) True   b) False   c) False   d) False   e) True

EXPLANATION

Renal failure
Opioids:

- *Avoid:* pethidine, dextropropoxyphene

- *Caution:* morphine, codeine, methadone, pentazocine, diamorphine
- *Low risk:* buprenorphine, fentanyl, alfentanil, sufentanil.

Renal impairment reduces excretion of most opioids leading to increased analgesia, sedation and respiratory depression. Some opiates are more problematical in renal failure than others.

Pethidine should be avoided in renal failure because it is broken down into norphethidine which is neurotoxic, can stimulate the CNS and may cause convulsions.

Morphine is primarily metabolized in the liver, while about 10% is excreted unchanged in the urine. However, 90% of the metabolites are excreted by the kidney, and one metabolite, morphine-6-glucuronide, is at least as active as morphine. Therefore morphine should be used with caution in renal failure.

Fentanyl, alfentanil and sufentanil are mainly metabolized in the liver and very little is excreted in the urine. They are relatively safe in renal impairment, as is buprenorphine the metabolites of which are relatively inactive.

NSAIDs. Prostaglandins cause vasodilatation and, because of their antiprostaglandin action, NSAIDs are potentially dangerous in renal impairment, causing reduction in renal perfusion and glomerular filtration. Prostaglandins also inhibit tubular reabsorption of water and sodium and can therefore cause oedema and hyperkalaemia which can cause problems in patients with hypertension, congestive heart failure, cirrhosis, and renal impairment. NSAIDs may be safe in patients with mild renal impairment, but renal function must be monitored closely. If there are signs of renal damage (i.e. decreased urine output, increased urea and creatinine), the NSAIDs should be discontinued. In the presence of more severe renal impairment (creatinine above 430 μmol/litre) NSAIDs should not be used at all, and the dose should be halved if creatinine is between 160 and 430 μmol/litre. NSAIDs can also cause interstitial nephritis and nephrotic syndrome. This is immunologically mediated and presents with haematuria, proteinuria and loin pain.

Liver failure

Opiates. Morphine is metabolized in the liver into the inactive morphine-3-glucuronide and the active metabolite, morphine-6-glucuronide. Liver damage reduces the rate of clearance of morphine and prolongs its half-life; therefore, doses should be reduced to avoid excessive sedation and respiratory depression. Similar caution with other opioids is also required.

NSAIDs. On the whole, hepatic toxicity, apart from mild asymptomatic rises in liver enzymes, is rare with NSAIDs. Because of the antiplatelet activity of NSAIDs, the risk of gastrointestinal bleeding is increased if these agents are given to patients with liver cirrhosis.

6.5   a) True   b) False   c) True   d) False   e) True

EXPLANATION

Problems in patients with spinal injury are numerous:

Respiratory complications. C3–C5 transection causes paralysis of abdominal, intercostal and diaphragmatic muscles. The only muscles which function during respiration are the accessory muscles (i.e. sternomastoid and scalenes) causing abdominal paradox. Pulmonary function tests are severely compromised in lesions at T7 or above, i.e. inability to cough and clear secretions, decreased vital capacity, flow, and pulmonary compliance, decreased functional residual capacity which encroaches on closing volume. These changes cause hypoventilation, alveolar collapse and ventilation-perfusion mismatch. Pneumonia is always a major hazard, and aggressive pulmonary toilet is of paramount importance.

Patients who have had cervical spinal injury present airway problems to the anaesthetist. During intubation the head should be kept in the neutral position and the patient may require awake fibreoptic intubation, tracheostomy, etc. (i.e. all the problems associated with difficult intubation).

Cardiovascular problems:

1. Acute, i.e. in the first few minutes following the injury. There is sympathetic discharge causing hypertension and increase in cardiac output. There is also increase in lung and cerebral water causing cerebral and pulmonary oedema.

2. Phase of spinal shock lasting days to a few weeks. Spinal (sympathetic) shock is characterized by flaccid paralysis. There is also vasodilatation, hypotension and bradycardia if the spinal injury is above T7 and these changes are due to sympathetic denervation.

3. Phase of autonomic hyper-reflexia. After a few weeks the spinal shock resolves, and the blood pressure returns to normal. However, many patients with transections above T7 experience episodes of autonomic hyper-reflexia, i.e. episodes of severe hypertension accompanied by headache, sweating, and muscle contraction. These episodes can be triggered by everyday stimuli, e.g. bladder or rectal distension, and the symptoms are due to increased sympathetic tone below the level of injury where higher sympathetic control is lost. These patients are also susceptible to cardiac arrhythmias, both brady- and tachyarrhythmias.

Genitourinary problems. Acute renal failure (together with chest infections) is a common cause of death due to sepsis, dehydration, hypotension, nephrotoxic drugs. Chronic renal failure is also common.

Thermoregulatory problems. These patients are likely to lose heat because of vasodilatation (sympathetic denervation), inability to shiver and impaired thermoregulation in the hypothalamus.

Other problems. Anaemia, hypercalcaemia, osteoporosis, hypovolaemia, frequent respiratory and urinary infections.

Anaesthetic management

The anaesthetic management should take into account all the possible changes mentioned above. There is also the problem of hyperkalaemia after the administration of suxamethonium. 20 mg of suxamethonium can result in a potassium concentration of 13.6 mEq/litre in some patients. Pretreatment with a non-depolarizing relaxant does not significantly block the hyperkalaemia.

6.6   a) False   b) False   c) True   d) True   e) False

EXPLANATION

Principles

A pulse oximeter depends on the proportion of light absorbed by the blood at two

129

wavelengths – red light at 660 nm and infrared light at 940 nm. The amount absorbed is also dependent on the concentrations of oxygenated and deoxygenated haemoglobin. Therefore a saturation reading of 90% indicates the presence of 10% desaturated normal haemoglobin (HHb). Because of the sigmoid shape of the Hb dissociation curve, saturation lags behind falls in PaO_2 if the latter is above 10 kPa (75 mmHg); therefore, there may be a significant fall in PaO_2 before saturation starts to decline. Below a PaO_2 of 10 kPa, a small reduction in PaO_2 produces a large decrease in saturation. For the above reasons, a pulse oximeter is not a reliable guide to patient disconnection, which is best detected either by a capnograph, which detects a sudden fall in end-tidal CO_2, or by a disconnection alarm, which is activated if the airway pressure falls below a preset minimum. A PaO_2 of 10 kPa corresponds to a saturation of 94%, and the lower alarm limit on the oximeter should thus be set at 94%.

Factors affecting saturation readings

1. PaO_2 levels. As stated above, when PaO_2 is above 10 kPa (75 mmHg), saturation lags behind arterial oxygen levels; below 10 kPa, a small drop in PaO_2 produces a large fall in saturation reading.

2. Blood flow. Cold, vasoconstriction and hypotension may stop flow through fingers and prevent detection of SaO_2; in these cases, one may restore oximeter detection by a finger block with 1% lignocaine, or use an ear probe instead.

3. Other haemoglobins:

- Carboxyhaemoglobin. At the wavelengths used in pulse oximeters, oxygenated haemoglobin is practically indistinguishable from carboxyhaemoglobin, and therefore a pulse oximeter would not detect the presence of COHb, even though the oxygen-carrying capacity is greatly reduced.
- Methaemoglobin. In methaemoglobinaemia (e.g. caused by prilocaine), methaemoglobin absorbs both 660 and 940 nm light and SaO_2 readings fall.

4. Dyes. Injected methylene blue (sometimes used for parathyroid detection in parathyroid surgery) and indocyanine green produce transient false falls in oxygen saturations. Low readings have also been observed with the use of fingerprinting ink, and henna which is a stain used on fingers and toes by Middle Eastern women.

Jaundice and anaemia have no effect on pulse oximetry.

6.7   a) False   b) False   c) True   d) False   e) False

EXPLANATION

The lower oesophageal sphincter is the lower 2–5 cm of the oesophagus which extends above and below the diaphragm. It helps to prevent regurgitation of gastric contents into the oesophagus because of its natural increased muscle tone compared with the rest of the oesophagus. If the sphincter becomes incompetent (e.g. hiatus hernia, increased abdominal pressure) gastro-oesophageal reflux may follow.

There are a number of factors which increase/reduce lower oesophageal sphincter tone:

1. *Mechanical.* Compression of oesophagus by diaphragm; acute angle of entry of oesophagus into the stomach, mucosal flap at oesophageal opening.

2. *Neural.* Vagal stimulation increases tone; reversed with atropine. Also increased with alpha stimulation and beta blockade; decreased with beta stimulation and alpha blockade.

3. *Drugs:*
- Increased tone: metoclopramide, domperidone, prochlorperazine, neostigmine, pancuronium, suxamethonium, antacids owing to increase in pH; drugs which cause alpha stimulation (e.g. noradrenaline) and beta blockade (e.g. propranolol).
- Reduced tone: anticholinergic drugs (e.g. atropine), opioids, i.v. induction agents and volatile anaesthetics, ganglion blockers, gut hormones (glucagon), progesterone, drugs which cause beta stimulation (e.g. dobutamine) and alpha blockade (e.g. phentolamine).

6.8   a) False   b) False   c) True   d) True   e) False

EXPLANATION

The pupil is normally 1–8 mm in size.
Miosis is caused by:

1. Parasympathetic stimulation and drugs which stimulate the acetylcholine receptors, such as acetylcholine, carbachol, pilocarpine, or acetylcholinesterase inhibitors such as neostigmine. Sympathetic block by stellate ganglion produces unilateral miosis.
2. Opioid analgesia drugs.
3. Pontine lesions.

Mydriasis is caused by:

1. Sympathetic stimulation, e.g. hypercapnia, awareness during anaesthesia, stress, and drugs which cause sympathetic stimulation (alpha but not beta stimulation causes pupillary dilatation, e.g. phenylephrine).
2. Anticholinergic drugs, i.e. antagonists of acetylcholine at muscarinic receptors (e.g. atropine, hyoscine, glycopyrrolate).
3. Head injury.

6.9   a) True   b) False   c) False   d) False   e) False

EXPLANATION
See Table 6.1.

6.10   a) False   b) False   c) True   d) False   e) True

EXPLANATION
When a patient who has a history of myocardial ischaemia is to undergo a general anaesthetic, it is important to try to determine the risks. About 25% of infarcts are

Table 6.1   Cardiomyopathies

	Types		
	Congestive (dilated)	**Hypertrophic (obstructive)**	**Restrictive**
Cardiac pathology	Decreased contractility of left or right ventricle causing cardiac failure	Mainly affecting the septum, but also the left ventricle with resistance to venous inflow causing diastolic failure	Rare. Endocardial or myocardial pathology, leading to reduction in ventricular distensibility, reduction in diastolic filling causing a picture of 'constrictive pericarditis'
Causes	Toxic – alcohol, lead; nutritional – vitamin deficiencies; metabolic – amyloid, glycogen storage disease, uraemia; infection – viral, bacterial; neurological – muscular dystrophies, myotonias; idiopathic	Autosomal dominant inherited disorder	Endocardial or myocardial disease
Clinical	Heart failure with ejection fraction often less than 0.4; compensatory increased peripheral resistance; arrhythmias; systemic embolism	Dyspnoea, dizziness, fainting, angina; usually patient in sinus rhythm, but arrhythmias possible and may cause sudden death. ECG: left ventricular strain and ischaemic changes. Systemic embolism	Heart failure; symptoms similar to constrictive pericarditis. There may be associated eosinophilia and thromboembolism if there is endocardial disease
Treatment	Diuretics; vasodilators to reduce raised peripheral resistance; ACE inhibitors; anticoagulants	Antiarrhythmic drugs, e.g. amiodarone; beta or calcium blockers; anticoagulants	Steroids; cytotoxics
Anaesthetic considerations	Myocardial depressants can precipitate cardiac failure and should be avoided – beta sympathetic drugs may be required; pregnancy puts extra strain on the heart especially in the third trimester when blood volume and coronary output are raised; arrhythmias are common with general anaesthesia; anticoagulant therapy may increase bleeding	Tachycardias and arrhythmias are common; can be caused by sympathetic stimulation (stress, intubation, pain, light general anaesthesia) and should be avoided; digoxin and beta drugs are contraindicated – increase outflow tract obstruction and further reduce cardiac output. Hypertension and vasodilators also reduce cardiac output and should be prevented – spinals should be used with great caution	Again myocardial depressants should be avoided, as well as hypotension and vasodilators. Avoid also changes in cardiac rate and rhythm. Diuretics should not be used because of blood volume depletion

silent, and in about a further 25% the ECG is inconclusive; only 25–50% of old infarcts can be detected on ECG. Therefore, a normal ECG does not rule out coronary artery disease. Stress ECGs are more likely to detect abnormalities, i.e. 52% of patients with myocardial ischaemia develop premature ventricular contractions and ST changes; 24-hour ECGs detect ventricular arrhythmias even more reliably.

The preoperative risk factors in a patient with coronary artery disease are:

- History: recent myocardial infarction (within the previous 6 months); crescendo angina

- Physical: hypertension; congestive heart failure
- ECG: 'Q' waves; left bundle branch block; complete heart block; left ventricular strain; arrhythmias
- Chest X-rays: cardiomegaly; congestive heart failure
- Catheter: two- and three-vessel disease; left main disease; valve disease; ejection fraction less than 50%.

In patients with myocardial ischaemia, left ventricular dysfunction is of major prognostic importance. In patients with ejection fractions of less than 40% the 1-year mortality is about 30%. Ejection fractions can be calculated by cardiac catheterization or echocardiography. The presence of dysrhythmias in patients with coronary artery disease is again of major prognostic significance. The worst arrhythmias are complex premature ventricular contractions and ventricular tachycardia, and conduction defects, especially complete heart block and left bundle branch block (right bundle block is of less significance). During anaesthesia, arrhythmias are usually supraventricular or preventricular contractions and usually associated with surgical stimulation, hypercapnia, hypoxia, potassium abnormalities, digoxin and specific anaesthetics. The incidence of dysrhythmias is increased threefold in patients with heart disease.

In patients with heart disease, etomidate and ketamine (sympathetic stimulation) cause least cardiovascular depression. Thiopentone and especially propofol are myocardial depressants and cause significant drops in cardiac output and blood pressure.

6.11　a) True　b) False　c) True　d) False　e) True

EXPLANATION
See Table 6.2.

6.12　a) False　b) False　c) True　d) False　e) False

EXPLANATION
It is a common misconception that femoral artery cannulation is associated with a high incidence of infection, because of proximity to the perineum, etc.; but this is not true. Both the radial artery and the dorsalis pedis are widely used for cannulation, because of ease of access and abundant collaterals. Thrombosis is uncommon, and dorsalis pedis cannulation has no higher incidence of infection than radial artery catheterization. Proximal arteries have a better collateral circulation than distal arteries, and therefore thrombotic and ischaemic complications are less likely with cannulation of larger arteries.

When cannulating an artery, one should always use the smallest possible catheter. Small catheters have the disadvantage of kinking, but the advantages include fewer vascular complications and a tendency to increase damping in an underdamped monitoring system.

Table 6.2   Available blood components

	Content	Indications	Volume	Shelf life
Red cells				
Whole blood	RBCs, WBCs, plasma platelet debris	To improve red cell volume and plasma volume	About 500 ml	Depends on anticoagulant used: ACD 21 days; CPD 28 days. Another advantage of CPD is levels of 2,3-DPG fall half as rapidly as with ACD
Packed cells	RBCs, WBCs, platelet debris	To improve red cell volume	200 ml RBCs	ACD 21 days; CPD 28 days
Platelets	Platelets, few WBCs, some plasma	Thrombocytopenia; platelet dysfunction	30–50 ml/unit	6–72 h
Fresh frozen plasma	Plasma proteins; all coagulation factors except platelets	Bleeding from coagulation deficiency; volume expansion	200–250 ml	Thawed: 2 h Frozen: years
Cryoprecipitate (Prepared by thawing 1 unit of FFP to 4°C and recovering the remaining cold precipitate which contains factors VIII, XIII, fibrinogen and von Willebrand factor)	Factors I (fibrinogen), VIII, XIII and von Willebrand factor	Haemophilia; von Willebrand's disease; fibrinogen deficiency, e.g. DIC	25 ml	Thawed: 4–6 h
Plasma protein fraction	Albumin and globulin (both alpha and beta globulins)	Volume expansion; to maintain oncotic pressure	260 ml	3–5 years
Albumin 20–25% (hypertronic)	Albumin	Volume; oncotic pressure	50 ml	3–5 years
Albumin 5% (isotonic)	Albumin	Volume; oncotic pressure	50 ml	3–5 years
WBC concentrate	WBCs; few platelets	Agranulocytosis	50–100 ml	12 h
Plasma serum globulin	Gamma globulin	Infections; prophylactic alpha-globulinaemia	Varies with weight	3 years

Key: ACD = acid citrate dextrose; CPD = citrate phosphate dextrose; 2,3-DPG = 2,3-diphosphoglycerate; FFP = fresh frozen plasma; RBC = red blood cell; WBC = white blood cells

The median nerve can be damaged by attempted brachial artery cannulation by direct injury. Radial artery catheterization can stretch the median nerve from wrist dorsiflexion or compression from a haematoma after traumatic cannulation.

6.13   a) False   b) True   c) False   d) False   e) True

EXPLANATION

Factors affecting renal blood flow include:

1. *Intravascular volume.* An adequate intravascular volume is required to prevent ischaemic renal damage. An adequate intravascular volume necessitates an adequate cardiac output and rate. Although vasopressin has a mild vasoconstrictor effect on renal arterioles, it increases intravascular volume and thus renal flow by conserving fluid. Aldosterone also causes fluid retention and increases blood volume.

2. *Autoregulation.* Autoregulation means 'a relatively constant blood flow over a wide range of perfusion pressures'. It operates within a systolic blood pressure range of 70–170 mmHg; thus at a systolic pressure of 50 mmHg, renal blood flow is reduced.

3. *Sympathetic control.* Alpha action (e.g. noradrenaline, methoxamine) causes vasoconstriction and reduced blood flow. Although beta-2 action relaxes the vascular musculature, it also stimulates renin release which diminishes renal blood flow. Drugs which act on dopaminergic receptors (e.g. dopamine) increase renal flow.

4. *Hormonal factors:*

- Renin-angiotensin: released from juxtaglomerular cells mainly by baroreceptor activity and beta-2 stimulation. They reduce renal blood flow.
- Prostaglandins: released from renal medulla and increase renal blood flow. Therefore prostaglandin inhibitors such as non-steroidal anti-inflammatory analgesics reduce renal flow and can precipitate renal failure in susceptible and compromised patients.

6.14   a) True   b) True   c) False   d) True   e) True

EXPLANATION

The adult trachea is normally 10–12 cm long but in deep inspiration lengthens by 3–5 cm. The diameter of the lumen is 2–5 cm while in an infant it is about 3 mm. The right main bronchus is more vertical and shorter (4–5 cm) than the left (5 cm).

The vocal cords lie just below the notch of the thyroid cartilage (Adam's apple). The muscles of the larynx are innervated by the vagal nerve through the superior and recurrent laryngeal nerves. If one recurrent laryngeal nerve is partially damaged, the affected vocal cord lies more medially but voice is not affected. With complete paralysis, the affected vocal cord lies in the cadaveric position, and hoarseness follows. This can be treated by Teflon injection onto the affected cord to give bulk and allow it to meet the opposite cord. In bilateral partial paralysis, the cords lie together because of the unopposed action of the adductor muscles, and the patient develops stridor. Complete bilateral paralysis causes a valve-like respiratory obstruction, because the slack vocal cords flap together.

In desperate situations, acute upper airway obstruction can be treated by tracheostomy, but for an anaesthetist, a safer and simpler way is cricothyroid puncture, or cricothyrotomy. The area between the thyroid cartilage and cricoid cartilage is soft and relatively avascular and respiratory obstruction can be relieved by inserting two large-bore needles, one connected to an inflating bag and oxygen supply, while the other vents expired air to the atmosphere. An alternative is to perform a cricothyrotomy, i.e. a small transverse incision in the cricothyroid membrane, and then insert a mini-tracheostomy tube or a 6.0 plain endotracheal tube.

6.15   a) True   b) True   c) True   d) False   e) False

EXPLANATION

Pancuronium increases the heart rate and shortens all nodal conduction because of vagolysis and sympathetic stimulation.

Sodium nitroprusside is widely used to induce hypotension, because of its rapid onset and short life. It acts by peripheral vasodilatation. One of its problems is that it induces a tachycardia, possibly by vagal nerve inhibition. This can offset the fall in blood pressure; therefore nitroprusside in anaesthesia is often combined with halothane because of the latter's vagal effect.

Cocaine is unique among local anaesthetics because of its sympathomimetic actions causing tachycardia, hypertension, bronchodilatation.

Classical signs of raised intracranial pressure are headache, vomiting and papilloedema; a rise in blood pressure and bradycardia accompany the rise in intracranial pressure.

During ophthalmic operations, traction on the extraocular muscles, or pressure on the globe may provoke bradycardia, which is mediated via the vagus nerve; intravenous atropine may be required if it occurs.

6.16   a) False   b) True   c) False   d) True   e) False

EXPLANATION

Local anaesthetics deny the entrance of sodium into axons; depolarization cannot take place and the axon remains polarized and therefore insensitive. A local anaesthetic is therefore a non-depolarizing block. The Cm of a local anaesthetic is the minimum concentration of local anaesthetic that will block impulse conduction within a specified time. It is a measure of potency, and is similar to the MAC (minimum alveolar concentration) of a volatile agent. Lignocaine is less potent than bupivacaine, and therefore has a higher Cm. Nerve fibres are blocked according to thickness, i.e. the thicker the nerve fibre, the less readily it is blocked. The first fibres to be blocked are the sympathetic fibres, followed by pain, temperature and touch, and the last to be affected is motor function; because motor fibres are thickest one needs a higher concentration of local anaesthetic to achieve motor blockage. As a local anaesthetic diffuses through a nerve trunk, anaesthesia spreads along the limb in a proximal to distal direction (i.e. arm to fingers); recovery occurs first distally and last proximally.

Hypersensitivity reactions to local anaesthetics are extremely rare and virtually limited to ester-linked agents, e.g. procaine; amide-linked agents, e.g. lignocaine, bupivacaine, are virtually free of allergic reactions.

6.17   a) True   b) True   c) False   d) True   e) True

EXPLANATION

Although very rare, any spinal postoperative neurological complications must be identified as soon as possible as surgical intervention may be necessary to avoid permanent neurological damage. Epidural and spinal needles and catheters frequently (3–11%) cause vascular trauma associated with minimal bleeding which usually resolves. However, in the presence of clotting problems there is an increased risk of epidural haematomas following even minor trauma. A patient with an epidural haematoma presents with sudden sharp back and leg pain and flaccid paralysis. Sensory loss is variable and late. Several reports have indicated that inserting epidural catheters prior to heparinization in patients undergoing minor vascular surgery is safe.

Anterior spinal artery thrombosis or spasm is often associated with arteriosclerosis and hypotension and use of vasoconstrictor agents. This presents with flaccid paralysis usually without backache and little or no sensory loss. Myelogram/CT scans are very useful in the differential diagnosis of epidural haemorrhage/anterior spinal artery syndrome. With the former there are signs of extradural compression which require surgical intervention.

Chronic adhesive arachnoiditis can cause cauda equina syndrome which can have variable clinical presentations, i.e. bowel and bladder dysfunction, sensory perineal loss, variable lower extremity paresis over days or weeks. Causative factors include bacteria; cord trauma; ischaemia; contaminants and neural toxins; and direct local anaesthetic toxicity, especially if too much local anaesthetic is used.

6.18   a) True   b) False   c) True   d) False   e) False

EXPLANATION

The hypothalamus regulates body temperature and responds to changes in temperature by initiating mechanisms which conserve or lose heat (i.e. vasoconstriction and shivering or vasodilatation and sweating). Anaesthesia eliminates these compensatory mechanisms, for example muscle relaxants prevent shivering, volatile agents cause vasodilatation; therefore hypothermia will develop in an environment that is normally well tolerated.

During general anaesthesia, hypothermia follows a typical pattern; there is a marked drop in the first hour (undressed in a cool environment, skin prepared with cold solution, while anaesthesia produces vasodilatation and decreases heat production). The temperature fall decreases slowly for 2–3 hours and then becomes constant. About 10% of heat is lost via respiration even when patients are ventilated with dry cool vapours, and airway humidification can prevent most of this loss. Large surgical incisions contribute to about 50% of skin heat loss by evaporation. Forced air-convective warming is the most effective method of preventing skin heat loss. Water blankets are not so effective, but are more efficient when placed over rather than under the patient. Cutaneous heat loss can also be diminished by covering skin with cloth, paper drapes, blankets, etc.

Postoperative shivering/tremors occur in about 40% of patients recovering from general anaesthesia. Apart from being associated with heat loss it increases metabolic rate by about 200% and therefore increases oxygen consumption and can contribute significantly to postoperative hypoxaemia. The tremors can be reduced by i.v. pethidine and possibly also with doxapram.

6.19   a) True   b) True   c) False   d) False   e) True

EXPLANATION

At least 75% of the liver has to be destroyed before liver function tests become abnormal.

Liver function tests aim to provide information on:

- bile metabolism
- plasma protein synthesis
- liver enzymes.

Bile metabolism

Bilirubin is formed by the breakdown of red blood cells. It becomes attached to albumin in the plasma, and when it reaches the liver it is conjugated to glucuronic acid. It is then passed by the bile ducts into the intestine, where bacterial action converts it into stercobilinogen. This is excreted in the faeces and on exposure to air converts into stercobilin making the faeces dark brown. Some of the stercobilinogen is reabsorbed into the bloodstream and excreted in the urine as urobilin. In severe obstructive jaundice there is no bilirubin in the intestine, and therefore no stercobilin in the faeces, which are therefore pale. There is also no urobilin in the urine; however there is a very high plasma bilirubin content which makes the urine dark.

Plasma proteins

Albumin and fibrinogen are synthesized in the liver, but not globulin, so in liver failure albumin falls while globulin remains unchanged, causing alteration in the normal 2 : 1 albumin/globulin ratio. Coagulation factors and prothrombin are also produced in the liver and require vitamin K for their synthesis. Without bile in the intestine, vitamin K is not absorbed and therefore in obstructive jaundice the prothrombin level is low and thus vitamin K is indicated before surgery.

Liver enzymes

Alkaline (not acid) phosphatase is removed from the blood by the liver and excreted in the bile; thus when the liver is diseased or bile ducts blocked, (obstructive jaundice) alkaline phosphatase is raised.

Serum glutamic pyruvic transaminase (SGPT) and serum glutamic oxaloacetic transaminase (SGOT) are raised in conditions leading to liver damage.

6.20   a) True   b) True   c) True   d) True   e) False

EXPLANATION

One of the main causes of mortality in severe liver failure is the increased bleeding tendency. This is due to a number of factors:

- thrombocytopenia and impaired platelet function
- decreased production of plasma clotting factors
- increased breakdown of plasma clotting factors
- formation of abnormal coagulation products.

Preoperatively the prothrombin time should be as normal as possible. Vitamin K should be given for at least 3 days preoperatively to stimulate synthesis of liver coagulation factors. Fresh frozen plasma corrects all coagulation factor deficiencies except for low fibrinogen levels which require cryoprecipitate. Platelets are required if the platelet count is less then 50 000/ml.

Patients with liver failure have an increased cardiac output and decreased peripheral resistance. Cardiac output can reach 14 l/min; PaO_2 is usually diminished because of increased lung perfusion so the ventilation/perfusion ratio is diminished. $PaCO_2$ is typically decreased causing a respiratory alkalosis.

These patients have increased renin-angiotensin levels and therefore there is a tendency towards water and sodium retention.

Alcoholic patients with minimal liver damage have increased tolerance of anaesthetic drugs, but if liver damage is severe there is increased susceptibility to drugs. This is due to a number of factors: abnormal blood-brain barrier, increased volume of distribution, decreased hepatic blood flow and decreased metabolism of drugs.

A patient in severe liver failure requiring an operation should be brought to theatre in the best possible condition, i.e. ascites should be controlled, nutrition improved, and prothrombin time corrected, together with albumin, bilirubin and electrolytic disturbances.

7.1 A 10-year-old girl is admitted to hospital with acute appendicitis and peritonitis. General anaesthesia is induced with propofol and suxamethonium, and maintained with halothane. The anaesthetist notices rigidity in the jaw muscle making intubation impossible. Tachycardia and ventricular ectopics are also noted but the temperature is no higher than the preoperative reading. After 3 minutes, the jaw is relaxed and intubation is possible. In these circumstances:

a) The patient has malignant hyperpyrexia
b) Anaesthesia should proceed with non-trigger agents and dantrolene prophylaxis
c) Fentanyl and a propofol infusion are appropriate agents with which to maintain anaesthesia after discontinuation of the halothane if the anaesthetist decides to carry on with the operation
d) A detailed anaesthetic family history and muscle biopsy from the girl are not necessary
e) Regional anaesthesia would be safe for this girl if she needed an elective operation in future

7.2 Factors determining cardiac output include:

a) Heart rate
b) Heart rhythm
c) Contractility
d) Length of myocardial fibre
e) Ventricular afterload

7.3 Premature labour can be inhibited with the following agents:

a) Beta blockers
b) Calcium channel blockers
c) Prostaglandins
d) Alcohol
e) Magnesium sulphate

7.4 With regard to beta and calcium channel blockers:

a) Out of the current commonly used calcium channel blockers, verapamil and diltiazem have anti-arrhythmic properties, while nifedipine does not
b) In ischaemic heart disease, beta blockers have an advantage over calcium channel blockers because they improve myocardial oxygen supply
c) As with beta blockers, calcium channel blockers must be used with great caution in patients with bronchospasm and vasospastic disease
d) Both can cause myocardial depression and aggravate congestive heart failure
e) Diabetics on beta blockers usually require more insulin to control their blood sugar

7.5 **With regard to anaesthesia and cardiac disease:**

a) In cardiac tamponade heart rate is usually decreased
b) With a transplanted heart, pulse rate increases when cardiac output needs to be augmented
c) Patients with aortic stenosis are very sensitive to changes in heart rate, rhythm and preload
d) Atrial fibrillation is common with both mitral stenosis and mitral insufficiency
e) Halothane induction in a child with cyanotic heart disease (e.g. Fallot's) is ideal

7.6 **After a dural puncture:**

a) The incidence of headache is reduced by using a pencil point spinal needle
b) The incidence of headache is reduced by bed rest for 24 hours
c) Headache always develops immediately
d) Headache is relieved with caffeine
e) The development of neckache, backache and pyrexia following an epidural blood patch almost certainly indicates meningitis

7.7 **With regard to blood and blood component transfusion:**

a) In normovolaemic patients a haematocrit of at least 50% or over is required to optimize oxygen transport
b) Metabolic complications of rapid transfusion of large volumes of blood include hypocalcaemia, metabolic acidosis and hyperkalaemia
c) Platelet concentrates contain solely platelets
d) Cytomegalovirus (CMV) infection is a particularly important problem in immunosuppressed patients
e) In patients receiving large transfusions, unexpected rapid decreases in platelet count and fibrinogen suggests a diagnosis of consumption coagulopathy (disseminated intravascular coagulation (DIC))

7.8 **With regard to AIDS/hepatitis:**

a) Transmission rate with hepatitis B is twice as high as HIV after needle exposure to hepatitis B virus or AIDS virus
b) Three doses of hepatitis B vaccine protects 50% of healthy adults
c) 80% of HIV-positive patients eventually develop full-blown AIDS within 1 year
d) Patients with acute HIV infection will develop HIV antibodies within 2 weeks of contamination
e) In the UK most cases of post-transfusion hepatitis are due to hepatitis B virus

7.9 With regard to anaphylactic drug reactions:

a) The severity of cutaneous manifestations correlates well with cardiovascular changes
b) When a reaction occurs after a barbiturate and a muscle relaxant have been given intravenously in rapid sequence, it is more likely that the barbiturate is at fault
c) Tachycardia after a suspected drug allergic reaction should be treated with a beta blocker
d) The immediate treatment of choice is intravenous hydrocortisone
e) Reducing the speed of administration of a drug attenuates the effects of a possible drug reaction

7.10 Placental transfer of a local anaesthetic increases:

a) If it is highly protein bound
b) If its pK_a is high
c) If it is highly lipid soluble
d) In the presence of fetal acidosis
e) On the addition of bicarbonate

7.11 With regard to hilar and mediastinal lymphadenopathy on chest X-ray:

a) The commonest cause in the UK is tuberculosis
b) Sarcoidosis typically causes bilateral hilar lymphadenopathy
c) Mediastinal and hilar lymphadenopathy with clear lung fields in a young adult suggests a lymphoma
d) Carcinoma of the bronchus usually causes bilateral hilar and mediastinal lymphadenopathy
e) Hilar lymphadenopathy with a positive Mantoux test is diagnostic of tuberculosis

7.12 During pregnancy:

a) There is an increase in functional residual capacity
b) The oxyhaemoglobin dissociation curve is shifted to the left
c) Anaemia is usually due to a fall in red cell mass
d) There is a decrease in plasma protein, especially albumin
e) If drugs are administered, the most dangerous period for teratogenesis is between 15 and 50 days

7.13 With regard to non-depolarizing relaxants:

a) A T4/T1 ratio of greater than 0.7–0.75 is assumed to be evidence of adequate reversal
b) The action of a non-depolarizing relaxant is shortened by hypothermia
c) Histamine release is more likely to occur with atracurium than tubocurare
d) Both atracurium and vecuronium undergo spontaneous degradation through Hofmann elimination
e) Mivacurium is metabolized by pseudocholinesterase

7.14 With regard to perioperative electrocardiography:

a) The detection of a Mobitz type II heart block in a preoperative electrocardiogram (ECG) contraindicates elective surgery
b) A perioperative ECG showing significant ST depression or elevation indicates probable myocardial ischaemia
c) Occasional premature ventricular contractions on an intraoperative ECG need urgent treatment
d) Wolff–Parkinson–White syndrome discovered on a perioperative ECG does not warrant any treatment
e) The presence of right or left bundle branch block indicates serious organic heart disease

7.15 With regard to hepatitis:

a) Compared to the short incubation period with hepatitis A, the incubation period for hepatitis B is long (1–5 months)
b) A person punctured by an infected hepatitis B needle should have both active and passive immunization
c) Active hepatitis B immunization normally provides protection for 2 years
d) Whereas hepatitis B can lead to a carrier state, patients infected with hepatitis A or C do not become carriers
e) Spread of hepatitis B virus is by the faecal or intravenous route

7.16 With regard to postoperative nausea and vomiting:

a) Ondansetron reduces nausea and vomiting by acting on 5-HT (5-hydroxytryptamine) receptor antagonists
b) Phenothiazines (e.g. prochlorperazine) and butyrophenones (e.g. droperidol) have antiemetic properties resulting primarily from antidopaminergic actions
c) Metoclopramide and cyclizine have primarily anticholinergic actions
d) It is more common in females than males and more common in intra-abdominal compared to abdominal wall surgery
e) Propofol causes more postoperative nausea and vomiting than thiopentone

7.17 An obese chronic smoker with a long history of chronic obstructive airways disease presents in casualty. He is cyanosed and breathless. An arterial blood gas obtained breathing air shows PaO_2 = 34 mmHg (4.5 kPa); $PaCO_2$ = 72 mmHg (9.5 kPa); pH = 7.35; HCO_3 = 35.8 mmol/l. After breathing oxygen for 3–4 hours he appears pink, less breathless and very drowsy. At that time PaO_2 = 470 mmHg (62 kPa); $PaCO_2$ = 82 mmHg (10.8 kPa); pH = 7.30; HCO_3 = 39 mmol/l. This information shows that:

a) He is getting the appropriate treatment
b) Assuming respiratory quotient (R) is 1, the alveolar-arterial oxygen tension difference when the patient was breathing air is 14 mmHg
c) The acid-base derangement while breathing air is a chronic respiratory acidosis with almost fully compensated metabolic alkalosis
d) FEV_1/FVC figures of 2.5 litre/3.0 litre are compatible with the clinical picture
e) His blood pressure and pulse were likely to be high throughout the 3–4 hours of treatment

7.18 **With regard to neurological disease:**

a) If a patient with Parkinson's disease on large doses of L-dopa presents for general anaesthesia, halothane should be avoided
b) Patients who present for a general anaesthetic within 6 weeks of a spinal injury are at risk of massive potassium release with the use of suxamethonium
c) Patients with myasthenia gravis are sensitive to suxamethonium and resistant to non-depolarizing relaxants
d) Patients with muscular dystrophy have a high incidence of cardiac arrhythmias when given a general anaesthetic
e) Thiopentone is the ideal induction agent in a patient with porphyria

7.19 **Of the agents used to induce hypotension:**

a) Trimetaphan reduces blood pressure by its direct vasodilator effects on capacitance and resistance vessels
b) Sodium nitroprusside acts by reducing the cardiac output
c) Nitroglycerine causes hypotension by directly dilating the capacitance vessels
d) Labetalol reduces blood pressure by peripheral vasodilatation and negative inotropic and chronotropic effect
e) Halothane, enflurane and isoflurane hypotension is due to varying degrees of myocardial and peripheral vascular depression

7.20 **With regard to tissue oxygenation:**

a) The quantity of oxygen transported to tissues (available oxygen) is approximately 1000 ml/min
b) Arterial hypoxaemia dilates the cerebral vessels
c) In one-lung anaesthesia, the hypoxia in the atelectatic lung dilates the pulmonary vessels in that lung
d) A decline in arterial PO_2 to 76 mmHg (10 kPa) produces markedly increased ventilation
e) Postoperative hypoxaemia occurs after all operations under general anaesthesia but not after regional techniques

7.1   a) False   b) True   c) True   d) False   e) True

EXPLANATION
This patient has masseter muscle rigidity (MMR) but not malignant hyperpyrexia as such. It is, however, possible though not proven conclusively that MMR may precede malignant hyperpyrexia. MMR is more common in children and much more common than malignant hyperpyrexia. It is said to have a 1% incidence in children when halothane and suxamethonium are used. It is not accompanied by hyperpyrexia but an elevated creatinine phosphokinase and myoglobinuria are common with masseter muscle rigidity. If one encounters this problem, it is advisable to treat it as malignant hyperpyrexia; therefore if the operation is elective, anaesthesia should be terminated. However, in an emergency situation (as with this case) the operation should proceed with dantrolene prophylaxis (1–2 mg/kg) and all triggering agents avoided. Suxamethonium, isoflurane, halothane, enflurane and desflurane are all unsafe; while local anaesthetics, barbiturates, propofol, ketamine, benzodiazapines, narcotics, vecuronium, pancuronium, atracurium, and probably nitrous oxide are safe. With this case, a detailed family history should be obtained and the girl should be subjected to a muscle biopsy. At present the only diagnostic test for malignant hyperpyrexia is the halothane-caffeine contracture test where 1–2 g of muscle is tested for a contracture response to halothane and caffeine. Patients with malignant hyperpyrexia will display a contracture to halothane and a left-shifted dose response to caffeine; 50% of patients with masseter muscle rigidity give a positive halothane-caffeine contracture test. It is possible that masseter muscle rigidity is merely an exaggerated response to suxamethonium, i.e. suxamethonium regularly causes a subclinical transient increase in jaw muscle tone; in MMR this response is increased to obvious jaw rigidity.

7.2   a) True   b) True   c) True   d) True   e) True

EXPLANATION
Heart rate. Cardiac output equals stroke volume times heart rate, and factors which reduce heart rate, e.g. mitral stenosis, severe heart failure, reduce cardiac output. A severe tachycardia (over 180 beats/min) also reduces cardiac output by limiting diastolic filling time and thus reducing ventricular preload.

Rhythm. Rhythm disturbances again reduce ventricular preload and thus cardiac output.

Contractility and preload. Increases in myocardial fibre length (preload) cause a linear increase in myocardial work (i.e. contractility – Starling's Law). Normally, increases in preload (e.g. exercise, thyrotoxicosis) increase cardiac work and cardiac output and possibly blood pressure (depending on peripheral resistance). Common causes of diminished preload encountered by the anaesthetist include hypovolaemia, venodilatation, cardiac tamponade and right ventricular failure, and all these factors reduce cardiac output. Contractility itself is diminished by anaesthetic drugs, ischaemia, bradycardia and tachycardia, dysrhythmias; again all these factors can reduce cardiac output.

Ventricular afterload (i.e. peripheral resistance). The variables in peripheral resistance are vascular tone and blood viscosity (this determined principally by temperature and haematocrit). Common anaesthetic factors which increase afterload and thus reduce cardiac output include light anaesthesia, hypertension and pulmonary emboli.

Therapy to improve cardiac output
- Increase heart rate: anticholinergic; beta sympathomimetic; pacemaker
- Reduce heart rate: vagal stimulating drug; beta blocker
- Eliminate dysrhythmias: correct cause, e.g. low or high K^+, high Mg, ischaemia; antiarrhythmic drugs; pacemaker
- Increase contractility: eliminate cardiac depressant anaesthetics; relieve ischaemia; inotropic drugs; cardiopulmonary bypass
- Increase preload: position patient to increase venous return; infuse fluids/blood; relieve tamponade; augment right ventricular output by increasing central venous pressure, reducing peripheral vascular resistance or using an inotrope
- Decrease afterload: with a vasodilator, intra-aortic balloon pump; or increase peripheral resistance by eliminating vasodilating factors, using vasoconstrictors and correcting anaemia.

7.3   a) False   b) True   c) False   d) True   e) True

EXPLANATION
Methods to suppress labour are becoming less common because nowadays premature infants have such a low morbidity that the risks associated with suppression of labour are often not justified. The most commonly used agents for labour suppression are:

1. *Ethanol.* Alcohol acts mainly by inhibiting oxytocin release from the posterior pituitary, though other mechanisms such as myometrium depression and prostaglandins inhibition also apply. It is given as a 10% solution in dextrose and should be given for short-term use as its maternal side-effects are very unpleasant, i.e. intoxication, sedation, hyperacidity, vomiting, hypoglycaemia, metabolic acidosis. Moreover, if the mother requires an anaesthetic, there are the anaesthetic problems of intoxication, hyperacidity and electrolytic imbalances. Alcohol also affects the fetus, causing depression, acidosis and hypoglycaemia. For all these reasons alcohol is not used any longer for suppression of labour.

2. *Beta-adrenergic agents.* Agents with predominantly beta-2 actions (myometrial inhibition, vaso- and bronchodilatation) are widely used for inhibition of premature labour. These agents are initially given parenterally and if successful, oral therapy is continued until required. Complications are due to beta actions, i.e. hypotension from vasodilatation, tachycardia, anxiety, restlessness, hyperglycaemia and hypokalaemia.

3. *Magnesium sulphate.* This is one of the safest ways of suppressing labour. It acts as a membrane stabilizer resulting in myometrial depression. Magnesium causes some vasodilatation and mild hypotension and, with prolonged administration, CNS depression in both mother and fetus. If the mother is having a general anaesthetic, it must be remembered that magnesium potentiates both depolarizing and non-depolarizing muscle relaxants.

4. *Prostaglandins inhibitors.* Awareness of the role of prostaglandins in initiation of labour has led to the possibility of using inhibitors (e.g. aspirin) to inhibit labour.

147

However, these agents have not been used clinically because of risks of premature closure of the ductus arteriosus.

    5. *Calcium blockers*. These agents are also myometrial inhibitors and the calcium blocker most investigated is nifedipine. Calcium blockers can cause cardiovascular depression and potentiation of muscle relaxants.

7.4   a) True   b) False   c) False   d) True   e) False

EXPLANATION
See Table 7.1.

Table 7.1   Comparisons and differences between beta and calcium channel blockers

	Beta blockers	Calcium channel blockers
Mode of action	1. Act on beta-1 receptors to reduce cardiac rate and contraction 2. Block beta-2 receptors to cause vascular, bronchial and uterine smooth muscle contraction. Also block beta-mediated glycogenolysis in muscle and liver causing hypoglycaemia	Interfere with the inward flow of calcium ions through cell membranes affecting mainly myocardial and nodal cells, and cells of vascular smooth muscle
Main uses	Ischaemic heart disease; arrhythmias; hypertension	Ischaemic heart disease; cardiac arrhythmias; hypertension. Increase coronary flow and improve myocardial oxygen supply; so may be more useful than beta blockers in ischaemic heart disease
Other uses	Obstructive cardiomyopathies; thyrotoxicosis; phaeochromocytoma; tremors; anxiety; headaches	Because of vasodilatation have been used in pulmonary hypertension and eclampsia (especially nifedipine); bronchospasm; to treat premature labour
Side-effects	CVS depression especially in patients with congestive heart failure; bradycardia; bronchospasm; hypoglycaemia in diabetics	Cardiovascular depression especially in patients with congestive heart failure; A–V block

7.5   a) False   b) False   c) True   d) True   e) False

EXPLANATION

Patients with cardiac tamponade (e.g. trauma, metabolic disorders) attempt to improve cardiac output by increasing the pulse rate and when anaesthetizing such a patient one should be careful not to induce a bradycardia as this will aggravate the cardiogenic shock.

A transplanted heart lacks sympathetic and parasympathetic innervation. Therefore a patient with a heart transplant cannot adjust heart rate to augment cardiac output and relies on circulating catecholamines and appropriate preload and afterload to maintain cardiac output. These (i.e. preload, afterload and possibly inotropes) are the factors which should be monitored carefully to maintain adequate cardiac output when anaesthetizing such a patient.

Patients with aortic stenosis have an enlarged left ventricle which is extremely vulnerable to ischaemia because of increased myocardial work and oxygen consumption. Maintenance of preload and avoidance of tachycardia, bradycardia and rhythm changes are essential to keep an adequate cardiac output.

Patients with both mitral stenosis and mitral insufficiency often have atrial fibrillation and careful digitalization is required before a general anaesthetic.

Children with cyanotic heart disease (e.g. Fallot's transposition of the great vessels, ventricular septal defect with pulmonary stenosis) have too little blood flowing to the pulmonary artery, and are therefore hypoxaemic. They usually have a left-to-right shunt and it is vitally important to avoid factors which increase pressure on the right side of the heart causing a right-to-left shunt with worsening hypoxaemia and cyanosis. Such factors include increased pulmonary resistance due to straining, crying, etc. or decreased systemic vascular resistance, e.g. caused by halothane.

7.6   a) True   b) False   c) False   d) True   e) False

EXPLANATION

Post-dural puncture headache is the most frequent complication of spinal anaesthesia. It may occur several hours after the puncture but nearly always within 2–3 days. The incidence depends on the size of the cerebrospinal fluid (CSF) leak and therefore on the size of the spinal needle. The incidence after inadvertent puncture during epidural analgesia is 33–40%. The incidence is reduced by using finer spinal needles and using a pencil point needle. Bed rest does not reduce the incidence but once it occurs bed rest relieves the symptoms. The headache is made worse by factors which increase the leak, e.g. coughing, head movements. The symptoms (i.e. pain in the neck, occiput and shoulder areas) are also improved by caffeine sodium benzoate (500 mg i.v.). Caffeine may act by cerebral vasoconstriction and reduced cerebral blood flow, or because of increased CSF production. An epidural blood patch is the most effective method to relieve the headache and the mechanism of action is twofold, i.e. transiently increasing the subarachnoid pressure and sealing the puncture by forming a fibrous plug. Following an epidural blood patch there is a 35% incidence of backache, pyrexia (5%) or neck pain (1%) which may last 24–48 hours.

7.7   **a) False**   **b) True**   **c) False**   **d) True**   **e) True**

EXPLANATION

If normovolaemia is maintained with crystalloids or colloids, healthy individuals can tolerate haematocrits of 20% or less. With normovolaemia, oxygen transport is optimal at haematocrit levels near 30% because oxygen transport improves with decreasing blood viscosity.

Complications following transfusion of large volumes of blood include hypocalcaemia and metabolic acidosis. Hypocalcaemia is due to calcium binding to citrate, and can lead to cardiovascular depression, and hyperkalaemia. Stored blood has a K^+ content of about 20 mEq/litre at 30 days and hyperkalaemia is then a real possibility.

Cytomegalovirus infection is a particular post-transfusion problem in blood recipients who are immunocompromised, such as transplant patients, patients on immunosuppressant drugs, neonates and splenectomized patients.

If a patient is receiving massive transfusions and unexpected falls in platelets and fibrinogen (below 100 mg/100 ml) occur, it is likely that DIC has set in. In these cases fresh frozen plasma is indicated.

It appears that patients receiving over 15 units of red blood cells without whole blood will require platelets and about 50% of these will also require fresh frozen plasma (FFP). Platelet concentrates contain significant amounts of FFP, i.e. about four units of platelet concentrate is equivalent to one unit of FFP somewhat lacking in factors V and VIII.

7.8   **a) False**   **b) False**   **c) False**   **d) False**   **e) False**

EXPLANATION

Following an HIV contamination injury the risk of developing AIDS is about 0.3–0.5%; with hepatitis B, however, the risk is considerably higher – about 30%. Patients with acute HIV infection may carry the virus for several weeks before developing antibodies; therefore a patient who is tested as HIV-negative may still be infectious. Eventually, 50% of patients develop symptoms of AIDS within 1 year; 80% within 3 years.

Hepatitis B has an incubation period of 2–6 months. Initially it was thought that it could only be contracted via the parenteral route; however, it is also possible to become infected after eye splashing or ingestion of infected material. Individuals presenting an increased risk include drug addicts, haemophiliacs, homosexuals, renal patients, tattooed patients, and patients with a recent history of jaundice. Having contracted hepatitis B, the majority recover normally, and are antigen free after about 4 weeks; a few develop chronic liver disease and possibly hepatic carcinoma, while others become chronic carriers of the hepatitis B antigen. Carriers may have a low infectivity; some, however, are highly contagious. Anyone who accidentally suffers a needle-stick injury from an infected patient should be screened immediately. If there is evidence of immunity, nothing further is necessary; if not, passive immunization is required within 24–48 hours, and after 4 weeks. Active immunization can be administered at the same time.

In order to prevent contracting hepatitis B, all anaesthetists should be vaccinated. The vaccination involves three i.m. injections, following which 95% of healthy adults develop antibodies. The antibody status should be assessed 6 weeks after the third dose to ensure immunity, absence of which necessitates a booster vaccine.

In most developed countries donor blood is routinely screened for hepatitis B surface antigen. It is also screened for alanine aminotransferase (ALT), an antibody to hepatitis core antigen, to detect non-A, non-B hepatitis. Because these latter two tests are not specific, over 90% of post-transfusion hepatitis is non-A, non-B and in most cases is hepatitis C. In many countries, donor blood is now screened for hepatitis C antibody. At present there is no vaccine for hepatitis C.

7.9   a) False   b) False   c) False   d) False   e) True

EXPLANATION
Cutaneous manifestations frequently occur as a result of histamine release, or from other causes, without causing cardiovascular changes.

When a reaction occurs after rapid administration of a barbiturate and a relaxant, it is seven times as likely to be caused by the relaxant. Allergic reactions to barbiturates occur but are very rare. When they occur they are usually very severe, possibly because the compensatory mechanisms of increased cardiac output are hampered by the depressant effects of barbiturates.

Histamine has a short half-life and its effects last up to 5–10 minutes. Giving a drug over several half-lives of histamine in incremental doses rather than by an immediate bolus can significantly attenuate the effects.

The immediate treatment of choice in a severe reaction is adrenaline (0.2–0.4 mg in an adult). Hydrocortisone takes about 6–8 hours to exert its maximum effect.

Histamine causes an inotropic and chronotropic effect on the heart and a tachycardia may occur. The fall in blood pressure after an allergic reaction is due to massive vasodilatation. Histamine is also a potent releaser of adrenaline and noradrenaline and if beta blockers are given to reduce the tachycardia, beneficial effects of adrenaline are counteracted. This is one of the few cases where a severe tachycardia mandates the use of adrenaline.

7.10   a) False   b) False   c) True   d) False   e) True

EXPLANATION
The transfer of drugs across cell membranes is determined by:

- lipid solubility
- protein binding
- pK_a.

Membranes contain lipoprotein, and local anaesthetics with high lipid solubility pass through them easily. Local anaesthetics with high protein-binding capacity will stay in protein receptors for a longer time. pK_a is defined as the pH at which 50% of the local anaesthetic remains in the uncharged form, 50% in the charged form. Agents closest to the body's pH (7.4) will cross membranes more easily as there is a higher uncharged proportion. Lignocaine has a pK_a of 7.7, so at a pH of 7.4, 35% of

151

this agent is uncharged and crosses the placenta easily. Bupivacaine with a pK$_a$ of 8.1 will only have 15% in the uncharged form at a pH of 7.4, and this takes longer to cross. In the presence of fetal acidosis, the local anaesthetic will transform into the charged form and will not be able to cross the placenta and accumulate in the fetus (ion-trapping phenomenon).

Local anaesthetics are supplied at a low pH to prolong the shelf life. Addition of bicarbonate increases the pH. Increasing the pH increases the proportion of uncharged form which facilitates placental transfer.

7.11   **a) False**   **b) True**   **c) True**   **d) False**   **e) False**

EXPLANATION
The commonest causes of hilar and mediastinal lymphadenopathy are tuberculosis (which, although increasing in incidence, is not the commonest cause in the UK), sarcoidosis, lymphoma and carcinoma of the bronchus. The clinical features helpful in differential diagnosis are given in Table 7.2.

7.12   **a) False**   **b) False**   **c) False**   **d) True**   **e) True**

EXPLANATION
The functional residual (FRC) capacity decreases by 20% during pregnancy. This is

Table 7.2   Clinical features helpful in the differential diagnosis of tuberculosis, sarcoid, lymphoma and carcinoma of the lung

	Tuberculosis (TB)	Sarcoid	Lymphoma	Carcinoma of the lung
Age	Any	20–30	20–30	50+
Hilar lymphadenopathy – one or both	One	Both	Both	One
Mediastinal	+	+	+	+
Pressure symptoms (e.g. superior vena cava obstruction, recurrent and phrenic nerve palsies)	–	–	+	+
Fever	+	–	+	+
Weight loss	+	+ or –	+	++
Finger clubbing	–	–	–	+
Lung fields infiltrated	+ or –	+	+ or –	Mass lesion
Kveim test	–	+ (75%)	–	–
Mantoux test	++	–	+ or –	+ or –
Response to anti-TB drugs	+	–	–	–
Alveolitis (pulmonary involvement)	–	+	–	–

important because at times the FRC is less than the closing capacity, so the terminal airways close and alveoli are perfused but not ventilated; deoxygenated blood is shunted causing arterial hypoxemia.

Because cardiac output increases, the oxyhaemoglobin curve is shifted to the right facilitating oxygen unloading to the fetus.

Blood volume increases but the plasma volume increase is greater than the increase in red cell mass so a dilutional anaemia occurs especially in the second trimester and iron and folic acid are required to restore haemoglobin levels.

Plasma protein decreases, especially albumin; therefore the albumin/globulin ratio decreases. This is clinically important in that drugs that are highly protein bound (e.g. bupivacaine) are released into the blood more readily; therefore pregnant women having epidurals need relatively less bupivacaine.

Most organs develop between 15 and 50 days and it is the period when drugs are most likely to cause congenital abnormalities. Organ development and maximum sensitivity are as follows:

Brain	18–38 days
Heart	18–40 days
Eyes	24–40 days
Limbs	24–36 days
Gonads	37–50 days
Male genitalia	45–70 days
Female genitalia	40–50 days.

Teratogenic drugs

- ACE inhibitors – skull defects.
- Alcohol, hallucinogens (e.g. LSD) – fetal alcoholic syndrome: CNS growth dysfunction; craniofacial, cardiac, liver and renal abnormalities.
- Androgens and anabolic steroids – masculinization of female fetus.
- Antiepileptics – carbamazepine, valproic acid and other antiepileptics – neural tube defects.
- Antithyroid drugs – thyroid abnormalities; aplasia cutis in the neonate.
- Cytotoxic drugs – craniofacial and other congenital anomalies; growth retardation.
- Cocaine – abortions; premature labour; congenital abnormalities.
- Coumarin anticoagulants – fetal abnormalities especially bony; fetal death.
- Diethylstilboestrol – vaginal carcinomas; urogenital abnormalities.
- Isotretinoin; vitamin A derivatives used for acne, psoriasis, etc. – congenital anomalies.
- Lead.
- Lithium – congenital malformations; fetal goitre.
- Mercury.
- Streptomycin and other aminoglycosides but mostly with streptomycin – auditory or vestibular nerve damage.
- Thalidiomide – limb abnormalities from limb absence to anomalies of thumbs or toes; depressed nose; ocular and facial palsies; spinal abnormalities; congenital heart problems; absent ears, small ears with deafness; bowel, urological and gynaecological defects.

7.13   a) True   b) False   c) False   d) False   e) True

EXPLANATION

A classic method of monitoring the degree of neuromuscular blockade is to observe the train of four, utilizing four consecutive stimulations at a frequency of 2 Hz and comparing the fourth twitch with the first. A T4/T1 ratio greater than 0.7–0.75 indicates adequate reversal.

The action of non-depolarizing relaxants is prolonged by a number of factors including hypothermia, respiratory acidosis, metabolic alkalosis, electrolyte abnormalities, inhalational agents such as isoflurane and some antibiotics.

Out of the non-depolarizing relaxants, tubocurare causes most histamine release followed by slight histamine release with atracurium (and suxamethonium) and virtually none with vecuronium, pancuronium, mivacurium or gallamine.

Atracurium undergoes spontaneous degradation through Hofmann elimination which is pH and temperature dependent. This accounts for 50% of elimination. The rest is probably eliminated by liver and/or kidney; however, the duration of action is not prolonged in renal failure. 50% of vecuronium is eliminated in the bile and 15% in the kidney; its duration is not altered significantly in liver and renal disease.

Mivacurium is a new non-depolarizer introduced in early 1992. It is short acting, lasts about 20 minutes and is hydrolyzed by plasma cholinesterase. Reversal agents are not usually required.

7.14   a) True   b) True   c) False   d) False   e) False

EXPLANATION

Mobitz (Wenckebach) type I heart block is a progressive prolongation of PR followed by a dropped P wave. With this type of block the heart recovers readily, but Mobitz type II is much more serious. A series of P waves are not conducted and such a patient can very quickly develop asystole; elective cases should thus have their surgery postponed. If emergency surgery is required, cardiac pacing should be available.

Newly appearing depressed ST segment (more than 1 mm) indicates significant myocardial ischaemia; new ST elevation greater than 1 mm indicates severe ischaemia, even if the patient has no cardiac pain (silent myocardial ischaemia). This is often found in diabetic patients.

Wolff-Parkinson-White syndrome (short PR with slurred QRS and ST and T abnormalities) is due to aberrant conduction via intra-atrial pathways. It is important to recognize, because it can predispose to serious supraventricular tachyarrhythmias during general anaesthesia. Procainamide is very useful in treating these tachyarrhythmias.

Right bundle branch block can be found in completely normal hearts. Left bundle branch block is almost always associated with serious organic heart disease and is usually indicative of severe ischaemia.

7.15   a) True   b) True   c) False   d) False   e) False

EXPLANATION

The incubation period of hepatitis A is about 2–3 weeks; hepatitis B 1–5 months; hepatitis C in between. The active immunization with hepatitis B vaccine requires 3 (0, 1, 6 months) or 4 (0, 1, 6, 12 months) injections and provides protection for about 5 years in over 90% of people. If a person is punctured by an infected needle, an immediate injection of immune serum globulin should be given (passive immunization) plus hepatitis vaccine (active immunization). Hepatitis B virus is spread by the intravenous route, e.g. blood transfusion, contaminated needles, sexual intercourse. The virus can also be found in semen and saliva and one of the most common forms of transmission is from mother to child during pregnancy. Hepatitis A is usually transmitted through the faecal route. Following infection with hepatitis B, about 5–10% of patients will become carriers and most of them never develop antibodies and remain carriers; they have an increased risk of developing chronic hepatitis and cirrhosis and hepatic carcinoma. Hepatitis A infection does not cause a carrier state. Hepatitis C is responsible for the majority of post-transfusion hepatitis in all countries where blood is tested for hepatitis B and in many countries blood donors are now screened for hepatitis C. A carrier state can occur with hepatitis C and a hepatitis C vaccine has recently been developed.

7.16   a) True   b) True   c) False   d) True   e) False

EXPLANATION

Drugs cause vomiting by acting directly on the vomiting centre (area postrema in the lower part of the fourth ventricle); their effects are either central or peripheral. Drugs such as opiates and general anaesthetics cause vomiting primarily by central effects. Peripheral factors, such as mechanical distension of the gut, irritants and toxins, stimulate gut receptors, which transmit signals to the vomiting centre by the vagus nerve. Antiemetics act by a number of mechanisms:

- Antidopaminergic actions (e.g. metoclopramide, domperidone, phenothiazines such as prochlorperazine, butyrophenones such as droperidol). These antiemetics can cause extrapyramidal side-effects.
- Anticholinergic (antimuscarinic) actions (e.g. hyoscine and atropine). Antihistamines such as cyclizine also reduce vomiting by anticholinergic (atropine-like) actions. Anticholinergic drugs cause their antiemetic action by a central effect.
- 5-HT receptor antagonists (e.g. ondansetron). Metoclopramide also has this action. Pure 5-HT receptor antagonists do not cause any of the side-effects caused by the other groups, i.e. extrapyramidal symptoms, or the atropine effects – sedation, dryness, urinary retention – caused by the anticholinergic antiemetics.

Postoperative nausea and vomiting occur in about 25% of patients, are two to three times more common in females and more common in adults than in infants.

The following factors increase the incidence of nausea and vomiting: delayed gastric emptying; anxiety; intra-abdominal surgery (probably due to vagal stimulation); adenotonsillectomy (blood in stomach); eye surgery especially squint; gynaecological operations; mask ventilation (air in stomach); gastric suction;

postoperative fluids or food given too early; analgesics (especially opioids, buprenorphine); induction agents – most with methohexitone, etomidate; less with thiopentone; least with propofol; anaesthetic vapours/gases especially cyclopropane/ether, much less with modern agents; spinal anaesthesia especially with a high block and hypotension, presence of postoperative pain.

7.17   **a) False**   **b) False**   **c) True**   **d) False**   **e) True**

EXPLANATION

When this gentleman was given oxygen it improved the PaO_2 but not the hypercapnia and respiratory acidosis, which indicates the original presence of a hypoxic drive to ventilation. He is therefore having too much oxygen and careful titration of inspired PO_2 is required.

The normal alveolar-arterial oxygen difference breathing air is 5–25 mmHg, depending on age as PaO_2 falls with age. In a healthy adult, $P_AO_2 = 101$ mmHg and $PaO_2 = 95$ mmHg, giving an alveolar-arterial oxygen difference of 6 mmHg. Any ventilation/perfusion imbalance is best measured by calculating the $P_AO_2 - PaO_2$ difference which is done as follows:

$P_AO_2 = (\% \ FiO_2 \times 713 \ \text{mmHg}) - PaCO_2$ (NB: 713 mmHg = normal air pressure minus water vapour pressure, i.e. $760 - 47 = 713$ mmHg). When this gentleman was breathing air, $P_AO_2 = (0.21 \times 713) - 72$, i.e. 77 mmHg; $PaO_2 = 34$ so the $P_AO_2 - PaO_2$ difference is $77 - 34 = 43$ mmHg. In other words this gentleman has significant venous admixture due to hypoventilation.

On breathing air he has a respiratory acidosis (high $PaCO_2$) which is compensated by a metabolic alkalosis (high bicarbonate) bringing the pH to near normal levels.

His FEV_1/FVC figures should show an obstruction pattern, i.e. FEV_1/FVC percentage would be less than the normal 75%, which it is not with these suggested values.

Hypercapnia causes drowsiness and sympathetic stimulation, so the gentleman is likely to be sweaty and show a tachycardia and a high blood pressure.

7.18   **a) True**   **b) True**   **c) False**   **d) True**   **e) False**

EXPLANATION

Parkinson patients do not usually present anaesthetic problems; however, since Parkinson's disease is associated with dopamine deficiency, they are often on large doses of dopamine and the combination of dopamine and halothane can cause arrhythmias, so halothane is best avoided in such patients. Butyrophenone drugs (e.g. droperidol) antagonize the action of dopamine and should also be avoided.

For the first 6 weeks after a spinal injury there is an exaggerated potassium release with the use of suxamethonium, enough to cause arrhythmias or even cardiac arrest. This is not prevented by pretreatment with non-depolarizing muscle relaxants.

Myasthenia gravis is thought to be an autoimmune disease resulting in destruction of acetylcholine receptors. Anticholinesterase drugs can provide symptomatic relief but excess use can cause a cholinergic crisis. These patients are usually resistant to depolarizing agents and sensitive to non-depolarizers. If a relaxant is required, a small (about one-third normal) dose of atracurium is the drug of choice because it is broken down spontaneously by Hofmann degradation.

Muscular dystrophy is characterized by atrophy of a number of muscles including cardiac and respiratory muscles. There is therefore a high incidence of arrhythmias; suxamethonium causes greater K^+ release than normal, while there is increased sensitivity to non-depolarizing agents. Patients with motor neuron disease are also unduly sensitive to depolarizing and non-depolarizing drugs.

Porphyria is due to a defect in porphyrin metabolism and an excess production of porphyrin precursors; barbiturates are contraindicated because they may exacerbate the disease.

7.19   a) False   b) False   c) True   d) True   e) True

EXPLANATION

The agents mentioned in the question are the ones most commonly used to achieve controlled hypotension during anaesthesia. Halothane, isoflurane and enflurane depress the myocardium and cause peripheral vasodilatation, halothane and isoflurane more so than enflurane. The fall in blood pressure (BP) is more profound if the inspired concentration of these volatile agents is increased.

Trimetaphan is a short-acting ganglion blocker which blocks both the parasympathetic and sympathetic systems. The latter effect results in resistance and capacitance vessel relaxation and a reduction in BP. Since the parasympathetic system is blocked more than the sympathetic system, tachycardia usually follows which offsets the drop in BP. Combining trimetaphan with halothane reduces the tachycardia.

Sodium nitroprusside is one of the most commonly used agents because of its short half-life and maintenance of organ blood flow and oxygen supply even at systolic pressures of 40 mmHg. Nitroprusside dilates peripheral vessels, especially veins, and does not affect cardiac output. As with trimetaphan, rebound tachycardia can occur together with cyanide intoxication if large doses are administered.

Labetalol is an alpha and beta blocker and causes vasodilatation by alpha blockade and a decrease in cardiac output and heart rate by beta blockade.

Nitroglycerine (glyceryl trinitrate) directly dilates capacitance vessels, has a short half-life and no toxic metabolites, and is therefore another popular hypotensive agent in anaesthesia and intensive care.

7.20   a) True   b) True   c) False   d) False   e) False

EXPLANATION

Available oxygen is 1000 ml/min which is dependent upon cardiac output, haemoglobin and saturation. Because oxygen consumption is only 250 ml/min, the available oxygen is four times the amount needed; therefore if oxygen saturation drops to 40% the oxygen available is 400 ml/min, but if this is associated with marked anaemia the necessary 250 ml will not be reached.

A low PaO_2 dilates the cerebral vessels in an effort to maintain normal flow and brain oxygenation. The dilatation is in response to the accumulation of vasodilator metabolites which appear with hypoxia, i.e. kinins, lactic acid, histamine, etc. In one-lung anaesthesia, however, hypoxia constricts the pulmonary vessels. The collapsed lung is not being ventilated and, if the pulmonary vessels remain dilated, there will be considerable shunting; therefore by constricting the pulmonary vessels the blood is diverted to the ventilated lung.

Marked stimulation of respiration by hypoxia only occurs when the PO_2 is less than 60 mmHg. This stimulation is achieved by increased discharge in the carotid and aortic chemoreceptors. A number of chronic bronchitics have a hypoxic drive to ventilation, and increasing their FiO_2 may improve oxygenation but may reduce ventilation to cause hypercapnia.

Postoperative hypoxaemia occurs after all operations, especially thoracic and upper abdominal procedures, and occurs even after regional techniques. It is more marked in the aged and after prolonged operations and it can last for 24 hours or more. Immediate postoperative hypoxia may be due to diffusion hypoxia as a result of expired nitrous oxide diluting the alveolar O_2; hypoventilation due to anaesthetic drugs, restlessness and shivering which increases oxygen consumption. Delayed hypoxaemia is due to ventilation/perfusion mismatching which occurs during anaesthesia.

8.1 **With regard to renal protection during anaesthesia:**

a) Oliguria can be defined as a urine flow less than 0.5 ml/kg/hour
b) In the absence of hypovolaemia loop diuretics such as frusemide are useful in treating oliguria and improving renal function
c) Mannitol reduces the risk of renal damage in abdominal aortic surgery
d) Nephrotoxicity with use of fluorinated anaesthetics increases in the following sequence: enflurane < isoflurane < methoxyflurane
e) The non-depolarizing relaxants least dependent on renal function for elimination follow this sequence: gallamine < pancuronium < tubocurare < vecuronium < atracurium

8.2 **In aortic regurgitation:**

a) Arrhythmias especially atrial fibrillation are a common presentation
b) There is a loud systolic murmur, best heard at the lower left sternal margin or cardiac apex
c) Collapsing pulse is a typical sign
d) Electro- and echocardiography show an enlarged left ventricle in severe cases
e) Aortic valve replacement is indicated when symptoms become severe

8.3 **With regard to vaporizers:**

a) If a patient is breathing spontaneously through a closed circuit with the vaporizer within the circle (VIC), manual ventilation on the rebreathing bag reduces the inspired concentration of the vapour
b) The carrier gases to a copper kettle vaporizer originate from the two flow meters, usually oxygen and nitrous oxide, on the anaesthetic machine
c) Halothane or isoflurane can be used with a simple Boyle's vaporizer
d) A Fluotec Mark III vaporizer can be incorporated within the circuit through which the patient is breathing
e) If two or more vaporizers are used in series on an anaesthetic machine, their sequence is unimportant

8.4 **With regard to regional blocks:**

a) The 3 in 1 block for the lower limb aims to block the lateral cutaneous nerve of thigh, the femoral nerve and the obturator nerve
b) Infiltration of local anaesthetic and adrenaline at the base of the penis is a good technique to use to provide analgesia following a circumcision
c) Axillary nerve block is a suitable block for operation on the upper arm
d) The ilioinguinal and iliohypogastric nerves arise from L1
e) Intercostal blocks block both somatic and sympathetic nerve pathways

8.5 **Complications of right-sided subclavian vein cannulation include:**

a) Injury to thoracic duct
b) Pneumothorax
c) Dysrhythmias
d) Chylothorax
e) Haemothorax

8.6 **With regard to carbon dioxide carriage in the blood:**

a) 55% is as bicarbonate
b) Carbonic anhydrase is contained in red cells and plasma
c) The amount carried as carbamino compounds depends on $PaCO_2$
d) The amount dissolved depends on PaO_2
e) As bicarbonate is transferred from red cells to plasma, it is replaced by chloride

8.7 **With regard to rotameters:**

a) Their accuracy is affected by static electricity
b) The flow should be read at the bottom of the float
c) They do not need to be altered at altitude
d) At high flows the calibration is mainly dependent on the viscosity of the gas passing through it
e) Their cross-section is uniform throughout

8.8 **With regard to the Sander's injector:**

a) It operates on the Venturi-Bernoulli principle
b) It delivers 100% oxygen with a respiratory rate of 20/min
c) The driving oxygen pressure is 410 kPa
d) Increasing ventilation to 100 respirations per minute (high-frequency jet ventilation – HFJV) reduces air entrainment
e) Its use is contraindicated with laser surgery

8.9 **With regard to position on the operating table:**

a) In the lateral posture, functional residual capacity is increased in the dependent lung, and decreased in the non-dependent lung
b) Sitting is best for respiratory stability, worst for the cardiovascular system
c) The peroneal nerve is at risk from damage in the lithotomy position
d) Ventilation/perfusion inequalities are more marked in the supine than in the lateral position
e) The neck is safer in the neutral, face-up position than rotated to one side

8.10 **Increased levels of 5-hydroxytryptamine are associated with:**

a) Administration of ergotamine
b) Depression
c) Reduced gut motility
d) Administration of ondansetron
e) Carcinoid syndrome

8.11 Epidural facts include:

a) A sensory block up to T10 should be sufficient for a caesarean section done under epidural anaesthesia
b) Segmental spread of local anaesthetic through an epidural increases in the elderly
c) Excluding caudals in adults, the L2/L3 and L3/L4 interspaces are usually the easiest places to enter the epidural space
d) The incidence of post-surgical thromboembolic phenomena is reduced with epidurals
e) Epidurals are contraindicated in patients on prolonged non-steroidal anti-inflammatory analgesics

8.12 Of the drugs that reduce gastric acid secretion:

a) Both omeprazole and ranitidine inhibit gastric acid secretion by the same action
b) Both omeprazole and ranitidine inhibit the action of warfarin
c) Omeprazole is more effective than ranitidine in the treatment of reflux oesophagitis
d) Misoprostol is a prostaglandin analogue which inhibits gastric acid secretion
e) Oral ranitidine acts within 2 hours and lasts about 6 hours

8.13 With regard to stellate ganglion block:

a) A successful stellate ganglion block causes miosis, ptosis, enophthalmos and absence of sweating on the opposite side of the face
b) A unilateral stellate ganglion block relieves the pain associated with intractable angina
c) Bilateral stellate ganglion blocks should be avoided
d) A stellate ganglion block can be very effective in relieving long-standing arm pain due to post-herpetic neuralgia
e) Convulsions are most probably due to injection of the local anaesthetic into the vertebral vein

8.14 In oxygen therapy:

a) Carbon dioxide rebreathing is significant with a nasal catheter delivering oxygen at 2 l/min
b) With Venturi-type masks an oxygen flow of 4 l/min gives optimal performance
c) A child's oxygen headbox requires high oxygen flow rates
d) With a Hudson or MC mask the fractional inspired oxygen concentration (FiO_2) is not patient dependent
e) Normal oxygen consumption at rest is 250–300 ml/min

8.15 With regard to anaesthesia and respiratory disease:

a) Patients with restrictive lung disease develop more respiratory complications than those with obstructive lung disease
b) Postoperative respiratory complications are more common with upper abdominal than with lower abdominal operations
c) Functional residual capacity is increased in both obstructive and restrictive lung disease
d) Prophylactic temporary postoperative positive ventilation reduces the incidence of postoperative respiratory complications
e) Reduction of smoking in the perioperative period markedly reduces the incidence of postoperative complications

8.16 Physiological changes in the elderly are such that:

a) There is increased closing volume
b) In general an elderly person requires the same drug dosage per kilogram weight as a young fit adult
c) Cardiac output is the same as in a fit young adult
d) There are increased serum creatinine levels even in the absence of renal disease
e) There is increased heat loss under general anaesthesia compared to a fit young adult

8.17 With regard to hyperthyroidism:

a) Antithyroid drugs act by increasing the iodine uptake by the thyroid gland
b) Presentation may be as an acute abdominal emergency
c) Tachyarrhythmias are a common problem with thyrotoxicosis
d) It is a very unlikely complication after treating thyrotoxicosis with radioactive iodine or subtotal thyroidectomy
e) Thyroid hormone levels may be low following cardiopulmonary bypass

8.18 Physiological changes associated with hypothermia include:

a) Vasoconstriction and tachycardia in mild hypothermia; vasodilatation, bradycardia and fall in cardiac output in severe hypothermia
b) Reduced blood viscosity
c) Respiratory and metabolic acidosis in severe hypothermia
d) Hypoglycaemia
e) Ventricular fibrillation occurring below 28°C; respiration ceasing at 24°C, and coma at 30°C

8.19 Bronchospasm is improved with:

a) Histamine (H_2) antagonists
b) Edrophonium
c) Nebulized lignocaine
d) Morphine
e) Hypocapnia

8.20 The following drugs can be given via the routes indicated:

a) Papaverine intra-arterially
b) Suxamethonium intramuscularly
c) Clonidine by the epidural route
d) Metronidazole rectally
e) Depomedrone (methylprednisolone acetate) intrathecally

EXPLANATION

If intraoperative urine flow drops below 0.5 ml/kg/hour, diagnosis and treatment of the oliguria are necessary. Once mechanical obstruction of the urinary catheter is excluded, one should evaluate the fluid input/output. If a fluid challenge of 250–500 ml of saline produces a diuresis, hypovolaemia is confirmed. One should also evaluate the haemodynamic status. If despite a patent urinary outflow tract, haemodynamic stability and adequate hydration oliguria persists, incipient acute renal failure is likely and should be treated with mannitol and dopamine. Loop diuretics, such as frusemide, are often used to improve oliguria without much logic. If pulmonary oedema is present frusemide is indicated; otherwise it may enhance the damage done by renal insults. If hypovolaemia is the cause of the oliguria, frusemide will dehydrate the patient further. Mannitol, freely filtered by the glomerulus, is considered protective in certain high-risk situations. Low-dose dopamine (beta effect and dopaminergic effects) causes renal vasodilatation; however, high-dose causes alpha effects with unwanted vasoconstriction. In emergency abdominal aortic surgery 40% of patients suffer some renal damage, from which the mortality is 80%. Dopamine and mannitol are protective in this situation.

Fluorinated anaesthetic agents can cause renal damage; especially methoxyflurane, possibly with enflurane but very unlikely with isoflurane. Renal damage is related to fluoride metabolites which are highest with methoxyflurane. Renal damage from fluoride toxicity presents with polyuria and the syndrome lasts 10–20 days and may be permanent.

In the presence of renal failure, one should use a non-depolarizing relaxant which is least dependent on renal function for elimination. Less than 10% of atracurium is eliminated via the kidney and it is the relaxant of choice in this situation. The percentage dependence on the kidney for elimination of muscle relaxants is as follows:

Greater than 95%	suxamethonium (if pseudocholinesterase is low); gallamine
60–90%	pancuronium
40–60%	tubocurare
10–20%	vecuronium
Less than 10%	atracurium

EXPLANATION

The most common causes of aortic regurgitation (incompetence) are rheumatic fever and infective endocarditis. The presenting symptoms are often angina and signs of left ventricular failure which is confirmed with ECG and echocardiography. Arrhythmias (unlike in mitral stenosis) are a relatively uncommon presentation. The signs are those of left ventricular enlargement and hyperdynamic circulation (i.e. collapsing pulse causing a wide margin between systolic and diastolic blood pressures; capillary pulsation in nail beds; nodding head with each heart beat; and a systolic bruit over the femoral arteries). On auscultation there is a high-pitched diastolic murmur best heard at the lower sternal margin or cardiac apex. Because symptoms do not develop until the myocardium fails and because the myocardium does not recover fully after surgery, it is important to operate before significant symptoms appear. The timing of the valve replacement is best determined by haemodynamic values and echocardiography.

8.3   **a) False**   **b) False**   **c) False**   **d) False**   **e) False**

EXPLANATION
With a vaporizer inside a circle (VIC), apart from the fresh gas flow, the patient's expired gas also passes through the vaporizer. Therefore increasing the ventilation causes the gas in the closed circuit to pass more frequently through the vaporizer and the inspired vapour concentration rises considerably. Increase in fresh gas flow dilutes the vapour concentration in the circuit. The reverse is true with a vaporizer outside the circuit (VOC). Here an increase in ventilation reduces the vapour concentration in the circuit while an increase in fresh gas flow increases it.

With a copper kettle vaporizer, a separate flow of oxygen from a separate flow meter passes through the vaporizer and becomes fully saturated. This fully saturated vapour then gets diluted as it joins the fresh gas flow from the nitrous oxide and oxygen flow meters.

Halothane, isoflurane and other modern volatile agents have too high a vapour concentration and therefore one needs a vaporizer in which the concentration of the vapour can be controlled and in which the calibration takes account of changes of temperature and the level of the liquid agent within the vaporizer. Agents such as ether, which is much less potent, can be used safely with a simple Boyle's bottle where the actual vapour concentration is not actually known.

Most modern vaporizers have too high a resistance to be used within a patient's breathing circuit and require the carrier gases to pass through the vaporizer under pressure. An example of a low-resistance vaporizer which can be included in a breathing circuit (draw-over vaporizer) is the EMO vaporizer.

The order of placing vaporizers in series is important to minimize contamination of one vaporizer by another. This problem can be eliminated completely by having vaporizers in parallel (popular in America). If vaporizers are in series when two agents are equipotent, the agent with the higher boiling point (i.e. lower saturated vapour pressure) should be placed distal to the patient. If both agents have similar vapour pressures, the less potent agent should be distal.

8.4   **a) True**   **b) False**   **c) False**   **d) True**   **e) False**

EXPLANATION
The 3 in 1 block utilizes the fascial envelope around the femoral nerve as a conduit to carry local anaesthetic to the lumbar plexus. Thus it provides anaesthesia of the femoral, obturator and lateral femoral cutaneous nerve of thigh. In combination with sciatic block one can perform all operations on the lower limb. A 22-gauge needle is inserted 0.5 cm below the inguinal ligament (which stretches between pubic tubercle and anterior superior iliac spine) one finger's breadth lateral to the femoral artery.

165

The needle is inserted in a slightly cranial direction. Paraesthesia of the femoral nerve should be obtained before giving the local anaesthetic (20–30 ml of 0.5% bupivacaine).

Infiltration of local anaesthetic around the nerves at the base of the penis provides excellent anaesthesia and analgesia for operations on the penis. As in digital ring blocks it is imperative that the local anaesthetic is free of adrenaline because, like the digital arteries, the penile arteries are end arteries and vasoconstriction can be catastrophic. The penile nerves are located within Buck's fascia to the right and left of the dorsal vessels of the penis. The needle is inserted at 10.30 and 1.30 positions about 3–5 mm below the skin surface.

Axillary nerve block is suitable for operations on the forearm but not on the arm. For arm operation a supraclavicular or interscalene brachial plexus block is required. For an axillary block, the needle is inserted in the axilla just above the axillary artery to enter the perivascular sheath. With a supraclavicular block the needle is inserted 1 cm above the clavicle and lateral to the subclavian artery and directed backward, inward and downward (BID) until contact is made with one of the divisions of the brachial plexus (causing paraesthesia) or with the first rib, in which case the needle is moved along the rib until paraesthesia is elicited.

An interscalene block is performed by inserting the needle in the interscalene groove at the level of the cricoid cartilage and directing it backwards, inwards and downwards (BID) to the transverse process of C6. In all techniques about 30 ml of bupivacaine is used.

The ilioinguinal and iliohypogastric nerves derive from L1 and supply the cutaneous innervation of the scrotum, root of penis and area above the inguinal ligament. A 25-gauge needle is inserted 1 cm above and medial to the anterior superior iliac spine and directed downwards and laterally until it strikes the inside of the ilium. As the needle is withdrawn, local anaesthetic is injected along this line. The needle is then reinserted at the same point but directed downwards and medially in the direction of the inguinal ligament. The external oblique fascia is penetrated with a click, and the local anaesthetic is deposited in several fan-like sweeps.

Paravertebral blocks are more effective than intercostal blocks, because both somatic and sympathetic pathways are blocked, while intercostal blocks only achieve somatic analgesia. Intercostal blocks are performed posterior to the mid-axillary line, otherwise the anterior branch which innervates the anterior part of the chest is missed. The needle is directed onto the lower border of the rib, then withdrawn slightly and reinserted just below the rib. After aspiration, to exclude intercostal vessel puncture, the local anaesthetic (3 ml) is injected in the subcostal groove. With a paravertebral block the needle is introduced two finger breadths from the spine and directed perpendicularly onto the transverse process of the relevant vertebra. The needle is then withdrawn slightly and redirected slightly upwards and inwards to glance past the upper border of the transverse process and 5 ml injected after a negative aspiration test.

8.5	a) False	b) True	c) True	d) False	e) True

EXPLANATION

Techniques. The most common techniques for subclavian vein puncture are: (1) supraclavicular; (2) infraclavicular.

Supraclavicular. Identification of the clavisternomastoid angle which is just medial to the midpoint of the clavicle is the key to the success of this procedure. In the obese, identification is made easier on tensing the muscle by raising the head from the bed against the resistance of a hand on the forehead. With the patient supine and head down the needle is inserted at the clavisternomastoid angle, at an angle of 45 degrees to the sagittal plane and slowly advanced through the deep clavicular fascia to enter the subclavian vein at a depth of about 1 cm from skin.

Infraclavicular. The needle is inserted just lateral to the midpoint of the lower border of the clavicle and directed towards the sternoclavicular joint. The needle enters the vein at a depth of about 4 cm.

Complications. These are numerous and it is not a procedure to be taken lightly.

1. Mechanical problems. The catheter can migrate upwards into the neck with the infraclavicular technique or across to the contralateral subclavian vein. Other mechanical problems include: loss of the introducer wire with a possible exploration to remove it, and arrhythmias if the wire or catheter lies in the heart; the catheter finding its way out of the vein causing hydrothorax if the catheter is attached to the drip.
2. Thrombophlebitis.
3. Infection. Central catheterizations should only be used in the presence of infection after careful consideration, as the tip may act as a focus of sepsis with resultant spread in the bloodstream and septicaemia.
4. Pneumothorax. This is more common with the supraclavicular approach. If subclavian puncture fails on the one side, one should think very carefully about attempting puncture on the other side because of the possible disastrous consequences of bilateral pneumothorax.
5. Haemothorax, hydrothorax and chylothorax (only on left side if the thoracic duct is punctured).
6. Air embolism especially in shocked patient with a low central venous pressure. Therefore puncture should be attempted with a head-down tilt.
7. Subclavian artery puncture causing a large chest haematoma. Bleeding can be catastrophic if a subclavian artery is punctured on a patient who has a coagulation disorder because one cannot apply direct pressure to stop the arterial bleed (unlike if the carotid artery is punctured when attempting internal jugular puncture).
8. Pericardial effusion and tamponade.
9. Brachial plexus injuries.

8.6	a) False	b) False	c) False	d) False	e) True

EXPLANATION

Tissues produce CO_2 and this passes via the capillaries into the blood. On reaching the pulmonary capillaries the PCO_2 in venous blood is 46 mmHg, while the alveolar PCO_2 is 40 mmHg so there is a gradient of 6 mmHg which drives CO_2 out. CO_2 is distributed in the blood in three manners:

- *Dissolved CO_2 in the plasma* (6%).
- *As bicarbonate* (70%). Most of the CO_2 passes to the red cells where the enzyme carbonic anhydrase aids its rapid hydration into H_2CO_3. Carbonic anhydrase is only present inside the cell; it is destroyed by heat and cyanide. There are only

small amounts in infants who therefore have to rely on adequate ventilation to get rid of CO_2. Carbonic anhydrase accelerates the reaction $H_2O + CO_2 \leftrightarrow H_2CO_3$ in both directions. The H_2CO_3 in the red cell dissociates into H^+ and HCO_3^- and the H^+ is buffered by haemoglobin (Hb). The decline in oxygen saturation of Hb as the blood becomes venous blood increases its buffering capacity because reduced Hb is a better buffer and therefore a better carrier of CO_2 than oxyHb. Inside the red cell there are HCO_3^- and K^+ ions, whereas Na^+ ions abound in the plasma. As HCO_3^- starts to increase in the cell, equilibrium is disturbed so that HCO_3^- passes into the plasma and is replaced by Cl^- (chloride shift). The HCO_3^- in the plasma reacts with Na^+.

In the lung capillaries there is a pressure difference of 6 mmHg which allows quick interchange of CO_2. At first the small percentages of dissolved CO_2 is eliminated creating a CO_2 gradient between cell and plasma which encourages elimination of CO_2 from the red cell. This occurs in a process that is the reverse of that described above. The $NaHCO_3$ in the plasma breaks down into Na^+ and HCO_3^-; HCO_3^- enters the red cell and Cl^- replaces it. In the red cell, H^+ reacts with HCO_3^- to form H_2CO_3 and then the enzyme carbonic anhydrase accelerates the breakdown of H_2CO_3 into H_2O and CO_2, so that CO_2 passes into the plasma and then across the alveolar membrane.

● *As a carbamino compound* (24%). Some of the CO_2 in the red cells combines with the amino group of Hb to form carbamino compounds. $CO_2 + HbNH_2 \leftrightarrow$ $HbNHCOOH$. At CO_2 values above 10 mmHg the amount of carbaminoHb formed is constant because the tendency to form more as the CO_2 increases is offset by the formation of more H^+ which ties up $HbNH_2$ to form $HbNH_2^+$. Again, deoxygenated Hb forms carbamino compounds more readily than oxyHb so the carriage of O_2 in venous blood is facilitated.

| 8.7 | a) True | b) False | c) False | d) False | e) False |

EXPLANATION
The commonest flow meter used is the bobbin flow meter (rotameter). The tube tapers downwards, and the pressure across the bobbin remains relatively constant producing a force which is equal to the force of gravity on the bobbin. As the flow rate increases, the bobbin rises higher in the tube and the size of the gap between it and the walls of the tube increases. At low flow rates the narrow space between the bobbin and the wall behaves like a tube and the calibration is mainly dependent on the viscosity of the gas passing through it. At high flow rates the width of the gap is large relative to the height of the bobbin and the annular space (gap round the bobbin) behaves like an orifice and the calibration is dependent on the density of the gas passing through it. Therefore flow meters must be calibrated for individual gases. Readings are taken from the top of the bobbin in a rotameter. The bobbin contains slits which cause it to rotate. This rotation reduces friction errors; accuracy (up to 35%) is also affected by static electricity, which can cause sticking especially at low flows. This can be minimized by covering the flow meter tubes with a thin layer of tin oxide.

8.8   a) **True**   b) **False**   c) **True**   d) **True**   e) **False**

EXPLANATION

Facts about Venturi injectors

1. A Sander's injector was first described in 1967 and uses the Venturi-Bernoulli principle, i.e. oxygen from a high-pressure source (410 kPa) is injected intermittently through a narrow needle at the proximal end of a bronchoscope or laryngoscope. When the oxygen flows through the needle constriction, velocity increases, which in turn causes a drop in pressure and a sucking effect, so that air is entrained.

2. The original Sander's system can be improved by connecting the side arm of the bronchoscope to an anaesthetic circuit, so that the injector then entrains oxygen and anaesthetic gas mixture, and by replacing the 16-gauge oxygen needle with a larger jet to deliver higher inflation pressures.

3. Besides ventilating at ordinary respiratory rates, one can employ high-frequency jet ventilation (HFJV), where rates of 60–150 respirations per minute provide adequate alveolar ventilation with lower intratracheal pressures. Because the tidal volumes generated are small, chest movements are not observed; on the other hand there is less movement of the tracheobronchial tree giving better surgical access.

4. Because of air entrainment the FiO_2 delivered to the patient is not 100%, but probably closer to 40–50%.

5. When one employs the Venturi injector, aspiration of blood and debris into the distal tracheobronchial tree can be caused by the jet of gas.

6. Effective alveolar ventilation depends on chest wall compliance.

7. When a sucker is used down a bronchoscope, gases are sucked out causing a fall in functional residual capacity, and possibly predisposing to atelectasis.

8. If the bronchoscope tip is above an area of stenosis (e.g. bronchial stenosis), better blood gases are obtained with low-frequency jet ventilation than high-frequency jet ventilation, because the former technique generates higher pressures.

9. Surgical access to the distal airway is achieved with a rigid bronchoscope when the CO_2 laser is used. The risk of a laser fire with a Venturi injector is minimal because the FiO_2 is only about 40%. (Flammability of endotracheal tube with laser is a serious problem and of the three commonly used tubes – PVC, red rubber and silicone – PVC is the least flammable; however, PVC melts at a lower temperature and is therefore more easily penetrated by the laser beam especially at the cuff. In order to reduce flammability with endotracheal tubes, one can wrap the tracheal tube with metallic tape (but the cuff cannot be wrapped); or use metallic tubes with or without a cuff, or use PVC tracheal tubes and restrict the FiO_2 to 0.3 or less in helium.)

8.9   a) **False**   b) **True**   c) **True**   d) **False**   e) **True**

EXPLANATION
See Table 8.1.

Table 8.1 Effects of position on the operating table

Position	Respiration	Cardiovascular system
Supine	Functional residual capacity (FRC) reduced – diaphragm pushed up to impede ventilation to lower lobes. FRC falls by 24% in conscious state; 44% during general anaesthesia and in supine posture. Gravity improves ventilation and perfusion in dependent parts. In supine posture dependent parts rotate by 90° – ventilation/perfusion anomalies are minor	Change from erect to supine posture prevents gravitational forces causing venous pooling – thus very little CVS changes in this position
Prone	FRC reduction less than in supine or lateral position	Heart at higher level than head and legs – thus venous pooling is possible with falls in BP. Abdominal pressure causes engorgement of perivertebral venous plexuses
Lateral	Compression of dependent lung by mediastinal and abdominal contents reduces FRC of dependent lung. Ventilation preferential to non-dependent lung; perfusion preferential to dependent lung especially with intermittent positive-pressure ventilation causing marked ventilation/perfusion anomalies	Insignificant cardiovascular effects
Semi-supine (supine with a slight head-up tilt)	FRC reduced less than in supine position because head-up tilt keeps abdominal contents away from the diaphragm	Insignificant cardiovascular effects
Semi-prone (jack-knife)	Same as prone position FCR less then supine	Legs dependent; thus venous pooling likely causing reduction in preload
Lithotomy	Chest supine – thus effects on FRC similar to those in supine position	Legs above heart level; thus no venous pooling or drop in BP

Proper placement	Comments
Table level; head neutral position facing upwards and slightly elevated on pillow; knees slightly flexed; arms on side with hand pronated or on padded board with moderate abduction; elbows padded; heels protected	Brachial plexus and ulnar nerves may be injured if arms extended, fully abducted and externally rotated
Table slightly head up; chest and pelvis supported on a frame allowing abdomen to hang, improving diaphragmatic position and pulmonary ventilation; arms at side or over head; elbows, knees, ankles protected; avoid pressure on eyes, ears, breasts, male genitalia; table may be flexed to open intervertebral spaces for back surgery	Movements of neck can reduce blood supply to brain and spinal cord causing cerebral/cervical ischaemia. Prone position probably most prone to this. When head is extended, flexed, rotated to one side, vertebral/carotid flows especially in aged or patients with vascular anomalies, osteophytes or arthritis
Patient on side; dependent leg flexed and non-dependent leg extended with pillow between them; pad distal to axilla to avoid pressure on axilla; upper arm padded or placed on a special holder; lower arm in neutral position	Eye injuries probably most likely with lateral/prone position. Trauma/pressure from face mask can cause periorbital oedema, supraocular or infraocular nerve palsies; reduced retinal flow may cause blindness. Cornea easily abraded because of reduced lacrimation during general anaesthesia. Eyes taped to avoid corneal damage
Table flexed; head-down position; knees slightly flexed; arm by side or on a padded board with safe abduction and hand pronated	Used for neck operations. Probably position which least disturbs CVS and respiratory physiology
Body flexed at hips and buttocks uppermost; head of table tilted down. Same precautions as in prone position	Used for rectal operations, e.g. pilonidal sinus
Hips flexed; knees bent; legs suspended by stirrups; patient supine; arms across chest; if tucked at sides avoid catching patient's fingers when foot of table is elevated	Peroneal nerve can be damaged by compression between fibula and stirrups, internal rotation of the thigh stretching the nerve at the head of the fibula

Table 8.1 (*Cont'd*)

Position	Respiration	Cardiovascular system
Sitting	Little ventilatory dysfunction because abdominal contents are pushed away from diaphragm and upright posture keeps alveoli open – thus ventilation/perfusion and FRC anomalies minimal and only related to anaesthesia	Peripheral vasodilatation leads to fall in pulmonary artery wedge pressure; fall in cardiac output; reflex increase in rate and systemic vascular resistance. Cerebral blood flow initially falls; then there is compensatory autoregulation
Trendelenburg (head-down)	FRC markedly reduced owing to upward diaphragmatic displacement on lungs	CVS stability maintained because venous return is improved

8.10   a) False   b) False   c) False   d) False   e) True

EXPLANATION

Synthesis

The synthesis of 5-hydroxytryptamine (formerly called serotonin) is very similar to that of noradrenaline, i.e. its precursor is tryptophan rather than tyrosine. Tryptophan is converted to 5-hydroxytryptophan by tryptophan hydroxylase, and is then decarboxylated to 5-HT. The carboxylase is non-specific, and is also involved in the synthesis of noradrenaline and histamine. The breakdown of 5-HT is catalyzed by monoamine oxidase, again similar to noradrenaline catabolism. The main metabolite is 5-hydroxyindoleacetic acid (5-HIAA), which is excreted in the urine, and its measurement provides a reliable indicator of 5-HT activity.

Distribution

- Gut – 90% of body 5-HT is present in the chromaffin cells in the stomach and small intestine.
- Blood, i.e. in platelets.
- Central nervous system – 5-HT is a transmitter in the CNS, and is present in neurons in the raphe nuclei, pons, medulla with projections to the cortex, hypothalamus and spinal cord.

Effects

1. Autonomic and endocrine function. 5-HT pathways inhibit the hypothalamic control on pituitary secretions. There is some evidence suggesting that 5-HT is involved in temperature regulation and 5-HT levels are increased by cold.
2. Nervous system. CNS effects include:
- 5-HT can cause hallucinations.
- Sleep and mood control – 5-HT abolishes sleep, and tryptophan has been used for treatment of insomnia with doubtful results. It is also mood enhancing, and

Proper placement	Comments
Legs wrapped or compression boots to reduce venous pooling; neck flexed to 2 cm off chest to avoid cervical vein obstruction; protect ulnar and peroneal nerves; use head holder; knees placed at heart level	Best position for respiratory stability, but worst for cardiovascular physiology. Risk of air embolism detected by fall in end-tidal CO_2, doppler or echocardiography
Patient may have to be restrained to avoid slipping off table	Commonly used for pelvic or leg surgery, e.g. varicose veins

has been administered as an antidepressant. Many antidepressants act partly by increasing 5-HT metabolism or release.

- Analgesia – 5-HT has an inhibitory effect on pain transmission both in the spinal cord and brain. Depression of 5-HT antagonizes the analgesic effect of morphine, while inhibition of 5-HT uptake, e.g. tramadol, is associated with analgesia.

3. Gut. Increases gut motility.

4. Platelets. Causes platelet aggregation.

5. Blood vessels. 5-HT causes vasoconstriction of large vessels, arteries and veins; in the microcirculation arterioles dilate while venules constrict causing a rise in capillary pressure and fluid escape. 5-HT also inhibits the release of noradrenaline, which tends to cause vasodilatation.

5-HT receptors
There are basically three types of 5-HT receptor:

- 5-HT_1 – mainly in CNS, blood vessels, stomach. Stimulation of these receptors is mainly inhibitory in nature.
- 5-HT_2 – mainly in CNS, smooth muscle and platelets, and responsible for increased smooth muscle activity and platelet aggregation.
- 5-HT_3 – peripheral nervous tissue especially in pain-transmitting sensory neurons and on autonomic reflexes. These effects are predominantly excitatory in nature.

Drugs which are 5-HT agonists or 5-HT antagonists
Agonists. There are no agonist drugs which are of therapeutic use. Lysergic acid diethylamide (LSD) is a specific agonist at 5-HT_2 receptors.
Antagonists:

- 5-HT_1 antagonists, e.g. quipazine, methiothepin.
- 5-HT_2 antagonists, e.g. ketanserin, mianserin, which have been used as vasodilators in vasospastic conditions such as Raynaud's disease.
- 5-HT_3 antagonists, e.g. ondansetron, an effective antiemetic especially with nausea and vomiting caused by cytotoxic drugs.

Drugs such as phenothiazines, butyrophenones and some bronchodilators also have 5-HT antagonistic actions.

Conditions involving 5-HT secretion

Migraine. Vascular spasm in migraine is thought to be due to 5-HT release, and levels of 5-HIAA are elevated during an attack. 5-HT causes vasoconstriction, and a local inflammatory response with local release of other mediators, such as bradykinins and prostaglandins which produce a pain response by acting on the nociceptive nerve terminals. Many of the antimigraine drugs are 5-HT antagonists, e.g. ergotamine and methysergide which are both 5-HT$_2$ antagonists, while recently the 5-HT$_3$ antagonist ondansetron has been claimed to be effective in the treatment of migraine.

Carcinoid syndrome. Carcinoid tumours secrete a variety of hormones, but principally 5-HT, causing flushing, diarrhoea, bronchospasm and hypotension. The syndrome can be diagnosed by measuring urinary levels of 5-HIAA, the main metabolite of 5-HT. The level can be 20 times normal, and is high even during asymptomatic periods. 5-HT$_2$ antagonists, such as cyproheptadine are effective in controlling many of the symptoms of carcinoid syndrome. Another useful agent is somatostatin which suppresses 5-HT secretion from the chromaffin cells.

8.11   a) False   b) True   c) True   d) True   e) False

EXPLANATION

In the past, sensory block at T8–T6 was considered adequate for caesarean sections. Nowadays a T4 block is required because a low transverse skin incision is used and a bladder flap is raised which requires much retraction. Moreover, the uterus is exteriorized for repair. Any sensory block below T4 is therefore associated with pain, nausea, vomiting and retching. Perineal surgery requires a block of up to L5. Lower extremity surgery and cervix, testicle and bladder operations with bladder distension require a T10 block; and vaginal hysterectomy a T4 block because of peritoneal traction.

Intra-abdominal surgery – T2–T4

Age is one of the most important factors influencing the spread of local anaesthetics which increases with ageing so that an 80-year-old patient requires about half that in someone aged between 20 and 40. Pregnancy also reduces the local anaesthetic requirement by about 30%.

In general L2–L3 and L3–L4 spaces are the easiest spaces to get into because the epidural space is widest (4–5 mm). Moreover the ligaments are firm and give clear loss or resistance and the epidural veins are least concentrated in the medial aspect of these spaces making venepuncture less likely.

The incidence of post-surgical thrombosis and embolism is reduced especially in vascular and lower leg surgery. Other advantages of epidurals include greater protection from surgical stress, greater cardiovascular stability, earlier return of gastrointestinal function, reduced fluid shifts during surgery and they can be used postoperatively for analgesia with reduction of respiratory complications.

NSAIDs and prophylactic mini-heparin with normal partial thromboplastin time do not contraindicate epidurals. Absolute contraindications are patient refusal, uncooperative patients, gross neurological disorders, marked hypovolaemia, gross coagulopathies, septicaemia or infection near the site of injection.

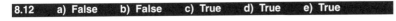

8.12   a) False   b) False   c) True   d) True   e) True

EXPLANATION

Drugs which reduce gastric acid secretion are mainly of three types:

- H_2 receptor antagonists, e.g. cimetidine, ranitidine
- Proton pump inhibitors, e.g. omeprazole
- Prostaglandin analogues, e.g. misoprostol.

Drugs such as cimetidine and ranitidine are histamine H_2 antagonists, while the newer omeprazole inhibits gastric acid by blocking the hydrogen-potassium-adenosine triphosphatase enzyme system (proton pump) of the gastric parietal cell. Both H_2 antagonists and omeprazole (Losec) are beneficial in the treatment of peptic ulcers but omeprazole is supposed to be more effective than ranitidine (Zantac) for reflux oesophagitis. Both omeprazole and ranitidine inhibit the action of liver metabolic enzymes and therefore enhance the action of oral anticoagulants and antiepileptic drugs.

When given orally, ranitidine acts within 2 hours (1 hour i.v.) and lasts about 6 hours. Therefore when used as prophylaxis of acid aspiration in labour it should be given at the onset of labour (150 mg) and repeated every 6 hours during labour. One disadvantage of H_2 blockers is the possible increased incidence of postoperative pneumonia, because raising gastric pH allows Gram-negative bacterial colonization of the stomach and oropharynx.

Misoprostol (Cytotec) is a prostaglandin analogue and since NSAIDs are prostaglandin inhibitors, it is used mainly to protect against NSAID-associated peptic ulcers. Ranitidine and omeprazole can also be used for this purpose.

8.13   a) False   b) False   c) True   d) False   e) False

EXPLANATION

A stellate ganglion block blocks the sympathetic pathways to head, neck, chest and upper limbs. A successful block causes Horner's syndrome on the ipsilateral side (i.e. miosis, ptosis, enophthalmos and absence of sweating).

Anterior approach

With the patient flat and neck extended, a mark is made $1\frac{1}{4}$ inches (two finger breadths) lateral to the midline of the jugular notch and $1\frac{1}{4}$ inches above the clavicle. A long needle is inserted backwards and medially through the mark until the transverse process of the 6th vertebra is hit, usually at a depth of 2-2.5 cm. The needle is then withdrawn slightly and after careful aspiration the local anaesthetic (5 ml 0.25% bupivacaine) is injected.

Complications:

1. Block of nearby nerves:
- Recurrent laryngeal nerve block causes hoarseness, feeling of lump in the throat, subjective shortness of breath. Bilateral stellate ganglion blocks should be avoided because bilateral blocking of the recurrent laryngeal nerves can result in loss of laryngeal reflexes and respiratory embarrassment.
- Phrenic nerve block causes temporary diaphragmatic paralysis with possible respiratory problems, especially in patients with poor respiratory reserve.
- Brachial plexus block may occur if the needle is placed too posteriorly, allowing the local anaesthetic to spread along the prevertebral fascia.

2. Intraspinal or epidural injection – causing total spinal block which may require ventilation and cardiovascular support for approximately 2 hours.

3. Intravascular injection – usually occurs in the vertebral artery, causing the local anaesthetic to go directly into the vasomotor centre, causing fits, apnoea, coma and possibly hypotension. If the quantity of drug injected is small, recovery is usually quick.

4. Pneumothorax – possible even with the anterior approach, because if the needle is inserted too caudally it can puncture the dome of the lung.

5. Cerebral air embolism – if air is injected from the syringe.

Indications:

1. Pain: reflex sympathetic dystrophy and causalgia; shingles and early post-herpetic neuralgia.(not effective when the pain is long-standing); phantom limb pain; neoplastic pain; intractable angina pectoris (also requires block of the upper five thoracic sympathetic ganglia to be effective).

2. Vascular insufficiency: Raynaud's disease; vasospasm; occlusive or embolic vascular disease; scleroderma.

3. Other indications: hyperhidrosis; sudden blindness associated with spasm of the optic arteries, e.g. quinine overdose.

8.14   **a) False**   **b) False**   **c) True**   **d) False**   **e) True**

EXPLANATION

Oxygen availability (oxygen flux) is dependent on haemoglobin and cardiac output and is normally 1000 ml/min. Only about 700 ml oxygen is actually available, while oxygen consumption at rest is 250–300 ml/min.

The methods used to deliver oxygen have the following requirements:

- control of FiO_2 (i.e. inspired oxygen)
- prevention of CO_2 rebreathing
- minimal resistance to breathing
- efficient use of oxygen
- acceptance by patients.

Oxygen devices can be classified into:

- fixed performance systems, i.e. FiO_2 not patient dependent
- variable performance systems, i.e. FiO_2 dependent on oxygen flow, device factors and patient factors.

68

Fixed performance systems. High-flow Venturi masks (Ventimasks) – high-flow
oxygen (6–8 l/min) entrains air by the Venturi principle to deliver an accurate fixed   *50ml/i.*
FiO_2, i.e. 24%, 28%, 35%, 40%. The oxygen entrains air so the total flow rate is
about 50 l/min. Because of this high flow rate rebreathing does not occur and
humidification is not necessary because of the presence of the entrained room air.
  Variable performance systems:

  1. Small capacity systems, e.g. nasal catheters. Here oxygen is delivered at
2–3 l/min to give an oxygen concentration of up to 30% with maximum comfort and   *2-3*
no CO_2 rebreathing. MC or Hudson masks are other examples; with these masks,
rebreathing of CO_2 occurs, so FiO_2 is set at 4–6 l/min to give an oxygen   *4-6*
concentration of up to 70%. Tracheostomy masks are another example of this
system.
  2. Large capacity systems. Here significant oxygen and CO_2 storage (i.e.
rebreathing) occurs; thus high oxygen flows are required (8–15 l/min), e.g.
polymasks, pneumomasks, oxygen headbox, oxygen tent and incubators.

8.15   a) False   b) True   c) False   d) False   e) False

EXPLANATION
Patients with chronic respiratory disease have a very high incidence of postoperative
pulmonary complications (collapse and pneumonia); the incidence is 80% in chronic
bronchitics compared with 7% in lifelong non-smokers. During evaluation of the
patient one should enquire about exercise tolerance, cough and sputum production.
Auscultation may reveal wheezes or rhonchi. It is important to distinguish whether a
patient has obstructive (e.g. asthma, bronchitis, emphysema), or restrictive lung
disease (interstitial fibrosis, obesity). On the whole, patients with restrictive lung
disease get fewer problems than patients with obstructive lung disease, since cough
and ciliary action are intact. On the other hand, restrictive disease is rarely reversible
(apart from obesity) while a number of measures can be employed to reduce
obstruction (i.e. steroids, beta agonists, anticholinergic drugs). Differential diagnosis
between restrictive and obstructive lung disease is therefore important and this is
best done from the history and pulmonary function tests (Table 8.2).
  There is no evidence that prophylactic postoperative intermittent positive-pressure
ventilation prevents atelectasis; in fact the reverse is true, because intubation
interferes with mucociliary function and provides a route for the introduction of
infections.
  The incidence of postoperative complications is much higher after thoracic and
upper abdominal operations (63%) compared to lower abdominal operations (9%).
  Theoretically, cessation of smoking in the perioperative period should reduce
pulmonary complications because of improved mucociliary function, decreased
sputum production and lower carboxyhaemoglobin levels, but in fact a number of
studies do not bear this out.

Table 8.2 Pulmonary function tests in the differential diagnosis of obstructive and restrictive lung disease

	Obstructive	Restrictive
Total lung capacity	No change or increased	Decreased
Functional residual capacity	Increased	Decreased
Residual volume	Increased	Decreased
Vital capacity	No change or decreased	Decreased
FEV_1	Decreased	No change or decreased
FEV_1/FVC	Decreased	No change or increased
Diffusing oxygen capacity	No change or decreased	Decreased

8.16   a) True   b) False   c) False   d) False   e) True

EXPLANATION

Drug pharmacokinetics. Lower doses are usually required in the elderly for a number of reasons: reduced plasma protein levels; decreased hepatic enzyme activity; reduced excretion of metabolites or, with non-metabolized drugs, decreased renal perfusion; reduced number of drug receptor sites; delay in drug redistribution because of decreased body mass and increased fat.

Anatomy. Decreased reactivity of protective airway reflexes could be a problem because of the likely presence of hiatus hernias. Cervical osteoarthritis may complicate intubation. Vertebral-basilar insufficiency may be present, and thus head extension can compromise the cerebral circulation. Senile atrophy and collagen skin loss cause more problems with skin trauma from pressure, warming blankets, infusions, etc., while degenerative bony changes often cause complications unless great care is taken to position these patients.

Respiratory changes. Chest wall stiffer; calcification of costal cartilages; pulmonary vasculature undergoes fibrosis; parenchymal tissue degenerates. Vital capacity, peak flows and FEV_1 are reduced; physiological dead space increases; increased ventilation-perfusion abnormalities due to increased airway closure and reduced cardiac output; increased closing volume which encroaches on functional residual capacity and exceeds it at age 45. All these changes help to reduce PaO_2.

Circulatory changes. Blood pressure rises owing to increased peripheral resistance; cardiac output falls because of increased afterload and reduced preload; autoregulation is reduced and there is a reduced sympathetic response to stress causing increased heat loss during anaesthesia. Arrhythmias are common.

Renal function. Degenerative changes in renal circulation cause a fall in renal perfusion; fall in glomerular filtration rate; decreased concentrating ability and less ability to handle an acid load because of distal tubular dysfunction. There is reduced creatinine clearance but because muscle mass is reduced creatinine levels remain more or less static unless there is underlying renal disease.

Summary

- *Drug:* usually less required.
- *Anatomy:* hiatus hernias; arthritic changes; skin and positional trauma more common.

- *Respiratory:* falls in vital capacity; peak flows and FEV_1; more ventilation-perfusion abnormalities; increased dead space; increased airway closure; stiffer chest wall and cartilages; pulmonary vasculature fibrosis; all leading to reduced PaO_2.
- *Circulatory:* reduced cardiac output, increased blood pressure; arrhythmias; reduced autoregulation and sympathetic response to stress; increased heat loss.
- *Renal:* fall in renal perfusion and glomerular filtration rate.

8.17   a) False   b) True   c) True   d) False   e) True

EXPLANATION

Thyrotoxicosis is usually due to the presence of a long-acting thyroid-stimulating (LATS) drug which stimulates the production of thyroid hormone. Thyroid hormone is produced by iodization of thyroglobulin in thyroid cells. Antithyroid drugs (e.g. thiocyanate) act by interfering with iodide binding, while radioactive iodine is trapped in the gland where it destroys glandular function. Patients treated with radioactive iodine or subtotal thyroidectomy often (over 10% incidence) develop hypothyroidism and require thyroxine.

Symptoms of thyrotoxicosis include tremors, tachycardia, arrhythmias, heart failure, weight loss, fatigue, sweating, exophthalmos. Gastrointestinal symptoms can also occur including nausea, vomiting, diarrhoea and severe abdominal pain which may suggest an underlying abdominal emergency. Many of these symptoms mimic sympathetic overactivity although the actual plasma levels of adrenaline/noradrenaline are normal. Beta blockers, however, improve a lot of the symptoms and signs of thyrotoxicosis.

Recent studies indicate that reduced thyroid levels may be partly responsible for myocardial depression after cardiopulmonary bypass and in organ donors awaiting transplantation; and thyroid hormone administration can improve myocardial performance. The cardiovascular effects of thyroid hormone are increased heart rate, cardiac index, myocardial and systemic oxygen consumption; decreased circulation time and arteriovenous oxygen difference and increased peripheral vascular resistance. Thyroid hormone levels may be low after cardiopulmonary bypass because of reduced protein levels, increased levels of glucocorticoids released by stress, and reduction of thyroid hormone production due to the presence of contrast media used in perioperative angiography. There have been some studies which showed improved cardiac output and myocardial performance when thyroid hormone had been administered before a patient came off bypass. Similarly, thyroid hormone has been used to improve cardiac function of potential organ donors.

8.18   a) True   b) False   c) True   d) False   e) True

EXPLANATION

Causes and predisposing conditions of hypothermia include:

- Accidental: exposure; immersion
- Drugs: prolonged anaesthesia, alcohol, sedatives

- Infection: pneumonia, sepsis
- CNS: cerebrovascular accidents, head injury, mental deterioration
- Cardiovascular: heart failure, infarcts, shock
- Renal: uraemia
- Endocrine: hypopituitarism, myxoedema, hypoadrenalism, diabetes
- Nutrition: malnutrition.

Physiological changes of hypothermia

1. Cardiovascular: initial sympathetic stimulation causes vasoconstriction, tachycardia, increased cardiac output; eventually there is vasodilatation with bradycardia and fall in cardiac output. Atrial fibrillation occurs below 30°C and ventricular fibrillation below 25°C: the ECG shows an extra J wave at the QRS/ST junction.

2. Respiration: depressed and ceases at 24°C. Oxygen consumption is reduced due to decreased basic metabolic rate (BMR).

3. Metabolic: acidosis both respiratory (due to hypercapnia) and metabolic (due to lactic acid accumulation). Initial shivering raises the BMR but then it falls by 6% per degree centigrade.

4. Blood: increased viscosity (due to dehydration), increased cardiac enzymes, hyperglycaemia (due to decreased insulin release and impaired utilization of glucose).

5. Kidney: decreased renal perfusion, decreased glomerular filtration rate and delayed clearance of drugs.

6. Liver: liver function including detoxification is depressed, prolonging action of drugs (non-depolarizing relaxants).

7. CNS: cerebral depression and reduced cerebral blood flow. Coma and pupil dilatation at 30°C.

8.19   a) False   b) False   c) True   d) False   e) False

EXPLANATION

1. *Premedication.* H_1 antagonists have sedative and drying properties which are useful in asthmatics.

2. *Induction agents.* Thiopentone does not cause bronchospasm; however, because it only provides a light plane of anaesthesia, airway instrumentation can trigger off bronchospasm. Propofol has no effect on peripheral airways, and is supposed to be preferable to thiopentone and methohexitone. Ketamine causes bronchodilatation through its sympathomimetic action, and is the induction agent of choice in a wheezing patient. Although etomidate does not cause histamine release, unlike propofol, it does not prevent a bronchoconstrictive response to airway introduction.

3. *Inhalation agents.* Halothane is a better bronchodilator than isoflurane or enflurane but the latter two are also acceptable in asthmatic patients.

4. *Muscle relaxants.* Most muscle relaxants cause histamine release and possible bronchoconstriction, especially tubocurare and suxamethonium, but also atracurium and pancuronium. Vecuronium causes no histamine release and is the relaxant of

choice in asthmatics. Cholinesterase inhibitors such as neostigmine and edrophonium promote airway constriction by inhibiting the destruction of acetylcholine. These effects are prevented and reversed by muscarinic receptor antagonists (e.g. atropine).

5. *Analgesics*. Morphine and other narcotics cause histamine release and potentially can cause bronchospasm but this is probably prevented by the narcotics blocking off airway reflexes. Non-steroidal anti-inflammatory analgesics trigger off an asthmatic attack through their action on prostaglandin inhibition.

6. *Other factors:*

- Local anaesthetic agents either systemically or as aerosols have been used to treat bronchospasm. Their modes of action include direct effects on smooth muscle; inhibition of mediator release and interruption of reflex arcs. Lignocaine (1–2 mg/kg i.v.) given prior to intubation is useful for preventing reflex bronchoconstriction caused by airway instrumentation.

- Vagal nerve stimulation and hypocapnia (by reducing sympathetic drive) can also cause bronchoconstriction.

- Regional anaesthesia. It is sometimes stated that spinals and epidurals should be avoided in asthmatics, because a high block may cause a sympathetic blockade, and therefore bronchospasm; furthermore a high block may impair accessory respiratory muscle activity, with reduction in expiratory reserve volume and inability to cough. These fears are unfounded; the major trigger to bronchospasm is airway stimulation.

8.20   a) True   b) True   c) True   d) True   e) False

EXPLANATION

Papaverine relaxes vascular spasm and has been used to dilate blood vessels where embolization or local damage has occurred, e.g. intra-arterial injection of papaverine to dilate the brachial artery when 5% thiopentone has accidentally been injected intra-arterially.

Suxamethonium can be given by the intramuscular route especially in neonates. It acts within 3 minutes (2 mg/kg) but the dose should not be repeated because of possible prolonged action.

Clonidine is an adrenergic agonist which is used to treat hypertension, and beta agonists have been used successfully by the epidural/intrathecal route to treat cancer pain.

Metronidazole is used widely for the prevention of anaerobic sepsis following abdominal surgery. It is usually given intravenously but it can be given just as successfully rectally and the latter route is considerably less costly (500 mg suppository = 70 p; 500 mg i.v. in 100 ml bag = £3.50).

Depomedrone (methylprednisolone acetate) is used widely in epidurals to treat chronic backache. It is potentially neurotoxic and has been blamed for causing arachnoiditis and should therefore not be used intrathecally. Many pain specialists will not use it by the epidural route either, because of the possibility of the above complications.

9.1 **Transoesophageal echocardiography:**

a) Detects myocardial wall motion and wall thickening
b) Is less sensitive than electrocardiography in detecting ischaemic myocardial changes
c) Permits continuous monitoring of preload and contractility
d) Is associated with complications that are frequent and serious
e) Allows continuous monitoring of the cardiac output

9.2 **With regard to myocardial ischaemia:**

a) Preoperative ischaemic changes in the electrocardiogram (ECG) are less predictive of postoperative myocardial ischaemia than preoperative arrhythmias
b) A normal resting preoperative ECG does not exclude coronary artery disease, but a preoperative exercise ECG almost certainly does
c) Intraoperative ECG ST depression indicates myocardial ischaemia
d) One of the most valuable indictors of myocardial ischaemia is increase in pulmonary artery pressures
e) High levels of creatinine phosphokinase and lactate dehydrogenase 4 hours after a cholecystectomy almost certainly indicate a myocardial infarct

9.3 **With regard to fluid management:**

a) In a 70-kg adult the total body water is 42 litres and represents 60% of total body weight
b) Sodium is primarily distributed in the intracellular volume
c) Maintenance water requirements increase in an adult compared to a neonate
d) A patient undergoing a cholecystectomy requires only maintenance fluid to maintain cardiovascular stability
e) Severe trauma causes water and sodium accumulation and peripheral oedema

9.4 **Fat embolism:**

a) Occurs in 50% of patients with major orthopaedic trauma
b) Is less common if the fracture is properly immobilized
c) Can occur with arthroplasties and use of methylmethacrylate (bone cement)
d) Is not associated with skin and retinal petechiae which occur with air embolism
e) Incidence is markedly reduced if patients with major orthopaedic trauma are given prophylactic oxygen

9.5 A 60-year-old man is admitted into hospital for a transurethral resection of the prostate. He has bad chronic obstructive airways disease, and has a history of chronic atrial fibrillation, for which he takes oral anticoagulants, which were stopped 2 hours prior to surgery. Because of his respiratory problems the anaesthetist decides to conduct the anaesthesia under a single shot local anaesthetic lumbar epidural. The operation is uneventful; however, 12 hours postoperatively the patient complains of sharp transient back and leg pain and flaccid paralysis but no sensory loss. The most likely diagnosis is:

a) Anterior spinal artery syndrome
b) Cauda equina syndrome
c) Epidural haematoma
d) Motor paralysis associated with bony secondaries from a primary prostatic carcinoma
e) Epidural abscess

9.6 With regard to anaesthetic cylinders:

a) An oxygen cylinder has a black body and black and white shoulder, while an air cylinder has a black body with a white shoulder
b) Liquid oxygen in UK hospitals is stored in a pressurized container at a temperature of −100°C
c) Entonox in a full cylinder is in a gaseous state, while nitrous oxide in a full cylinder is a liquefied gas
d) As a full nitrous oxide cylinder empties, the pressure of the nitrous oxide falls in proportion to the reduction in volume
e) The pressure in a full oxygen cylinder at 15°C is 2000 pounds/square inch

9.7 With regard to hypertension:

a) Patients with uncomplicated hypertension have a normal cardiac output and a high peripheral resistance
b) Both endotracheal intubation and extubation can cause significant increases in heart rate and blood pressure in such patients
c) An elderly patient presenting for elective surgery with a high systolic but normal diastolic pressure should have surgery postponed
d) Absence of left ventricular changes on electrocardiography rules out ventricular hypertrophy
e) A patient presenting with hypertension due to an aldosterone-secreting tumour will have accompanying hypokalaemia

9.8 In a patient undergoing anaesthesia for renal transplantation:

a) If the haemoglobin is less than 4 g/ml it is preferable to treat this with human erythropoietin than with a blood transfusion
b) Rejection of the new kidney is more likely if the patient is given a blood transfusion
c) Pancuronium or alcuronium is an appropriate long-acting relaxant
d) Enflurane is preferable to isoflurane
e) Morphine can be used without any extra precautions for postoperative pain relief

9.9 **In head injury:**

a) A computerized tomography scan on a patient with a severe head injury is very useful in determining the location and extent of a focal lesion
b) Steroids should be given immediately to a patient with raised intracranial pressure
c) A Glasgow coma score of 5 indicates minimal brain damage
d) A patient who,when admitted to the intensive care unit of a district general hospital following a severe head injury is flaccid, apnoeic and has no motor response, should immediately be transferred to a neurological centre for treatment
e) Hypocapnia and hypothermia are preferable to hypercapnia and a high temperature

9.10 **With regard to anaesthesia in muscle disease:**

a) Patients with muscular dystrophy often have respiratory and cardiac impairment
b) Because atracurium is degraded by Hofmann elimination the dose requirements in a myasthenic patient are the same as in a normal patient
c) Patients with myaesthenic syndrome are resistant to both depolarizing and non-depolarizing muscle relaxants
d) The weakness of myaesthenic syndrome is improved with anticholinesterase
e) Patients with muscle sclerosis respond normally to normal doses of non-depolarizing relaxants

9.11 **With regard to postoperative central nervous system disturbance:**

a) The duration is not related to the duration of anaesthesia
b) As with ketamine, recovery from propofol anaesthesia can be associated with dreams and hallucinations
c) Midazolam's amnesic effect is of considerably shorter duration than that of diazepam
d) Both hypoventilation and hyperventilation can lead to postoperative delirium
e) Postoperative delirium thought to be due to an anticholinergic drug, can be reversed with physostigmine

9.12 **With regard to local anaesthetics:**

a) Spread and depth of epidural and spinal anaesthesia are increased during pregnancy
b) Bupivacaine carbonate compared to bupivacaine hydrochloride has a longer onset of action and less intense block
c) The shortest duration of action of local anaesthetic follows intrathecal or subcutaneous administration, the longest durations follow major peripheral nerve blocks
d) Prilocaine is more toxic to the cardiovascular and central nervous systems than lignocaine
e) The amino amide agents (e.g. lignocaine, bupivacaine) are metabolized primarily in the liver

9.13 Xenon:

a) Can be used to measure cerebral blood flow
b) Can be used for ventilation/perfusion scans of lung
c) Is more potent and insoluble than nitrous oxide
d) Has myocardial depressant properties
e) Has poor analgesic properties

9.14 With regard to sleep:

a) Benzodiazepines produce sedation by blocking the GABA (gamma-aminobutyric acid) receptor
b) It is associated with increased activity in the ascending reticular activating system
c) It is induced by serotonin
d) Dreaming tends to occur in the non-rapid eye movement stage (NREM)
e) Functional residual capacity is reduced while responses to hypoxia and hypercarbia are impaired during sleep

9.15 With regard to neurolytic agents:

a) Phenol is hypobaric to cerebrospinal fluid while alcohol is hyperbaric
b) High concentrations of local anaesthetics can be neurotoxic
c) Both extreme heat and extreme cold have neurolytic actions
d) Sciatic nerve block with a neurolytic agent is safer than intrathecal phenol injection in a patient with leg pain due to malignancy, because motor block is less likely
e) Coeliac plexus block with neurolytic agents may relieve pain associated with gastric carcinoma

9.16 Obstructive sleep apnoea:

a) Is more common in the obese patient
b) Can be caused by nasal obstruction
c) Is unlikely to be accompanied by significant oxygen desaturation
d) Can be a cause of pulmonary hypertension
e) Can be due to adenotonsillar hypertrophy in children

9.17 Problems with drugs of abuse include:

a) Respiratory and cardiovascular depression is more likely with barbiturates than with benzodiazepines
b) Cannabis often causes nausea and vomiting
c) A 'cannabis' abuser requires less anaesthetic in the 'acute' intoxication stage; more in the chronic stage
d) A neonate born to a diamorphine (heroin) addict is likely to show respiratory depression at birth followed by tachypnoea
e) Tolerance to cocaine is marked, so the 'user' requires ever increasing doses

9.18 Intrapleural regional analgesia:

a) Is no more effective than intercostal nerve blocks for postoperative analgesia
b) Provides very effective analgesia after thoracotomies
c) Should use 0.75% rather than lower concentrations of bupivacaine
d) Requires entry into the interpleural space to be identified with the 'loss of resistance' technique with the epidural needle
e) Does not block the sympathetic system

9.19 With regard to acquired immunodeficiency syndrome (AIDS):

a) Low levels of T lymphocytes are typical in full-blown case
b) *Pneumocystis carinii* is an AIDS-related pneumonia primarily caused by cytomegalovirus
c) Unlike hepatitis B, a patient infected with the AIDS virus never develops immunity to it
d) Kaposi's sarcoma and lymphomas are typical tumours in AIDS patients
e) Blood is the only body fluid in which the AIDS virus can be detected

9.20 With regard to steroids and anaesthesia:

a) The anti-inflammatory action of steroids is due to inhibition of prostaglandins synthesis
b) Steroid therapy causes adrenal suppression which lasts 2–12 months after cessation of therapy
c) Combinations of dexamethasone and ondansetron are less likely to be effective in reducing postoperative nausea and vomiting than ondansetron alone
d) Hypoalbuminaemia significantly increases the levels of circulating cortisol
e) Mineralocorticoids tend to cause hypokalaemia and sodium and water retention

9.1   **a) True**   **b) False**   **c) True**   **d) False**   **e) False**

EXPLANATION

There is obviously a lot of interest in introducing new non-invasive monitoring techniques and transoesophageal echocardiography is potentially the most informative cardiovascular monitor ever introduced. Its most useful intraoperative applications are assessment of haemodynamic function and detection of myocardial ischaemia. Ventricular function is assessed by measuring ejection fractions, ventricular volume and wall shortening, and permits continuous monitoring of preload and contractility. Myocardial ischaemia is accompanied by wall thickening and wall movement, both of which are detected by transoesophageal echocardiography well before 'ST' changes occur on the ECG. Since the procedure is relatively non-invasive, complications are rare and minor. Transoesophageal echocardiography uses intermittent ultrasound pulses at 2.5–7.5 million cycles/second. The transducer is 4 cm long, 1.5 cm wide and 1 cm thick and is mounted on the tip of a gastroscope. The disadvantages of this method are cost, the large size of the instrument and difficulty in accessing information.

Transoesophageal echocardiography cannot produce a continuous measurement of cardiac output; however, other non-invasive methods can:

- Thoracic bioimpedence. This measures the change in thoracic electrical impedance caused by change in thoracic blood volume.
- Doppler estimation of cardiac output. Here a single ultrasound beam is projected on to the aorta. The velocity of blood flow is estimated by measuring the change in frequency (Doppler shift) of the reflected ultrasound that is induced by the red blood cell movement. One can either use an oesophageal transducer to transmit a beam on to the descending aorta, or a transducer mounted on the endotracheal tube to project the beam on the ascending aorta. The maximum measured blood flow velocity is then multiplied by the assumed cross-sectional area of the aorta to estimate flow and cardiac output.

Continuous non-invasive blood pressure monitoring is another interesting possibility. Methods available include:

- Arterial tonometry where a microtransducer partially compresses an artery (e.g. radial) and thus tracks the blood pressure continuously.
- Pulse wave velocity detection. Here two photometric sensors (as in pulse oximetry) at different sites (e.g. digit and forehead) detect the rate of propagation of the arterial pulse wave.

9.2   **a) True**   **b) True**   **c) False**   **d) False**   **e) False**

EXPLANATION

ECG changes associated with myocardial ischaemia include arrhythmias, Q waves, ST depression or elevation and T wave changes. The presence of an arrhythmia in a preoperative ECG is a better indicator of postoperative myocardial ischaemia than the presence of ischaemic changes (i.e. ST, Q and T wave changes). A normal resting preoperative ECG does not exclude coronary artery disease, but it is likely that patients who do not develop ischaemic changes with an exercise ECG will not develop cardiac ischaemia postoperatively.

Intraoperatively, ST depression does not necessarily indicate myocardial ischaemia. ST segment depression is quite common on intraoperative ECG monitors, where the frequency response is reduced to filter out distortion from muscle movement and electrical equipment. Myocardial ischaemia causes rises in pulmonary artery pressures, but these rises can occur with increase in afterload; so increases in pulmonary capillary wedge pressures are not valuable in diagnosing myocardial ischaemia.

Postoperative T wave changes are not uncommon even in the absence of myocardial ischaemia, therefore ECG diagnosis depends on ST/Q wave changes.

Lactate dehydrogenase (LDH) and creatinine phosphokinase (CPK) are used frequently to diagnose myocardial infarction, but LDH levels are raised postoperatively after biliary surgery and red cell haemolysis, while CPK rises after muscle trauma. CPK is a more valuable indicator than LDH and if CPK remains elevated 18 hours after surgery myocardial infarction is likely.

9.3   a) True   b) False   c) False   d) False   e) True

EXPLANATION

In a 70-kg adult, total body water (TBW) is about 42 litres and accounts for 60% of body weight. The TBW is divided into intracellular volume (ICV – 40%) and extracellular volume (ECV – 20%) where sodium is primarily distributed. The extracellular volume is further subdivided into interstitial fluid volume (IFV – 16%) and plasma volume (PV – 4%). The plasma volume, which is the volume we must keep normal to maintain cardiovascular stability, is primarily dependent on the colloid osmotic pressure between interstitial fluid volume and plasma volume. Albumin plays a major part in determining the osmotic pressure.

Severe trauma which includes some surgical procedures leads to sodium and water retention and peripheral oedema. This is due to sequestration of water, sodium and albumin into the surgical site. Water requirements during surgery are therefore greater than normal maintenance requirements. Thus for surgery with minimal trauma the intraoperative fluid infusion rates should be 4 ml/kg/hour; with moderate trauma (e.g. cholecystectomy) 6 ml/kg/hour; with major trauma (e.g. abdominal aortic surgery) 8 ml/kg/hour. When one is giving large volumes of fluid one must decide whether to use crystalloids or colloids. The relative merits of each are given in Table 9.1.

Different crystalloids are distributed as shown in Table 9.2.

Maintenance water requirements decrease with weight as follows:

1–10 kg:	4 ml/kg/hour
11–20 kg:	2 ml/kg/hour
Over 21 kg:	1 ml/kg/hour

For every litre of water, the sodium requirement is 30 mEq and potassium 20 mEq.

Table 9.1   Relative merits of crystalloids and colloids

	Advantages	Disadvantages
Colloids	Smaller infused volume Prolonged increase in plasma volume Less peripheral oedema Decreased thromboembolism (dextrans)	Expensive; allergic reactions Coagulopathy (dextrans) Decreased calcium levels (albumin) Decreased glomerular filtration rate Osmotic diuresis (low molecular weight dextrans) Pulmonary oedema
Crystalloids	Inexpensive Greater glomerular filtration rate Replace interstitial fluid volume	Short-lived expansion of plasma volume Peripheral oedema

Table 9.2   Colloid distributions

	Plasma volume	Interstitial fluid volume	Intracellular volume
5% dextrose 1000 ml	70 ml	280 ml	650 ml
Hartmann's 1000 ml	214 ml	786 ml	0
Normal saline 1000 ml	250 ml	1000 ml	−1000 ml
Hypertonic saline 7.5% 250 ml	−1000 ml	−375 ml	−375 ml
5% albumin 500 ml	375 ml	125 ml	0

9.4   a) False   b) True   c) True   d) False   e) False

EXPLANATION

Risk factors. Fat embolism syndrome occurs in 5–10% of patients who have had major orthopaedic trauma especially with long bone leg fractures and pelvic fractures. The incidence is less if the fracture is immobilized properly. It can also occur during the application of bone cement in arthroplasties, and this can be recognized by hypoxaemia. The incidence is probably not diminished with prophylactic oxygen but it is recommended that all patients who have had major bone trauma should be administered oxygen to prevent the hypoxaemia which occurs with fat embolism.

Clinical picture. Signs and symptoms may occur immediately, but there is usually a latent period of 24–48 hours. The main clinical features are in the lungs, brain and skin.

Lungs. The first sign is usually hypoxaemia and increased alveolar-arterial oxygen difference. This may be followed by dyspnoea, cyanosis, frothy sputum and tachycardia and possibly pulmonary oedema and respiratory failure. Chest X-ray reveals bilateral fluffy opacities, while the ECG may show a right ventricular strain pattern.

Brain. Mental changes, due to cerebral hypoxia, are restlessness, confusion and coma in severe cases.

Skin. A petechial rash appears relatively late – within 36 hours in approximately 50% of cases. It tends to occur in the skin folds of the upper half of the body, conjunctivae and mouth mucosa. The retina may show exudates and haemorrhages, as well as fat droplets.

Other signs. Pyrexia, anaemia, thrombocytopenia. Disseminated intravascular coagulation is a rare complication.

Diagnosis:

- Sputum and urine show fat globules.
- Retina – Fat exudates, haemorrhages.
- Blood gases – hypoxaemia acidosis, increased alveolar-arterial oxygen difference (over 100 mmHg).

Management:

- Early stabilization of fracture.
- Respiratory support – oxygen, intermittent positive-pressure ventilation with positive end-expiratory pressure in severe cases.
- Cardiovascular support
- ? steroids – high doses of steroids are often administered, but the benefit of this is debatable.

9.5   a) False   b) False   c) True   d) False   e) False

EXPLANATION

Although this patient has chronic obstructive disease, the anaesthetist made the wrong choice of anaesthetic technique and should have given him a general anaesthetic rather than an epidural. The oral anticoagulants should have been stopped at least 48 hours prior to the operation and hence an extradural technique was contraindicated because of the possibility of epidural haematoma which can develop even after minor trauma.

Bony secondaries can lead to major flaccid paralysis of the lower extremities, but this is likely to be slow to develop and progressive.

Epidural abscess: There is a previous history of infection; onset is 1–30 days; symptoms include fever, back pain, flaccid paralysis but minimal sensory involvement. Myelogram/CT shows signs of extradural compression, while CSF shows an increased cell count.

Epidural haemorrhage: Previous history of anticoagulant medication; sudden onset of sharp back and leg pain with initial flaccid paralysis followed by spastic paralysis and late sensory involvement. Myologram/CT shows signs of extradural compression.

   Anterior spinal artery syndrome: occurs in the elderly with a history of arteriosclerosis. There is a sudden onset of flaccid paralysis with little sensory involvement.

   Cauda equina syndrome (*Chronic arachnoiditis*): Can be caused by spinal contaminants e.g. toxins, bacteria, trauma. Onset is prolonged (days or weeks), and typical symptoms are perineal sensory loss with variable lower extremity paralysis and bladder and bowel dysfunction.

9.6   a) False   b) False   c) True   d) False   e) True

EXPLANATION

In the UK cylinders are primarily identified by their label, secondarily by their colour. An oxygen cylinder has a black body and white shoulder; Nitrous Oxide is all blue, air – black body and black and white shoulder; carbon dioxide – all grey; helium – all brown. The valve outlet of cylinders is the British Standard pin index system, which is designed in such a way that one cannot connect a cylinder to an incorrect yoke.

   In UK hospitals oxygen is stored in the liquid state in a sealed and pressurized vacuum container, away from the main buildings, because of fire hazard. The pressure inside the cylinder is 2000lbs/sq inch (1200KPa). In order to become liquid it must be below the critical temperature of oxygen (–119°C); the actual storage temperature is thus –150°C. (The critical temperature is the temperature at the critical point, which is the point when the pressure applied to a gas is sufficient to convert it to a liquid). Fresh supplies of liquid oxygen are pumped from a tanker into a hospital storage vessel, which rests on a weighing machine to measure the liquid mass. Reserve supplies of oxygen cylinders are kept, in case of supply failure. In the UK, oxygen cylinders come in four different sizes with capacities of 170, 340, 680, and 1360 litres.

   Oxygen, air, helium and entonox are in gaseous states in full cylinders; carbon dioxide, cyclopropane and nitrous oxide are partly in the liquified and partly in the gaseous state in full cylinders. During emptying the pressure in an oxygen cylinder falls in proportion to the volume left (Boyle's Law) so long as the temperature is constant. However with liquefiable gases (e.g. nitrous oxide) the pressure remains the same until all the liquid nitrous oxide is vaporized; then the pressure falls according to Boyle's Law. When the pressure starts dropping, there is about 30 minutes of nitrous oxide use left. Nitrous oxide cylinders are filled to a filling ratio of 0.75. (filling ratio equals ratio of weight of gas in the cylinder to weight of water it can hold.)

9.7   a) True   b) True   c) False   d) False   e) True

EXPLANATION

Hypertension is either secondary (10% of cases) or primary (essential 90%). Causes of secondary hypertension include: renal disease, where the hypertension is due to renin and angiotensin secretion; and endocrine diseases – Cushing's (hypertension due to sodium retention), aldosterone tumours (sodium retention and hypokalaemia) and phaeochromocytoma (hypertension due to excess secretion of adrenaline and noradrenaline).

By far the most common form of hypertension is primary or essential hypertension, and these patients have normal cardiac outputs and increased peripheral resistance. All drug therapy aims to reduce the increased peripheral resistance – by decreasing vasoconstriction, the blood flow and therefore the oxygen delivery to major organs is improved. Untreated hypertension affects mainly three organs: heart, kidney and brain. The heart eventually develops left ventricular hypertrophy which may be detected on echocardiography even in the absence of ECG changes. Angina and myocardial ischaemia may also be present. The kidney is also affected in that glomerular sclerosis can occur, as well as loss of glomerular filtration. Long-term hypertension also impairs autoregulation of the brain, i.e. for normal cerebral blood flow to occur a higher pressure is needed. Antihypertensive therapy restores normal autoregulation. Moreover ischaemic and haemorrhagic strokes are common.

Systolic hypertension is a disease that is related to the loss of elasticity in the arterioles with advancing age. Therefore patients with systolic pressures of 180 or 190 mmHg, but with normal diastolic pressures should present no anaesthetic problem. Diastolic hypertension is much more serious and elective surgery should be postponed on a patient presenting with a diastolic pressure of 110 mmHg or above. In such patients, intubations and extubations are accompanied by wild swings of blood pressure and pulse rate which may predispose to myocardial ischaemia or strokes. It is therefore prudent to minimize these swings with short-acting narcotics or antihypertensive agents. Hypertension is also common in the recovery room and this may have various causes, e.g. inadequate pain relief, hypoxia, hypercarbia, distended bladder or inaccurate monitoring, and all these have to be treated accordingly.

9.8   a) True   b) False   c) False   d) False   e) False

EXPLANATION
Patients in renal failure are usually severely anaemic because of decreased erythropoietin production, bone marrow depression, increased red cell haemolysis, etc. The anaemia causes a reduction in oxygen-carrying capacity which is compensated by an increased cardiac output and increased 2,3-diphosphoglycerate (2,3-DPG) and metabolic acidosis which shift the oxyhaemoglobin curve to the right, thus improving oxygen delivery to tissues. The question of preoperative transfusion to improve the anaemia is controversial. Disadvantages include possible pulmonary oedema especially with the increased cardiac output, reduction in 2,3-DPG and the risk of inducing anti-HLA cytotoxic antibodies; if this happens the patient becomes virtually untransplantable. One advantage of blood transfusion is that the transfusion depresses the autoimmune system and the kidney is less likely to be rejected. However, the same result can be obtained with cyclosporin. Rather than treat the anaemia with blood, it would be preferable to use human erythropoietin which improves exercise capacity, induces well-being and improves haemostatic function. However, it is very expensive (£5000/year per patient).

Muscle relaxants have to be carefully chosen in such a patient. Suxamethonium may be required but it should not be used if potassium is greater than 5 mmol/litre.

One should use the long-acting relaxants which are least excreted by the kidney. Thus with gallamine over 90% is renally excreted; alcuronium 60–90%; pancuronium 60%; D-tubocurare 25–60% (biliary excretion takes over in renal failure); vecuronium and atracurium less than 25%. Atracurium is the best relaxant to use in renal failure.

As regards volatile agents, methoxyflurane is contraindicated because of high fluoride levels. Enflurane also leads to lower levels of free fluoride production and should theoretically be avoided. Halothane does not cause this problem, while isoflurane and especially desflurane, because of their very limited metabolism, should be the ideal agents.

One should use morphine with caution in patients with renal failure because of the accumulation of morphine-6-glucuronide which prolongs the effect of morphine. Therefore infusions are dangerous, and it is better to give small regular doses. Most narcotics are on the whole safe as they are mostly metabolized in the liver except for phenoperidine of which 50% is excreted unchanged in the urine. Fentanyl is probably the drug of choice because its pharmacokinetics are unchanged in renal failure.

| 9.9 | a) True | b) False | c) False | d) False | e) True |

EXPLANATION

The Glasgow criteria for transferring patients to a neurological centre are:

- *Indications.* Deterioration in neurological status; skull fracture unless alert, orientated and asymptomatic; focal neurological signs; any impairment of consciousness greater than confusion; confusion that persists 6 hours after injury.
- *Contraindications.* Major injuries until resuscitated; patients over 70 in coma from time of injury; patients of any age who are flaccid, apnoeic and with no motor response.

The severity of the head injury can be evaluated from the Glasgow coma scale which assesses three functions – eye opening, best verbal response and best motor response – and assigns scores to each (see Table 2.4, p. 42).

Nowadays, diagnosis is obtained almost exclusively by CT scanning which is very useful in locating and determining the extent of the injury but shows very little in diffuse brain damage.

The principle of management is to keep the intracranial pressure low. There is no evidence that steroids are of any use in decreasing intracranial pressure. If intracranial pressure exceeds 3.3 kPa (25 mmHg) (normal is 0–2 kPa, 0–15 mmHg, with a supine patient) one should attempt to reduce it by giving mannitol, hyperventilation (intermittent positive-pressure ventilation) and possibly cerebrospinal fluid drainage. Factors which increase intracranial pressure must be avoided, i.e. convulsions (treat with phenytoin, phenobarbitone, thiopentone, etc.), pain (analgesics), hypercapnia, hyperpyrexia (tepid sponging, fanning, chlorperazine), avoidance of hypertension coughing and straining (therefore intubation should be performed with thiopentone and/or neuromuscular agents).

9.10   a) True   b) False   c) False   d) False   e) False

EXPLANATION
Patients with muscular dystrophy and dystrophia myotonica often have associated respiratory and cardiac impairment and arrhythmias.

Patients with myasthenia gravis are resistant to suxamethonium and sensitive to non-depolarizing relaxants. Because atracurium is broken down by Hofmann degradation it is probably the best non-depolarizing relaxant to use but the dose requirements should be reduced to about 20% of the normal recommended dose.

Malignant hyperpyrexia is inherited as an autosomal dominant disorder, and therefore children of known cases have a 50% probability of inheriting the disease susceptibility.

With all neuromuscular diseases including multiple sclerosis, suxamethonium should be used with care because hyperkalaemia is a distinct possibility in the presence of damaged muscle.

Myasthenic syndrome is probably an autoimmune disorder usually associated with oat cell lung carcinoma; occasionally there is no tumour. It causes weakness of thigh and pelvic muscles, while ocular muscles (unlike myaesthenia gravis) are usually unaffected. Autonomic dysfunction may be a feature causing hypotension, dry mouth, constipation and urinary retention. The weakness is not improved with anticholinesterase drugs, while there is increased sensitivity to both depolarizing and non-depolarizing muscle relaxants.

9.11   a) False   b) True   c) False   d) True   e) True

EXPLANATION
Postoperative delirium and confusion are common and it is important to diagnose the cause; it is commonly related to anxiety; pain; etc. Other causes include:

1. Anaesthetic agents. All agents used for premedication, induction and maintenance have prolonged CNS effects; even the shorter-acting agents. It has been shown that:
   - Midazolam's amnesic effect is similar in duration to that of diazepam
   - Anaesthesia with halothane/enflurane for 3½-minutes causes CNS disturbance for 5 hours and this is prolonged the longer the duration of anaesthesia
   - Although clinical recovery with methohexitone is rapid, psychomotor performance is altered for 12 hours
   - Propofol causes more rapid recovery than thiopentone or methohexitone but can cause vivid dreams and hallucinations
   - Sleep is disturbed for a few days after a general anaesthetic.
2. Specific factors:
   - Cerebral hypoxia is the most important cause of postoperative CNS dysfunction. This can be the result of hypo- or hyperventilation or hypotension and is usually easy to treat with supplemental oxygen
   - Specific drugs, e.g. ketamine, propofol (hallucinations and dreams), droperidol (anxiety, restlessness, and other extrapyramidal symptoms), other antiemetics and phenothiazines (extrapyramidal symptoms), anticholinergic agents (e.g. atropine, scopolamine) especially in the elderly (treatment is with

anticholinesterases, such as physostigmine which crosses the blood–brain barrier)
- Endocrine disorders, e.g. hyponatraemia, hypernatraemia, diabetes
- Perioperative cerebrovascular accident (CVA). The incidence is rare (about 0.01%). Probably hypertension is more prone to cause thrombotic episodes than intraoperative hypotension. Elective surgery should be delayed for 6 weeks following a CVA.

In conclusion, about 10% of patients are unrousable for 60 minutes in the recovery room and in the vast majority of cases this is related to drugs rather than neurological problems. If the delayed arousal is thought to be due to narcotics a small dose of naloxone is indicated. Neostigmine will reverse atropine- or scopolamine-induced CNS depression, while flumazenil will reverse the effects of diazepam or midazolam; it must be remembered, however, that flumazenil has a shorter duration of action than diazepam/midazolam, and therefore resedation is possible.

9.12   a) True   b) False   c) True   d) False   e) True

EXPLANATION

During pregnancy less local anaesthetic is required for epidural/spinal anaesthesia, possibly because of hormonal factors (increased progesterone levels) and dilatation of epidural veins during late pregnancy which decreases the diameter of the epidural and subarachnoid spaces.

Alkalinization (by addition of sodium bicarbonate) decreases the time before onset of block. Carbonation also provides a quicker onset of action and a more profound block. Alkalinization of the local anaesthetic increases the pH and thus increases the concentration of the drug in the uncharged base form. Carbonation of a local anaesthetic allows more rapid dissociation of the drug into the active base form.

Potency is directly related to lipid solubility because the site of action of local anaesthetics is the nerve membrane which is primarily lipid. Prilocaine is the least toxic of the amino amide local anaesthetics, and is particularly useful for i.v. regional anaesthesia since CNS toxic effects are rare even after early accidental release of a tourniquet.

The breakdown of local anaesthetics depends on their chemical structure. The esters (e.g. procaine) are hydrolysed in plasma by cholinesterase. The amino amide agents are metabolized primarily in the liver and breakdown is prolonged in hepatic failure.

9.13   a) True   b) True   c) True   d) False   e) False

EXPLANATION

Xenon is an inert gas and like krypton and argon has anaesthetic properties, but xenon is the only one that is anaesthetic under normobaric conditions. Xenon has many of the properties of an ideal anaesthetic agent and has been proposed as a carrier gas to replace nitrous oxide, which is probably the only anaesthetic agent which has not been superseded after many years of use. Xenon is more potent and insoluble than nitrous oxide. Induction and recovery are rapid. 60% xenon with 40% O_2 achieves anaesthesia within 5–6 minutes but full anaesthesia is not obtained; therefore like nitrous oxide it should really be employed as a carrier gas. Analgesia is better than with nitrous oxide and the stress response is also less. There is no myocardial depression with xenon. Cerebral blood flow is probably increased and, because xenon gas has a high density and high viscosity, airway resistance is slightly increased but this is not significant. The main drawback with xenon is its expense and it should thus be used in low flow anaesthesia.

Cerebral blood flow (CBF) can be measured by injecting a diffusible radioactive tracer. Radioactive xenon-133 in saline is injected as a bolus into the internal carotid artery and the rate at which radioactivity disappears from the head can be measured using extracranial radiation detectors. If CBF is high, the rate of washout will be fast and the slope of the washout curve steep; if CBF is low the washout rate is slow. Xenon-133 washouts are also used for ventilation/perfusion scans of the lung. The total number of counts over both lungs are obtained, and each lung is scanned separately through a split-function crystal and collimator. Ventilation and perfusion are reported as a percentage of overall function in each lung relative to the total number of radioactive counts taken over a specified period. Ventilation/perfusion measurements are important in patients having lung resections with borderline respiratory function. The predicted postoperative FEV_1 must exceed 800 ml to survive a pneumonectomy.

9.14   a) False   b) False   c) True   d) False   e) True

EXPLANATION
The human subject undergoes diurnal changes in sleep so that he is most awake in the early evening and most prone to sleep at night and in the early afternoon.

Sleep changes
Electroencephalograph. Normal sleep is divided into two phases depending on EEG changes – non-rapid eye movement (NREM) and rapid eye movement (REM) sleep. NREM sleep comprises four stages which are designated 1, 2, 3 and 4; 1 being the lightest and 4 the deepest sleep. In an awake subject the EEG activity is random and fast. In stage 1 NREM sleep there are low-frequency, low-amplitude theta waves. Stage 2 is characterized by large-amplitude biphasic waves and sleep spindles (short bursts of high-frequency activity). In deeper sleep (stages 3 and 4) there is further slowing and increased amplitude on the EEG (delta activity). In NREM sleep the brain is quiet and an electromyogram (EMG) shows activity in skeletal muscles. REM sleep is characterized by EEG activity similar to stage 1 of NREM sleep. The brain is active. REM sleep is associated with dreaming and there is no associated EMG muscle activity, although there may be involuntary periodic distal limb movement.

Chemical. Wakefulness is associated with activity in the ascending reticular activating system (RAS) so that increased activity in the RAS leads to wakefulness while decreased activity leads to sleep. There are a number of chemicals in the blood or acting as neurotransmitters which promote the 'awake state' or sleep. Arousal is induced by catecholamines, acetylcholine, histamine and substance P;

sleep by serotonin and GABA (gamma-aminobutyric acid). Barbiturates and benzodiazepines cause sedation by acting at the GABA receptor.

Respiratory. During sleep there is a slight reduction in minute ventilation and responses to hypoxia, hypercapnia airway obstruction and airway irritation are slightly impaired; functional residual capacity is reduced. With the onset of sleep, breathing is initially periodic and then becomes regular in NREM sleep. It again becomes irregular in REM sleep.

Cardiovascular system. Blood pressure and heart rate are normal during REM sleep but tend to decrease in NREM sleep.

9.15	a) False	b) True	c) True	d) False	e) True

EXPLANATION

In the past, agents such as ammonium salts, distilled water and hypertonic ice-cold saline were used as neurolytic agents, but they are rarely used now. The methods most commonly used today are:

- chemical with phenol, alcohol or glycerol
- physical with cryoanalgesia.

Nerve destruction procedures are mainly used in relieving chronic pain in terminal cancer patients and in relieving ischaemic pain by employing appropriate neurolytic sympathetic blocks. Ideally the neurolytic agents should disrupt pain pathways for many months without compromising other nervous pathways. Unfortunately neurolytic agents are non-selective; therefore in a mixed nerve with both sensory and motor components, such as the sciatic nerve, neurolytic destruction will be complicated by motor impairment. As might be expected the higher the concentration of the neurolytic agent, the more nerve damage it will cause. The chemical agents most commonly used are alcohol, phenol and glycerol. Alcohol is hypobaric and phenol hyperbaric to cerebrospinal fluid, and this must be taken into account when using these agents, especially when they are injected intrathecally. The nerve damage is not permanent, but lasts about 4–12 months. High concentrations of local anaesthetics can also be neurotoxic to nerve fibres.

Another problem of neurolytic injections is the formation of neuromas in damaged nerves. Axons can sprout out of the neuromas and, if these are sensory fibres, the patient complains of a burning pain (neurolytic neuritis) which can be just as incapacitating as the original pain. (e.g. genitofemoral neuritis causing a burning pain in the groin after a lumbar chemical sympathectomy).

Commonly performed procedures with chemical agents/physical destruction

Intercostal nerve blocks are useful in blocking somatic (superficial) pain associated with rib metastasis and pleural involvement. Several nerves have to be blocked because of dermatome overlap and intercostal neuritis from neuroma formation is a possibility. If the pain is transmitted through sympathetic pathways, a paravertebral block is more effective and this can be done at any level for pain secondary to neoplastic lesions. Visceral pain from stomach, pancreas, gall bladder and liver can be eased with coeliac plexus block. Sympathetic dystrophy and ischaemic pain of the lower limbs require lumbar sympathetic blocks. Intrathecal neurolytic injections is another method of controlling terminal cancer pain. Phenol is highly soluble in glycerine and diffuses slowly; for these reasons phenol is preferable to alcohol for intrathecal injections. Because phenol is hyperbaric, the patient lies with the painful area dependent and rotated backwards at 45 degrees so that the phenol spares the motor fibres. Sensory roots and ganglia can also be treated with neurolytic agents (e.g. gasserian ganglion block with glycerol for trigeminal neuralgia).

Apart from chemical agents, physical interruption to pain pathways can achieve the same effect. Cryoanalgesia is an example of this, and is used for the prolonged relief of post-thoracotomy pain. The exposed intercostal nerves are frozen by a tip cooled to −60° by high-pressure nitrous oxide.

9.16　a) **True**　b) **True**　c) **False**　d) **True**　e) **True**

EXPLANATION
Obstructive sleep apnoea (OSA) can occur both in children and adults. In children below 3 years of age, OSA is usually caused by adenotonsillar hypertrophy causing obstruction of the upper airway, hypoxaemia and alveolar hypoventilation; in severe cases it can lead to pulmonary hypertension and cor pulmonale. Adenotonsillectomy should be performed early to avoid complications. Premedication and analgesics should be used with caution in these patients. OSA can also occur in children with craniofacial abnormalities. In adults, smoking, alcohol and especially obesity are common factors associated with snoring and sleep apnoea. Weight loss is recommended in these patients and in some cases sleep splints to elevate the jaw, uvular palatopharyngoplasty and nasal continuous positive airway pressure to improve oxygenation may be indicated.

The obstruction can occur anywhere in the airway from the soft palate to the supraglottic region. Even nasal obstruction and insertion of nasal balloons can cause the syndrome.

Obstructive sleep apnoea is characterized by snoring with frequent sleep arousals. There are paradoxical movements of thorax and abdomen and hypoxaemia (oxygen saturations often below 85%) follows until arousal occurs, which is then followed by a snore in order for the subject to draw in oxygen. Sleep then returns. This sequence is repeated several hundred times during the night. The subject wakes up tired which, in children, can be detected as poor attention span, and poor school performance. Daytime somnolence, nocturnal enuresis and morning headaches are also possible. The persistent hypoxaemia increases myocardial work and in severe cases can lead to pulmonary hypertension and cor pulmonale.

9.17　a) **True**　b) **False**　c) **False**　d) **True**　e) **False**

EXPLANATION
See Table 9.3.

Table 9.3   Properties of addictive agents

Agents	Clinical	Withdrawal
Cocaine, amphetamines	CNS: stimulation – anxiety, agitation psychosis. CVS: tachycardia, hypertension, myocardial ischaemia, dilated pupils. Treatment: beta blockers. Ecstasy is a methylamphetamine which can cause fits, hyperthermia, hyperkalaemia, rhabdomyolysis, DIC	Agitation, insomnia, depression
Alcohol	Acute: agitation, disinhibition; then CNS, cardiac, respiratory depression; electrolyte abnormalities. Chronic: hepatic, pancreatic, gut damage, marrow depression – anaemia, leucopenia, thrombocytopenia; fits, polyneuropathy, dementia – Wernicke's and Korsakoff's syndromes, malnutrition with protein and vitamin deficiencies	Fits, delirium, hallucinations. Hyperadrenergic state: high BP, tachycardia, arrhythmias, cardiac failure. Treat with sedatives, beta blockers
Hallucinogens: cannabis, LSD, etc.	Acute stage: anxiety, panic, hallucinations due to increased catecholamine levels. CVS: tachy- or bradycardias, low BP. Respiratory system: bronchodilatation, respiratory depression, pulmonary oedema. Anticholinergic, antiemetic actions, depression of thermoregulatory mechanism	No withdrawal symptoms because there is no physical dependence

9.18   a) False   b) False   c) False   d) False   e) False

EXPLANATION

The aim of this procedure is to provide prolonged postoperative analgesia by inserting an epidural catheter between the visceral and parietal pleura and injecting repeated doses of local anaesthetic through the catheter. The local anaesthetic diffuses through the pleura to reach the intercostal nerves and the paravertebral space where the sympathetic chain is located. Neural blockade is strongly influenced by gravity, and the local anaesthetic will accumulate in the most dependent areas of the thorax. With intercostal nerve blocks only somatic analgesia is achieved; with intrapleural analgesia both the intercostal nerves and the sympathetic paravertebral chain are blocked, therefore visceral analgesia is also achieved.

Tolerance/dependence	Anaesthetic problems	Pregnancy
Limited tolerance Psychic dependence	Sympathetic effects make assessment of anaesthetic depth and blood loss and intravascular volume difficult	Sympathetic placental vasoconstriction decreases blood flow increasing incidence of abortion and premature labour. Higher incidence of congenital deformities
Steady tolerance. Liver enzyme induction causes cross-tolerance to sedatives	Acute: full stomach, raised intracranial pressure. Blood volume estimation masked by sympathetic stimulation. Lower doses of anaesthetic required Chronic: higher anaesthetic doses required because of enzyme induction. Possible liver damage (coagulopathy), low cholinesterase levels – action of suxamethonium prolonged	Increased incidence of abortion and abruptio placentae. Fetal alcohol syndrome: CNS and growth dysfunction, facial abnormalities causing difficult airway, possible cardiac, renal and liver problems
Rapid tolerance Psychic dependence	Acute stage: increased catecholamines – arrhythmias and increased anaesthetic doses. Chronic stage depletes catecholamines, thus less anaesthetic required	Similar to fetal alcohol syndrome (see above)

The patient is placed in the lateral position with the side to be blocked uppermost. After local infiltration with local anaesthetic, an epidural needle is inserted at the 6th, 7th or 8th rib in the mid-axillary line or more posteriorly. The needle is inserted until the rib is contacted and then it is 'walked off' the superior margin of the rib and advanced inwards. Puncture of the parietal pleura is identified by a distinct 'pop'. The epidural needle should be filled with saline, which is sucked in by the negative intrapleural pressure when the needle enters the interpleural space (hanging drop technique). Alternatively, the needle is attached to a syringe (without a plunger) filled with saline and, again, the saline is sucked into the interpleural space when it is entered. A third method is to attach the epidural needle to a syringe with a plunger containing 2 ml of air which is sucked in as the pleura is pierced. One should not rely on the 'loss of resistance' technique as with epidurals, because this leads to a high

Table 9.3 (Cont'd)

Agents	Clinical	Withdrawal
Narcotics: heroin, methadone, pethidine	Euphoria, lethargy, miosis (except pethidine – dilated pupils – atropine action), constipation, coma, depressed respiration, low BP	Cold turkey: lacrimation, yawning, sweating, goose flesh, fever, tachycardia, high BP, tachypnoea. Treatment: methadone, buprenorphine, clonidine and anticholinergic drugs to treat CVS signs
Sedatives: benzodiazepines, barbiturates	Disinhibition, agitation, progressive CNS depression and coma. Respiratory and cardiovascular depression but not with benzodiazepines	Fits, delirium, insomnia, headache, hypertension and tachycardia, fever. Treatment: sedatives
Volatile solvents: e.g. toluene (in glues), trichloroethane, butane, fluorocarbons in spray cans	Photophobia, eye irritation, diplopia, spots around mouth and nose, tinnitus, sneezing, cough, nausea, vomiting, diarrhoea, anorexia, myalgia, arrhythmias due to sensitization of heart to endogenous catecholamines which may cause sudden death especially with cardiac stimulation, e.g. exercise	No physical dependence

Key: BP = blood pressure; CNS = central nervous system; CVS = cardiovascular system; DIC = disseminated intravascular coagulation

Tolerance/dependence	Anaesthetic problems	Pregnancy
Marked tolerance and dependence with the mu agonist drugs. Partial agonists/antagonists have low dependence	Continue narcotics perioperatively. Advise detoxification with buprenorphine, methadone, clonidine	Increeased incidence of high BP in pregnancy. General anaesthesia in abusers complicated, with low BP if narcotics withdrawn. Fetus: increased incidence of poor growth, chromosomal abnormalities, decreased mental/neurological ability. Increased incidence of breech presentation, possible respiratory depression. Neonatal narcotic withdrawal – can last 4 months: tachypnoea, high-pitched cry, autonomic dysfunction. Treatment: sedatives, methadone, clonidine
Marked tolerance to sedation but not to other symptoms	Acute: additive with anaesthetics thus less required. Chronic: cross-tolerance due to enzyme induction – higher anaesthetic requirements	
Rapid tolerance	Possible hepatic, renal and bone marrow damage	

incidence of pneumothoraces. The catheter is then advanced 5–6 cm into the chest, secured and 20 ml of 0.25–0.5% bupivacaine injected. This should provide analgesia for 4–6 hours after which subsequent doses of local anaesthetic are administered.

Intrapleural analgesia has been used mostly to provide postoperative analgesia for cholecystectomy, mastectomy, nephrectomy, chest wall operations and rib fractures. It does not provide good results after thoracotomies because of loss of local anaesthetic through the chest drain; dilution of local anaesthetic by serum; rapid absorption of local anaesthetic through depleuralized areas; poor diffusion of local anaesthesia because of oedema.

Complications

1. Pneumothorax – high incidence if loss of resistance technique used, otherwise about 2%.
2. Local anaesthetic toxicity – large repeated doses of bupivacaine are usually employed and toxicity is not uncommon especially if 0.75% bupivacaine is used.
3. Others – pleural effusion; Horner's syndrome; phrenic nerve block.

9.19   a) True   b) False   c) False   d) True   e) False

EXPLANATION
First described in 1981, the causative agent of AIDS is a retrovirus termed the human immunodeficiency virus (HIV). The virus is surrounded by a protein envelope which attaches itself to a specific receptor on the host cell and the core viral material is then injected into the host cell, initiating the infection. Some individuals exposed to the virus develop an immunity to it, probably because a blocking agent at the receptor site prevents penetration of the virus into the host cell. The primary target of the virus is the T lymphocyte and slow destruction of the lymphocytes results in cell-mediated immunodeficiency with the development of serious infections and uncommon neoplasms. HIV also destroys cells of other organs – bowel, myocardium, adrenal cortex, neurons, haemopoietic cells – hence the multisystem nature of this infection.

Transmission is via contaminated blood and the high-risk groups include homosexuals, drug users, haemophiliacs, and infants of high-risk mothers.

Symptomatology
Acute stage. Most patients infected with HIV do not develop any clinical symptoms, a few develop a glandular-fever-type picture – fever, fatigue, rash and lymphadenopathy. These symptoms resolve while the virus continues to proliferate.

Asymptomatic stage. The patient now has serological evidence of infection and is capable of transmitting the disease, but can remain asymptomatic for many years.

Chronic lymphadenopathy stage. There is persistent generalized palpable lymphadenopathy. It usually lasts 3–5 years.

'Full-blown AIDS' stage. The cell immune deficiency continues over several years and is evidenced by falling T lymphocyte cell levels (less than 400 cells/ml). Different presentations occur during this stage and can be divided into five subgroups:

1. Subgroup A: fever, persistent diarrhoea, weight loss

2. Subgroup B: neurological disease, dementia, myelopathy, peripheral neuropathy tremors and extrapyramidal symptoms

3. Subgroup C: secondary infectious diseases, especially opportunistic infections:

- Viral: cytomegalovirus causing pneumonias, encephalitis, colitis, myocarditis, pericarditis; herpes simplex causing cutaneous, disseminated manifestations; Epstein–Barr virus causing oral hairy leucoplakia
- Fungal: *Candida* causing pharyngitis, oesophagitis, disseminated pathology, *Cryptococcus neoformans* causing meningitis, pneumonia, disseminated pathology; *Aspergillus* causing pneumonia, disseminated pathology.
- Protozoal: *Pneumocystis carinii*, the most common cause of pneumonia, complicated by viral and bacterial superinfection – presents with low pyrexia, tachypnoea, cough over a period of several weeks. Chest X-ray reveals bilateral infiltrates and restrictive lung disease. *Toxoplasma gondii* causing encephalitis, brain abscess, myocarditis
- Bacterial: mycobacteria causing enteritis, pneumonia, meningitis, disseminated manifestations; legionellae causing pneumonia; infections with non-opportunistic bacteria (e.g. tuberculosis, influenza, salmonellosis).

4. Subgroup D: secondary cancers, typically non-Hodgkin's lymphoma and Kaposi's sarcoma. About 50% of the lymphomas involve the CNS.

5. Subgroup E: other presentations not listed above, e.g. chronic lymphoid interstitial pneumonitis, other infectious diseases and neoplasms not listed above.

Diagnosis
Viral culture is difficult and not widely available. The primary detection test for AIDS is ELISA (enzyme-linked immunosorbent assay) which detects the presence of antibody to an extract of HIV grown in tissue culture. It is over 99% accurate; other confirmatory tests are available.

Anaesthetic evaluation
Pulmonary system. This is often compromised, especially by pneumonia caused by *Pneumocystis carinii*. Kaposi's sarcoma often involves the pulmonary system – causing pulmonary infiltrates – and the tracheobronchial area, which can cause tracheobronchial compression. Lung function tests: flow loops should identify the severity of the restrictive disease and tracheobronchial obstruction.

Cardiovascular system. Problems include myocarditis, pericarditis, pericardial effusions, and cardiomyopathies. Preoperative evaluation with electro- or echocardiography is important to discover cardiac involvement.

Central nervous system. CNS involvement affects over 50% of patients. Clinical presentation of encephalopathies includes dementia, motor weakness, tremors and peripheral neuropathies. There may be raised intracranial pressure due to tumours or cerebral abscesses. Magnetic resonance imaging is indicated.

Haemopoietic system. Problems include anaemia, thrombocytopenia and bleeding disorders. Zidovudine (AZT), radiation, chemotherapy and many antibiotics used to treat infections aggravate anaemia and thrombocytopenia. Packed red cells, platelets and fresh frozen plasma may be required especially before major surgery.

Gut. Problems include diarrhoea, oesophagitis leading to dehydration and electrolyte imbalance especially hyponatraemia, hypokalaemia.

Renal system. Hyponatraemia is present in 60% of AIDS patients. AIDS patients often develop renal disease – acute tubular necrosis, and HIV-associated nephropathy which often progresses rapidly to end-stage renal failure. The preoperative evaluation of renal function – creatinine and electrolyte measurements – is imperative.

The anaesthetic technique will depend on the preoperative evaluation. Droperidol and other drugs which can cause extrapyramidal symptoms should be avoided in patients who display a parkinsonism-like picture. Suxamethonium should be avoided in renal failure and myelopathy because of the risk of hyperkalaemia.

Transmission of AIDS to health care workers
Although HIV has been detected in many body fluids (blood, semen, vaginal secretions, urine, cerebrospinal fluid, breast milk, pleural effusions), by far the most infectious medium is blood. Every patient should be assumed to be contagious, and precautions should be adopted for all patients whether they are infected or not. The most likely source of HIV infection to a health worker is by an accidental needle-stick injury or exposure to secretions contaminated with infected blood. The risk of infection with a needle-stick injury from an infected patient is about 1% (with hepatitis B it is about 10%). Gloves should be worn for all patients whether infected or not. With AIDS patients, barrier precautions (gowns, protective eye wear, repeated washing of hands, great care in disposal of sharps and scalpels) must be used to prevent contamination by patients' blood or body fluids. If a worker suffers a stick injury from a contaminated needle, HIV testing should be performed immediately after the accident and again at 6, 12 and 24 weeks and at repeated intervals after that.

9.20   a) True   b) True   c) False   d) False   e) True

EXPLANATION

Physiology
Three groups of steroids are secreted by the adrenal cortex: glucocorticoids (cortisol), mostly produced from the central zona fasciculata; mineralocorticoids (aldosterone) mostly from the outer zona glomerulosa; sex hormones (mostly androgens) from the inner zona reticularis. Synthesis of adrenal corticoids is from cholesterol.

Glucocorticoids (cortisol)
Secretion of cortisol is under the influence of the hypothalamic-pituitary-adrenal axis. The hypothalamus secretes corticotrophin-releasing factor (CRF) which acts on the anterior pituitary gland for the latter to release adrenocorticotrophic hormone (ACTH). ACTH in turn stimulates the adrenal gland to release cortisol. There is a feedback mechanism so that the rising plasma cortisol levels inhibit release of CRF and ACTH, thus keeping plasma cortisol levels constant. There is a diurnal rhythm so that the greatest amount of cortisol is secreted in the morning. Glucocorticoid therapy suppresses ACTH secretion; this may eventually lead to atrophy of the adrenal gland which can last 2–12 months after treatment is stopped. Thus, when a patient is on steroid therapy in doses above the physiological secretion rate (above 30 mg hydrocortisone in 24 h) and the treatment is suddenly stopped, the secretion of ACTH may be suppressed and the response to stress impaired.

90% of the circulating cortisol is bound to cortisol-binding globulin (CBG); the rest to albumin. CBG is synthesized in the liver, and levels of CBG fall in liver disease as well as nephrotic syndrome, obesity and hypothyroidism. Levels of CBG are increased in pregnancy, hyperthyroidism, diabetes and with use of the contraceptive pill.

Pharmacological actions:

1. *Gluconeogenesis*, i.e. breakdown of proteins and their conversion to glycogen. Breakdown of protein causes reduction in muscle mass, growth retardation, thinning and ulceration of mucosa (possible peptic ulceration), osteoporosis, vertebral collapse, increased conversion into glycogen causing hyperglycaemia and predisposition to diabetes.

2. *Lymphoid tissue*. Glucocorticoids cause decreased activity in lymphoid tissue including thymus, spleen, tonsils and lymph nodes and decrease in circulating lymphocytes especially T lymphocytes. These effects cause reduction of antibody formation, thus accounting for the value of glucocorticoids in type I allergic reactions and as immunosuppressants (e.g. organ transplantation, autoimmune disease).

3. *Anti-inflammatory action*. This is due to the attachment of steroids to steroid receptors in target cells. Once attached to the receptor, an intracellular glycoprotein (lipocortin) is released which inhibits the enzyme phospholipase A_2 thus preventing the conversion of phospholipids into arachidonic acid; therefore the formation of prostaglandins is reduced. This anti-inflammatory effect may reactivate latent infections and activate peptic ulceration because the inhibition of prostaglandins synthesis leads to decreased gastric mucosal protection. The extent of anti-inflammatory action varies in different glucocorticoids. Hydrocortisone is the least potent; methylprednisolone and triamcinolone are about four times more potent, while dexamethasone is 30 times more anti-inflammatory.

4. *Fat mobilization*. Glucocorticoids mobilize fats from fat depots and convert them into ketones.

5. *Secondary effects*. Steroids are essential for other hormones (e.g. insulin, adrenaline) to exert their actions. Thus the hypotension and respiratory depression and delayed recovery from anaesthesia in adrenocortical insufficiency is probably due to diminished adrenaline action.

Mineralocorticoids (aldosterone)

The control of aldosterone release is the renin-angiotensin system. Renin secreted in the kidney acts on angiotensinogen in the liver to form angiotensin I which is converted to angiotensin II in the lung. Angiotensin II regulates the secretion of aldosterone from the adrenal gland. Aldosterone acts on the distal renal tubules to cause retention of sodium and water and release of potassium. Renin is synthesized in the juxtaglomerular cells in renal arterioles and these cells are sensitive to pressure changes within the arterioles. Thus, when the blood pressure is low, the drop in pressure in the arterioles releases renin which promotes the secretion of angiotensin (a potent vasoconstrictor) and aldosterone, causing vasoconstriction and water and salt retention to bring the blood pressure up again. Corticosteroids with marked mineralocorticoid activity (e.g. aldosterone, fludrocortisone) may cause oedema, hypertension and cardiac failure.

Indication for corticosteroids are numerous and include anaphylaxis, bronchial asthma, cerebral oedema, active chronic hepatitis, Crohn's disease, ulcerative colitis, haemolytic anaemia, malignancies (both for treatment and pain reduction from anti-inflammatory actions), nephrotic syndrome, rheumatoid arthritis, systemic lupus erythematosus, polyarteritis nodosa, temporal arteritis, fibrosing alveolitis, thrombocytopenic purpura, transplantation rejection, etc. They are also used by local application (and sometimes systemically) in a variety of skin conditions (eczema, discoid lupus erythematosus, lichen planus), in ear, nose and throat conditions (e.g. allergic rhinitis) and ophthalmic conditions (e.g. allergic conjunctivitis, keratitis, uveitis).

Side-effects

- Increased tissue breakdown – muscle wasting, growth stunting, myopathy, osteoporosis, vertebral collapse, thinning of skin mucosa and hair, bruising and petechiae, haemorrhages, impaired wound healing.
- Glycogenesis – hyperglycaemia, diabetes.
- Anti-inflammatory effects – suppression of immunological responses, diminished resistance to infection and reactivation of latent infection, peptic ulceration.
- Fat deposition – facial (cushingoid facies), truncal and supraclavicular obesity.
- Mineralocorticoid effects – salt and water retention causing oedema, hypertension, cardiac failure, hypokalaemia.
- Others – dependence, euphoria, depression psychosis, acne, peripheral neuropathy, cataract.

Anaesthesia and steroids

Apart from the side-effects of prolonged steroid intake, which may affect the choice of anaesthetic, there are some aspects of steroid therapy of anaesthetic interest.

Anaesthesia and stress response. One of the metabolic responses to stress in major surgery is the increase of secretion of hydrocortisone from 30 mg/day to 100–300 mg/day. If a patient is on steroid therapy, this response is suppressed because of adrenal atrophy. Therefore if these patients are not given supplementary steroids there is a danger of hypotension and cardiovascular collapse during surgery. This can be prevented by the administration of 100 mg hydrocortisone 8-hourly on the day of surgery with the dose reduced slowly postoperatively over 3–5 days. This regime should be instituted for every patient who has been on steroid therapy within 6–12 months of surgery, because adrenal suppression persists for a period of at least 2 months and possibly 12 months. During minor surgery, if a patient is on steroid therapy or has stopped taking steroid 3–12 months earlier, it is probably sufficient to give a single dose of hydrocortisone on the day of surgery.

Etomidate and adrenal suppression. There is evidence suggesting that even a single dose of etomidate can suppress adrenal function. In practice the only adverse effect from this adrenal suppression is in the intensive therapy unit set-up, where infusions of etomidate can cause an increased incidence of hypotension and mortality.

Steroids as antiemetics. In 1981 dexamethasone was reported as being an effective antiemetic in patients receiving chemotherapy. The mechanism of this antiemetic effect is not clear, but may be related to central inhibition of prostaglandins synthesis or decreased serotonin levels in the central nervous system. Dexamethasone has also been shown to be useful in reducing postoperative nausea and vomiting and some studies have showed combinations of ondansetron and dexamethasone to be more effective than ondansetron alone.

10.1 With regard to sympathetic dystrophy:

a) Causalgia is a sympathetic dystrophy associated with peripheral nerve damage
b) It may follow explorations on the lumbar spine
c) The skin is cold and white in the initial stage, warm and red in later stages
d) Sympathetic blocks are more successful if done in the early stages
e) A successful sympathectomy with phenol provides permanent pain relief

10.2 With regard to rheumatoid arthritis:

a) Mainly peripheral joints are involved
b) In patients with cervical spine subluxation, neck extension is usually more dangerous than flexion
c) Cervical subluxation is commonly at the atlantoaxial joint
d) Laryngeal joints are rarely involved
e) A patient with cervical spine rheumatoid arthritis is likely to have a Mallampati Class 1 score

10.3 With regard to factors affecting cerebral function:

a) The brain has large tissue stores of essential oxygen and glucose
b) A computed tomography (CT) scan is better at detecting cerebral ischaemia than magnetic resonance imaging (MRI)
c) A CT scan is better at detecting an intracranial haematoma than MRI
d) Both hypoglycaemia and hyperglycaemia can be harmful in neurosurgically compromised patients
e) By reducing metabolic demand, barbiturates improve the prognosis in patients with diffuse cerebral hypoxia

10.4 Of the fentanyls:

a) Sufentanil is preferable to fentanyl in renal failure
b) Accumulation with repeated doses/infusions is less of a problem with remifentanil than with fentanyl
c) Metabolism of remifentanil is similar to the other fentanyls
d) Duration of action from shortest to longest follows the sequence: remifentanil < alfentanil < sufentanil < fentanyl
e) Alfentanil is more lipid soluble than fentanyl

10.5 With regard to contaminants in breathing circuits:

a) Denitrogenation is 80% complete in a patient breathing 100% oxygen for 1 minute at normal tidal volumes
b) If the temperature within the soda lime is kept constantly low, production of carbon monoxide steadily increases during a prolonged operation
c) Presence of methane in breathing circuits can affect vaporizer readings
d) Plasma carboxyhaemoglobin levels are higher in a non-smoker anaesthetized with soda lime/sevoflurane, compared to a mild smoker who is not subjected to any anaesthesia
e) Bone cement can cause vasodilatation and hypotension

10.6 With regard to pulmonary oedema:

a) It is always bilateral
b) It is more likely to occur postoperatively than during surgery
c) Protein levels in oedema fluid are invariably high
d) Diuretics are always indicated
e) It can be a complication of respiratory obstruction and neurological insults

10.7 With regard to the gut and multiple organ failure:

a) High gastric intramural pH is a bad prognostic feature in critically ill patients
b) The administration of broad spectrum antibiotics to critically ill patients invariably diminishes bacterial invasion through the gut
c) Splanchnic hypoperfusion is characteristic
d) Noradrenaline is likely to be more beneficial than dopexamine
e) Nitric oxide therapy may help in reducing pathogenic invasion through the gut

10.8 With regard to gamma-aminobutyric acid (GABA):

a) It is an inhibitory neurotransmitter
b) Anaesthetics act on $GABA_A$ receptors
c) Barbiturates and benzodiazepines bind to the $GABA_B$ receptor
d) Drugs that act on GABA receptors tend to cause convulsions
e) Flumazenil competes with benzodiazepines for the binding site on GABA receptors

10.9 With regard to postoperative pain relief:

a) Postoperative pain is more severe following a craniotomy than after decompression laminectomy
b) Intercostal nerve blocks are more effective in relieving postoperative pain than paravertebral blocks
c) Adequate postoperative pain relief reduces the incidence of respiratory complications and thrombosis
d) Patient-controlled analgesia is safer than continuous opiate infusion
e) For relieving post-thoracotomy pain, epidural/intrathecal fentanyl inserted at the lumbar level is more effective than morphine injected at the same site

10.10 With regard to opioid analgesics:

a) Compared to adults, children between 6 and 12 months of age are more prone to respiratory depression after opioid administration
b) The metabolite of morphine – morphine-6-glucuronide – has very little morphine activity
c) Partial agonists are useful analgesics to treat postoperative pain in a heroin (diamorphine) addict because of their relatively low addictive potential
d) Absorption of diamorphine by the subcutaneous route is better than by intramuscular injections
e) The metabolite of pethidine – norpethidine – stimulates the central nervous system

10.11 With regard to anaesthetic injuries:

a) Maternal mortality is not reduced by performing caesarean sections under regional anaesthesia as compared to general anaesthesia
b) Brachial plexus injuries are most likely with arms fully abducted and externally rotated
c) Venous embolism tends to cause focal or generalized cerebral damage; arterial embolism causes reduction in cardiac output
d) Anaesthetic mortality is higher during anaesthesia than in the recovery period
e) The most common cause of anaesthetic mortality is hypoxaemia associated with hypoventilation

10.12 Laryngospasm:

a) Is more likely in young children than in adults
b) Is more likely with sevoflurane induction than with isoflurane
c) Incidence is reduced if patients stop smoking 24 hours prior to surgery
d) Tends to be caused more by thiopentone than by propofol
e) Incidence is not increased by upper respiratory tract infections

10.13 With regard to pacemakers during surgery:

a) Pacemakers threshold is not altered by electrolytic or pH changes
b) Monopolar diathermy is safer than bipolar
c) Ventricular demand pacemakers may diminish cardiac output, while atrial demand pacemakers tend to increase it
d) Halothane should be avoided
e) They can be a cause of ventricular fibrillation

10.14 With regard to the causes and prediction of difficult intubation:

a) The Cormack and Lahane classification predicts difficulty depending on the extent of laryngeal structures viewed with a laryngoscope
b) Intubation is likely to be difficult if the angle between maximal neck extension and flexion is less than $90°$
c) In Pierre Robin syndrome, intubation is likely to be difficult because of the possible presence of micrognathia and cleft palate
d) Laryngeal oedema is more prone to develop in the supraglottic region than in the subglottic area
e) In a patient with carcinoma of the tongue, intubation will almost certainly be easier after radiotherapy treatment

10.15   **With regard to anaesthetic problems among diabetic patients:**

a) Non-insulin-dependent diabetics are more likely to develop ketoacidosis compared to insulin-dependent diabetics
b) Diabetics with autonomic neuropathy often have prolonged QT intervals on the electrocardiography which make them more susceptible to arrhythmias
c) Insulin-dependent diabetics undergoing major surgery should be stabilized on a glucose/insulin infusion many days before surgery
d) Pulmonary function tests are normal in the vast majority of long-standing diabetic patients
e) Intubation may be difficult because of stiffness of the atlantoaxial joint

10.16   **In adult respiratory distress syndrome:**

a) Pulmonary wedge pressures tend to be elevated
b) Hypoxaemia is improved significantly by increasing inspired oxygen tensions
c) The condition can be caused by aspiration
d) High ventilator pressures should be employed during intermittent positive-pressure ventilation (IPPV) to increase tidal volumes
e) IPPV with hypercapnia can be beneficial

10.17   **With regard to awareness during anaesthesia:**

a) Pain stimulus is the modality most likely to be remembered
b) Awareness is more likely with nitrous oxide/oxygen/relaxant/vapour anaesthetic compared to nitrous oxide/oxygen/relaxant/opioids
c) The incidence of auditory awareness is increased with atropine
d) Over 80% of patients who have suffered awareness during anaesthesia develop post-traumatic stress disorders
e) It is most common with obstetric and cardiac anaesthesia

10.18   **Of the sympathomimetic drugs:**

a) Dobutamine selectively increases renal and mesenteric blood flow
b) Methoxamine is a drug of choice in treating hypotension following spinals especially in patients with cardiac problems
c) High-dose dopamine infusions cause more vasoconstriction and rises in blood pressure than high-dose dobutamine infusions
d) Dobutamine stimulates dopaminergic receptors
e) Noradrenaline has mild alpha and strong beta actions

10.19   **Anaesthetic implications of hepatic impairment include:**

a) The vast majority of oxygen delivery to the liver is derived via the portal vein
b) Halothane is the only anaesthetic vapour which reduces liver oxygen delivery
c) Pancuronium is preferable to rocuronium
d) There is a possibility of hyperdynamic circulation with increased blood volume and cardiac output
e) The albumin/globulin ratio is high

10.20 In a patient who requires ventilatory support after a severe head injury, the following would make a diagnosis of brain death unacceptable:

a) Residual activity on an electroencephalogram
b) Hypothermia
c) Limb movements
d) Pupils fixed but not widely dilated
e) No pupil reaction in response to irrigation of the ipsilateral ear with ice-cold water

EXPLANATION

Reflex sympathetic dystrophy

This is a syndrome of continuous limb pain, usually burning, secondary to injury or a noxious stimulus and characterized by sensory, motor, autonomic and trophic changes.

There are three stages of clinical presentation (Table 10.1).

Clinical tests to detect sympathetic impairment include measurement of skin temperature with thermometry/thermography, bone X-rays and scans, and response to sympathetic blockade.

Treatment:

1. *Sympathetic blocks.* If sympathetic blockade is started in the acute stage the chances of remission are high. Sympathetic blockade can be achieved in a number of ways:

- Repeated peripheral sympathetic blocks using drugs (e.g. guanethidine) which reduce alpha-adrenergic activity by blocking reuptake of noradrenaline. The technique is similar to a Bier's block, i.e. cuff inflated to above systolic pressure, i.v. guanethidine administered, cuff left inflated for 15–20 minutes. Recent studies have questioned the efficacy of this technique.
- Use of alpha-adrenergic blockers, e.g. phenoxybenzamine.
- Repeated stellate ganglion or lumbar sympathetic blocks with local anaesthetics. A few patients obtain complete relief with one block; others require repeated injections daily until symptoms improve.
- Continuous infusion of the sympathetic chain either by continuous sympathetic block or epidurals.
- Chemical sympathectomy with phenol or alcohol which can produce a sympathetic block of up to 12 months.

2. *Analgesic non-steroidal anti-inflammatory drugs (NSAIDs).* These are helpful in controlling inflammation, but narcotics should be avoided because of tolerance and addiction. Ketorolac has been used in intravenous regional blocks.

Table 10.1   Sympathetic dystrophy: stages of clinical presentation

Stage	Onset of symptoms	Pain	Skin
Acute	Immediately or several weeks after injury	Burning spontaneous pain and pain to a normally non-noxious stimulus – either mechanical or to cold (allodynia) or delayed pain after a stimulus (hyperpathia)	Warm; dry and red with slight oedema
Dystrophic	Weeks to 6 months after injury	Hyperpathia and allodynia more pronounced	Cyanotic, white, cold, brittle nails, oedema more diffuse. Increased sweating, osteoporosis
Atrophic	Within 6–12 months	Pain, hyperpathia and allodynia less pronounced	Cold, more atrophic changes with muscle atrophy and joint contractures

3. *Alternative medication.* Antidepressants may be helpful; oral or epidural clonidine has been tried as well as anticonvulsants, calcitonin and corticosteroids, and calcium blockers, all with variable results.

4. *Others.* Transcutaneous electrical nerve stimulation (TENS) and dorsal column stimulation may occasionally be beneficial. Since TENS is non-invasive it is worth a trial; however, in a few patients it may actually increase pain. Dorsal column stimulation may also be of benefit. Possible modes of action include stimulation of the large myelinated fibres blocking pain transmission in the spinal cord (gate theory); or else dorsal column stimulation releases endogenous opioids.

Causalgia

Causalgia is a specific sympathetic dystrophy associated with peripheral nerve injury. The picture is often similar to sympathetic dystrophy but without the clear-cut stages. The pain is severe, continuous and burning and occurs in the distribution of the injured nerve or may involve the entire limb. The treatment is the same as with sympathetic dystrophy. Surgical sympathectomy provides excellent relief in 85% of patients with causalgia.

10.2	a) True	b) False	c) True	d) False	e) False

EXPLANATION

Joints. All joints may be involved but mainly the peripheral joints. The synovium is primarily affected leading to fibrosis, joint destruction and deformity of the cervical spine. The temperomandibular and cricoarytenoid joints may be affected, making intubation difficult.

Cervical spine. The spine may be unstable or fused. Cervical spine instability occurs in 25% of patients with rheumatoid arthritis (RA). The commonest problem is atlantoaxial subluxation and possible migration of the odontoid peg backwards and upwards, which may compress the spinal cord. Compression is more likely to occur with neck flexion than extension. A lateral and flexion X-ray of the cervical spine will show the distance between the odontoid peg and posterior border of the anterior arch of atlas. If subluxation is present, this gap is greater than 3 mm in a flexion X-ray. Unless the rare complication of posterior atlantoaxial subluxation is present, gentle neck extension for tracheal intubation is usually safe. With severe subluxation, fibreoptic intubation may be required to minimize cervical manipulation. Rheumatoid arthritic patients may also have a fused cervical spine which again may make intubation difficult. (Mallampati intubation difficulty class is likely to be 3–4 in these patients.)

Temperomandibular joints. Involvement of these joints is very common (about 80%) in RA patients. Mouth opening is reduced making intubation very difficult.

Cricoarytenoid joints. Involvement of these joints occurs in 50% of RA patients. Inflammation of the joints can cause narrowing of the larynx, immobilization of vocal cords, possible change in voice, throat fullness and dyspnoea on exertion. Laryngeal narrowing may require a smaller endotracheal tube.

Extra-articular problems. These occur in over 50% of patients.

Pulmonary. Pleural effusions, pulmonary nodules, pulmonary fibrosis, and arteritis are all possible, causing impaired gas exchange, reduced diffusion capacity and pulmonary hypertension (due to arteritis).

Cardiac. Problems include pericarditis, myocarditis, endocarditis, coronary arteritis causing myocardial ischaemia, valve involvement, conduction defects.

Haematological. Problems include mild anaemia, thrombocytopenia,

Blood vessels. Infiltration of vessel walls with mononuclear cells predisposes to thrombosis and ischaemia. The vasculitis usually involves smaller arteries.

Kidney. 25% of patients die from renal failure which is due to vasculitis or amyloid disease.

Drugs. These patients are often on NSAIDs, gold salts, methotrexate. Increased bleeding, renal and adrenal insufficiency and fragile vessels may result from prolonged therapy.

Peripheral neuropathy. This is secondary to vasculitis. In mild cases there are distal sensory disturbances; in severe cases, sensory and motor problems.

10.3   a) False   b) False   c) True   d) True   e) False

EXPLANATION

The human brain weighs 1500 g (i.e. 2% of adult body weight) yet receives 15–20% of cardiac output. Thus the brain has a very high blood flow; on the other hand, there is little tissue storage of essential oxygen and glucose. The incidence of perioperative stroke during surgery is about 0.04% in patients below the age of 50; 0.2% in the elderly. The incidence increases in specific operations which predispose to strokes: 10% in carotid endarterectomy; 7% in cardiopulmonary bypass surgery and much higher in neurosurgical procedures. If a stroke is suspected, a CT scan should be done, although evidence of ischaemia may not be evident for many hours. MRI detects ischaemic damage earlier but a CT scan is much better at detecting an intracranial haematoma.

Factors affecting brain protection

Reduction in metabolic rate does not always provide cerebral protection.

Reduction of metabolic demand. It seems logical that the brain should be protected if metabolic demands are reduced and many anaesthetic agents reduce cerebral metabolic rate. However, the only anaesthetic drugs which have been shown to be of any benefit are barbiturates. It has been shown that during focal ischaemia barbiturate therapy improves outcome, but when the ischaemia is widespread, e.g. following hypoxia, barbiturates do not seem to be of any value. Other anaesthetic agents which are known to reduce cerebral metabolic rate (e.g. isoflurane, etomidate, midazolam, propofol) do not provide any protection.

Reduction of metabolic demand by hypothermia. Hypothermia reduces both cerebral metabolic rate and EEG activity. Infants undergoing cardiac surgery can withstand hypothermic circulatory arrest for 1 hour; adults for 45 minutes. Deep hypothermia is only used in open heart surgery, but it is likely that even moderate hypothermia to 33–34°C may offer protection in high-risk cerebrovascular procedures.

Glucose. Although the brain is dependent on endogenous glucose for maintenance of energy requirements, glucose administration to a patient with cerebral ischaemia is detrimental. In the absence of oxygen, energy is maintained by anaerobic glycolysis which leads to intracellular acidosis. Therefore glucose infusion in these conditions increases acidosis, which worsens the prognosis of cerebral ischaemia. If a patient undergoing a major neurological procedure or suffering from cerebral ischaemia is found to have hyperglycaemia, insulin should be considered to correct this.

Fluid administration. Traditionally patients who have had neurological insults are kept dry to reduce brain water content. Thus fluid is restricted or water excretion increased by the administration of mannitol and steroids (the benefit of the latter is doubtful). However, one must take into account that a fall in the intravascular volume may be accompanied by hypotension and a reduction in cerebral perfusion.

Osmolarity plays an important role in determining brain water content and reduction of plasma osmolarity significantly increases cerebral oedema. Therefore hypotonic solutions should be avoided in these patients. As explained above, dextrose infusion can be harmful as it causes acidosis; it also leaves the circulation rapidly and increases brain water content. The latter argument also applies to Hartmann's solution and, thus, isotonic saline is probably the best crystalloid for neurosurgically compromised patients, especially in the presence of hypovolaemia.

10.4	a) False	b) True	c) False	d) True	e) False

EXPLANATION
See Table 10.2.

10.5	a) True	b) False	c) True	d) False	e) True

EXPLANATION
Apart from fresh gas flow and anaesthetic vapour, there are a number of contaminants which can accumulate in breathing circuits and can have some detrimental effects on patients. The most important contaminants (and potential problems) are:

- nitrogen – hypoxia risk
- compound A – potential renal toxicity but not a clinical problem
- carbon monoxide – levels never high enough to cause a problem
- BCDFE – nil
- methane – can interfere with vapour analyser readings
- acetone – nausea, vomiting, sedation if levels above 50 mg/ml
- hydrogen – potentially explosive but not a clinical problem
- alcohol
- bone cement – vasodilatation and fall in blood pressure.

Nitrogen. The presence of nitrogen in the breathing circuit obviously reduces the concentration of inspired oxygen and one of the advantages of preoxygenation is to wash out the nitrogen. Denitrogenation is 80% complete if a patient breathes 100% oxygen for 1 minute at normal tidal waves. However, if the mask does not fit properly causing leakages, deoxygenation occurs rapidly. Preoxygenating a patient with 100% oxygen for 1 minute will maintain SaO_2 above 93% during apnoea for at least 3 minutes, while 3 minutes of 100% preoxygenation will double the period of 'safe'

Table 10.2 Properties of fentanyls

Agent	Potency	Onset/duration
Fentanyl	100 times more potent than morphine	Highly lipid soluble; thus rapid onset (30 s); half-life 200 min. 100 μg provides analgesia for 10–20 min; larger doses longer
Transdermal fentanyl	25 patch equivalent to 10 mg morphine sulphate twice a day	Four patch strengths available: 25, 50, 75, 100 providing 25–100 μg/hour over 3 days. Plasma fentanyl increases slowly over 12–18 to achieve constant levels for 3 days
Sufentanil	5–10 times more potent than fentanyl	Rapid analgesia. Duration less than fentanyl
Alfentanil	5–10 times less potent than fentanyl	Onset: 1–2 min. Duration: 5–10 min
Remifentanil	Similar to fentanyl. 15–30 times more potent than alfentanil	Onset of action similar to alfentanil (1–2 min), but shorter duration

Metabolism	Effects	Comments
By dealkalation, hydroxylation and hydrolysis to norfentanyl and despropionorfentanyl. Less than 8% excreted in urine – safe in renal failure	Usual miosis; nausea, vomiting. Marked respiratory depression and analgesia. Low sedation at low doses (1–2 μg/kg); at high doses sedation marked due to accumulation. Bradycardia especially with high doses. Sedation and CVS effects unlikely. Incidence of nausea and vomiting about 50%. Possible respiratory depression, muscle rigidity	Oral administration not feasible because of first pass metabolism and low availability (32%). However, transmucosal fentanyl increases bioavailability to 52%
		Advantages: decreased first pass metabolism; constant plasma levels; ease of administration. Drawbacks: inability to titrate dose to analgesic requirements; thus supplemental analgesics may be required; slow onset; residual analgesia after removal of patch
Rapidly metabolized in liver. Excreted equally renally and in gut. Some of the metabolites are active; thus it should be used with caution in renal disease	More sedating than fentanyl. Bradycardia, miosis, nausea, vomiting, respiratory depression	Has been used for patient-controlled and epidural analgesia. Highly lipid soluble – possibility of transdermal patch becoming available
Rapidly metabolized in liver. Action prolonged in liver failure. Safe in renal failure	Similar to other opiates, but of short duration	Less lipid soluble than fentanyl. Can be used epidurally or intrathecally.
Fentanyl derivative with an ester linkage. Ester linkage broken down by plasma esterases to inactive carboxylic acid derivative which is renally excreted but safe in renal and hepatic failure	Analgesia, respiratory depression nausea, vomiting – rarely a problem because of short duration. Since metabolism is rapid, accumulation is unlikely with repeated boluses or infusions	Formulated in glycine which is an inhibitory neurotransmitter; thus should not be used epidurally or intrathecally

219

apnoea to 6 minutes. Thus 3 minutes of 100% preoxygenation without leaks will 80% denitrogenate the patient within the first minute and keep SaO_2 above 90% for 6 minutes during apnoea.

Compound A (fluoromethyldifluorovinyl ether). Sevoflurane is absorbed and degraded by soda lime (calcium hydroxide 94%; sodium hydroxide 5%; potassium hydroxide 1%) and baralyme (calcium hydroxide 80%; barium hydroxides 20%). One of the breakdown products is compound A which has been shown to cause renal toxicity in rats. The concentration of compound A is dependent on temperature and the presence of water vapour, i.e. the concentration is higher with higher temperatures and if the soda lime is allowed to dry out. Heat production is greater with baralyme than with soda lime so the degradation into compound A is higher with the former. However, in clinical practice the concentration of compound A is well below the concentration achieved in rats and there is no evidence of renal damage in humans.

Carbon monoxide. Anaesthetic vapours containing a CF_2 group (desflurane, isoflurane and enflurane but not sevoflurane or halothane) can break down in soda lime and baralyme to produce carbon monoxide. As with compound A, the concentration increases with higher temperatures and with dry soda lime. Since the reaction of CO_2 and hydroxides produces water, the soda lime is likely to be driest at the beginning of an operation and the longer the operation lasts the less the formation of carbon monoxide. As with compound A, in clinical practice, the concentration of CO_2 is not high enough to cause clinical problems. To put it into perspective, even mild smokers have a higher concentration of carboxyhaemoglobin than that produced with dry soda lime.

BCDFE (bromochlorodifluoroethylene). This is produced by interaction between halothane and soda lime. It does not appear to cause any clinical problems and is not a causative agent of halothane hepatitis.

Methane. Methane is produced by gut bacteria and the amount generated is very variable because the numbers of bacteria differ considerably in different patients. Methane is very insoluble, is not absorbed by charcoal filters, is an inflammable gas and is cleared very rapidly in the lungs. The only clinical problem with the presence of methane in a breathing circuit is that it can interfere with vapour analyser readings. It has been shown that the presence of 1000 parts per million of methane gives a false reading on a halothane (and other vapours) vaporizer of +1%; therefore the inspired vapour concentrate may be less than the vaporizer setting, and there is then a danger of patient awareness during anaesthesia.

Acetone. This is generated by oxidative metabolism of free fatty acids and levels may be elevated with prolonged fasting, diabetes and alcoholism. Acetone is highly water soluble and is difficult to flush out of breathing systems even if fresh gas flow is increased. When blood levels rise to over 50 mg/ml there is an increased incidence of postoperative nausea and vomiting and prolonged sedation.

Hydrogen. Again a metabolite of gut bacteria, hydrogen is excreted by the lung, diffuses easily through rubber and silicone, and is a very insoluble gas which is therefore easy to flush out from breathing circuits. It is inflammable and therefore potentially explosive, although this is very unlikely to be a problem.

Alcohol. This may have been self-administered. Levels in the breathing system are secondary to plasma levels, and elimination is via the liver. Alcohol is highly soluble and therefore difficult to flush out of the system.

Bone cement (methylmethacrylate monomer). Bone cement, used for hip/knee replacements etc., is a highly volatile agent and remains volatile until fully polymerized; excretion is entirely in the lungs. It is rapidly absorbed, and toxic levels in the rat cause vasodilatation; this action probably explains the drop in blood pressure when the cement is used.

10.6   **a) False**   **b) True**   **c) False**   **d) False**   **e) True**

EXPLANATION
See Table 10.3.

10.7   **a) False**   **b) False**   **c) True**   **d) False**   **e) True**

EXPLANATION
There is increasing evidence to suggest that in critically ill patients breakdown of the intestinal protection barrier, which normally prevents bacterial and toxin invasion, has an important role to play in the development of multiple organ failure. Under normal conditions the intestinal barrier is maintained by the normal anaerobic flora in the gut, by gut secretions and peristalsis, by the action of immune cells in the gut; and by the integrity of the gut epithelium.

- Normal anaerobic gut flora: limit colonization by other potentially harmful organisms. If these anaerobic microbes are destroyed by broad spectrum antibiotics, pathogenic Gram-negative bacilli, Gram-positive cocci and fungi can take over.
- Gut secretions: mucins create a mucosal gel layer which protects against bacterial invasion. Mucins are also rich in antibodies.
- Immune gut protection: the length of the small intestine is lined with lymphoid tissue (Peyer's patches) which produces numerous immunoactive cells – lymphocytes, plasma cells, etc.
- Integrity of intestinal epithelium: the intestine is lined with columnar epithelium arranged into villi. If this epithelium is breached, the pathogenic and toxin invasion can follow.

Factors which interfere with intestinal epithelial integrity. The prime cause of breakdown of the intestinal barrier in critically ill patients is splanchnic hypoperfusion. Haemorrhagic and cardiogenic shock and sepsis all lead to mesenteric vasoconstriction in order to maintain adequate perfusion to vital organs. The splanchnic hypoperfusion is followed by increased glycolysis and anaerobic metabolism to maintain adequate energy levels, causing intestinal mucosal acidosis. Once the acidosis sets in, adenosine triphosphate (ATP) levels are depleted, oxidants and cytokines are released and intracellular calcium is increased. All these factors help to increase permeability. There is also evidence suggesting that nitric oxide maintains the intestinal barrier and the administration of nitric oxide may be of use in critically ill patients to reduce intestinal permeability. Other conflicting evidence, however, suggests that overproduction of nitric oxide can actually increase epithelial permeability.

Monitoring. Since mucosal acidosis is inevitable in these critically ill patients, pH measurement may be a useful monitoring tool; in fact low intragastric pH has been shown to be a bad prognostic sign in patients with multiple organ failure.

Table 10.3 Pulmonary oedema

	Pathogenesis	Causes
Cardiac	Increase in pulmonary capillary pressure because of high left atrial pressure	1. Increased left atrial pressure: mitral stenosis; mitral myxoma 2. Increased right atrial pressure: fluid retention or overload 3. Increased afterload, i,e. hypertension, vasoconstriction, mechanical obstruction 4. Reduced myocardial contractility: infarction; cardiomyopathy
Pulmonary	Increased permeability of pulmonary capillaries	1. Pulmonary aspiration 2. Pneumonias; septicaemias 3. Adult respiratory distress syndrome 4. Allergic reactions 5. Air and amniotic fluid embolism 6. Drugs: beta-2 agonists used to suppress premature labour
Neurological	Brain insult leads to massive sympathetic discharge causing intense vasoconstriction and increased afterload. Pulmonary capillary damage also causes pulmonary leakage	Head injury, tumours, cerebrovascular accidents; also naloxone reversal of opiates can rarely produce intense sympathetic discharge and pulmonary oedema
Relief of respiratory obstruction	Marked negative intrathoracic pressures due to inspiratory attempts against obstruction increase pulmonary capillary permeability and hypoxic pulmonary vasoconstriction	Croup; epiglottitis; laryngospasm; upper airway lesions; tumours, e.g. mediastinal. May be unilateral after lung is reinflated if collapsed by pneumothorax, effusion, tumour

Clinical	Treatment	Comments
Dyspnoea, cyanosis, high BP; sweating, pink frothy sputum; basal crepitations. Chest X-ray: cardiac enlargement. ECG: hypertrophy; arrhythmias; ischaemia	Sit up; oxygen; intermittent positive-pressure ventilation (IPPV). Morphine reduces agitation and causes venodilation; frusemide. Atrial fibrillation: verapamil; digoxin; inotropes if there is poor myocardial contractility	<u>More likely postoperatively than</u> during surgery, because <u>vasoconstriction is more</u> likely postoperatively owing to pain and withdrawal of anaesthetic agents
Same as above	Same as above	If due to leaking pulmonary capillaries, protein level in oedema fluid is high whereas in cardiac causes, protein levels are low
Clinical signs of pulmonary oedema together with intense vasoconstriction – <u>cold</u>, pallor sweating	Oxygen; IPPV;? positive end-expiratory pressure. Reduction of raised intracranial pressure with IPPV and perhaps surgery. Reduction of vasoconstriction best with alpha blockers, e.g. <u>phenoxybenzamine</u> ✳ or vasodilators – nitroprusside; diuretics if there is fluid overload	
Clinical features of pulmonary oedema preceded by severe respiratory obstruction. Chest X-ray: normal cardiac size	Oxygen; IPPV; diuretics not usually required	

Treatment. Since the primary problem in these patients is poor splanchnic blood flow, one should attempt to improve splanchnic perfusion, though, paradoxically, improved flow is not always associated with increased gastric pH. Any hypovolaemia should be corrected, while sympathomimetic amines are frequently used to improve organ perfusion. The alpha effects of dopamine, noradrenaline and adrenaline tend to cause splanchnic vasoconstriction; the effects of dobutamine depend on whether alpha or beta effects predominate, while dopexamine with its beta-2 and dopaminergic actions is likely to be the most beneficial sympathomimetic in improving splanchnic blood flow.

10.8	a) True	b) True	c) False	d) False	e) True

EXPLANATION

Gamma-aminobutyric acid (GABA) is an inhibitory neurotransmitter located throughout the central nervous system. There are two receptors for this neurotransmitter, $GABA_A$ and $GABA_B$ receptors. Drugs that act on these receptors have anticonvulsant properties. There is extensive evidence that barbiturates and benzodiazepines bind to specific sites on the $GABA_A$ receptor. It is thought that many anaesthetic agents including steroids and volatile agents (but not ketamine) act on the $GABA_A$ receptor. It is likely that there are subtypes of $GABA_A$ receptors; thus it is possible that the sedative effects of benzodiazepines are generated by different receptors from those causing anxiolysis. Therefore it might be possible to develop antianxiety drugs with no sedative effects. Drugs that compete with barbiturates and benzodiazepines for their binding sites tend to cause convulsions and have no clinical use. However, one useful agent is the imidazobenzodiazepine, flumazenil, which has no intrinsic actions; however, by binding to the benzodiazepine receptor on $GABA_A$ it reverses the sedation caused by benzodiazepines and possibly also by general anaesthetics. Unfortunately, since the half-life of flumazenil is short (about 1 h), resedation is likely. The $GABA_B$ receptor does not bind barbiturates or benzodiazepines. It is believed that baclofen, which is an analogue of GABA and is used to reduce muscle spasm, acts at the $GABA_B$ receptor.

baclofen

10.9	a) False	b) False	c) True	d) True	e) False

EXPLANATION

There are two types of post-operative pain:

- dull aching pain which persists at rest – easier to treat
- severe sharp pain produced by movement/coughing and caused by recently incised muscle – more difficult to treat.

Severity of pain is dependent upon:

- Psychological factors: motivation, anxiety, fear, preoperative preparation.
- Site: surgery in the upper abdomen, chest, major joints, back and anal region produces the most severe postoperative pain; head, neck and limb surgery is least painful as the operative site can be kept motionless.

- Age: the elderly and very young usually require less analgesia.
- Pain tolerance: differs between individuals.
- Response to analgesics.
- Pre-emptive analgesia: it is possible that the administration of analgesic drugs prior to the noxious stimulus reduces the effects of the stimulus. Lower amounts of pain mediators such as prostaglandins are produced from the wounded tissues; the hormone response to injury is reduced lessening tissue breakdown in response to injury.
- Management by surgeon and anaesthetist: surgical manipulation, trauma; amount of analgesia given by the anaesthetist during the operation.
- Balanced analgesia: i.e. administering drugs at several parts of the pain pathways at the same time.

Reasons for treating pain

- Humanitarian.
- Reduction in respiratory complications. Upper abdominal surgery reduces preoperative vital capacity by 65% in the first 24 hours; lower abdominal surgery by 45%. Hypoventilation leads to atelectasis, shunting, pneumonia. Treatment of pain increases vital capacity by at least 10%.
- Reduction in deep vein thrombosis (DVT). Patients in pain do not move and thus the incidence of DVT is increased.
- Hormonal changes. Increased levels of catecholamines lead to widespread peripheral vasoconstriction and pulmonary and renal vasoconstriction. This may be detrimental in patients with myocardial ischaemia. The associated rise in blood sugar may cause an osmotic diuresis, possibly predisposing to dehydration in children. The cerebral vasoconstriction may be associated with a rise in intracranial pressure which may be relevant in patients with head injuries or in a premature baby who is at risk of intraventricular haemorrhage.

Measurement of pain

- Visual analogue scale: 100-mm line without any numbers or words.
- Digital scale: 0–11.
- Verbal score: none (0), mild (1), moderate (2), severe (3).
- Movement-sensitive verbal score: the range is from no pain at rest or on movement; through mild then moderate pain at rest or on movement, to extreme or severe pain at rest or on movement.
- Graphic representation: used for children.
- Subjective criteria: any pallor, sweating, etc.
- Objective criteria: respiratory, reductions in functional residual capacity/peak flows measured by spirometry.

Methods available to treat postoperative pain

- Opioids.
- Other general analgesics.
- Regional techniques, surface analgesia, peripheral blocks, epidurals/spinals.
- Inhaled analgesia.
- Physical methods.
- Supportive measures.

Opioids:

1. *Intramuscular.* There are many variable factors: absorption of drug is very variable; blood levels are also very variable and not related to body mass; delayed onset of action; relative short peak and rapid tail-off.

2. *Subcutaneous.* Uptake from subcutaneous tissue is better than from muscle. Diamorphine is the best opiate to use by this route as it can be administered in a small volume.

3. *Oral/buccal/sublingual.* Oral opioid drugs undergo first pass metabolism. Postoperative gastric stasis makes this route unsuitable. The buccal and sublingual routes have less first pass metabolism but efficacy is variable.

4. *Transdermal.* At the moment the only patch available is fentanyl. Although analgesia is very prolonged, onset is also very slow (about 18 hours) and therefore unsuitable for acute pain. Sufentanil is more lipid soluble and absorption should be more rapid but a sufentanil patch is not available at present. Iontophoretic transfer may also show more rapid absorption.

5. *Intravenous.* Compared to the above routes intravenous administration is more predictable; plasma concentrations are more consistent and can be titrated to patients' needs. Table 10.4 compares continuous infusion and patient-controlled analgesia.

6. *Epidural/spinal opioids.* Following intrathecal/epidural administration, narcotics attach themselves to opiate receptors on the spinal cord. Onset and duration depend on lipophilicity of the opioid. A poorly lipid-soluble opioid (morphine) diffuses slowly; thus onset is slow (35 min to 1 h). On the other hand the cerebrospinal fluid concentration is high and the drug diffuses slowly upwards giving prolonged (18 h) wide segmental analgesia but also delayed respiratory depression as it reaches the medulla. With lipophilic fentanyl the onset is rapid (10 min) and duration is limited to 2 hours, while segmental and cephalic spread is also limited because the drug gets attached quickly to spinal receptors.

Advantages. Lack of motor, sensory and sympathetic block.
Disadvantages:
- Nausea, vomiting.
- Pruritus especially of the nose – reversed with naloxone.
- Urinary retention – 50% incidence.
- Respiratory depression – can be delayed and is more likely with the poorly lipid-soluble opioids; reversed with naloxone, but repeated doses may be required because naloxone lasts only about 1 hour.

Table 10.4 Intravenous analgesia: pros and cons of continuous and patient-controlled systems

	Pros	Cons
Continuous infusion	Constant level; useful for all ages	Widely variable effective rate; cost of pump; not good for episodic pain
Patient-controlled analgesia	Titratable; safer; patient control and patient satisfaction	Cost of pump; not suitable below age 5–7 years and in old, frail, confused patients

Other general analgesics

1. Non-steroidal anti-inflammatory drugs act by prostaglandin inhibition and are useful in mild to moderate pain, or to supplement opioids in more severe pain. Problems include gastric irritation, renal impairment and bleeding problems due to platelet dysfunctions.
2. Agonist-antagonists (e.g. buprenorphine, pentazocine, nalbuphine). Advantages claimed compared to opioids are potent analgesia with less respiratory depression and less addiction potential; however, they are not as effective as opioids; any respiratory depression may be difficult to reverse and side-effects are common – nausea, vomiting, sweating, drowsiness, dysphoria.

Regional techniques

- Surface analgesia/local infiltration. Long-acting local anaesthetics injected into the operated site can be effective, especially with superficial operations. Lignocaine gel can be effective after circumcisions.
- Intra-articular injections. Apart from the central nervous system, opioid receptors are also located on nerves in peripheral tissues. This discovery has led to the use of intra-articular administration of opioids for postoperative analgesia after orthopaedic surgery. Small, systemically inactive doses produce prolonged (up to 48 h) pain relief, without the side-effects of morphine. Analgesia is only achieved if the injection is in an area showing an inflammatory response.
- Peripheral nerve blocks. Intercostal blocks for thoracotomies/abdominal surgery are not as effective as paravertebral blocks because intercostal blocks only block somatic (superficial) fibres, while paravertebral blocks also block the sympathetic fibres from viscera and peritoneum. Some examples are:

Operation	Block
Circumcision, hypospadias	Dorsal penile block
Inguinal hernia, orchidopexies	Ilioinguinal, iliohypogastric
Femur osteotomy	3 in 1 block – femoral, obturator, lateral femoral cutaneous
Lacerations, toe/nail surgery	Digital block
Arm surgery	Brachial plexus block
Hand surgery	Wrist block
Foot surgery	Ankle block
Lower limb surgery	Sciatic nerve block
Thoracotomies, laparotomy	Intercostal, paravertebral blocks

Catheters can be employed in some blocks (e.g. brachial plexus) for continuous analgesia.

Epidural analgesia

This method is superior to all other techniques in providing postoperative pain relief. By using indwelling catheters the patient can be kept pain free by repeated boluses or infusions of local anaesthetics or mixtures of local anaesthetics and opioids. The catheter tip should be as close as possible to the dermatomes involved in surgery so that the dose can be reduced and thus the side-effects of hypotension and motor block reduced.

After thoracotomies or upper abdominal surgery, the patient is able to breathe deeply and cough effectively while early ambulation is possible, reducing the incidence of postoperative respiratory complications and deep vein thrombosis.

Contraindications to epidurals include sepsis at site or generalized septicaemia, history of neurological disorders, bleeding problems. (Subcutaneous heparin is not a contraindication.)

Inhaled analgesia
This may be of use for short painful procedures (e.g. drain removal).

Physical methods

- Transcutaneous nerve stimulation – doubtful value; possible placebo effect.
- Cryotherapy, e.g. of intercostal nerves or paravertebral nerves to provide postoperative pain relief for thoracotomies; laparotomies, etc. Can be performed percutaneously or at the time of surgery. Complications include neuroma formation and prolonged muscle weakness.
- Acupuncture.
- Alpha-2 agonists (e.g. clonidine) are powerful sedatives and analgesics; the latter effect is probably due to release of substance P. Clonidine has been used for postoperative analgesia especially by the epidural route. Epidural clonidine produces analgesia for about 5 hours without sensory or motor block. However, high doses can cause bradycardia, hypotension and sedation and thus it is often combined with local anaesthetics or opiates to reduce side-effects.
- Supportive measures, e.g. relief of flatulence, urinary retention, mobilization of fractures, etc.

Control of pain in patients with pre-existing disease
Renal impairment. Pethidine should be avoided because norpethidine can accumulate, is neurotoxic and can cause convulsions. Morphine is mainly metabolized in liver, but its metabolite, morphine-6-glucuronide, is excreted in the kidney. It is as active as morphine and can accumulate in renal failure. Fentanyl and alfentanil are metabolized in the liver and are safe in renal failure, as is buprenorphine.

Non-steroidal anti-inflammatory drugs (NSAIDs) cause reduction in renal perfusion because of prostaglandin inhibition and should be avoided in the presence of renal impairment.

Liver impairment. Morphine is metabolized in liver to morphine-6-glucuronide; therefore in liver impairment lower doses should be used. Similar caution is required with other opiates; the short-acting ones, e.g. fentanyl, are better tolerated. NSAIDs should be used cautiously because of the increased risk of bleeding in patients with hepatic cirrhosis.

Respiratory disease. Opioids should be used with caution in severe respiratory disease. In asthmatic patients, NSAIDs should only be administered if patients have no reactions to aspirin.

Cardiovascular disease. Most opiates cause bradycardia (except pethidine – atropine-like actions). High levels of circulating catecholamines associated with acute pain increase cardiac work and predispose to myocardial ischaemia; therefore adequate analgesia is essential.

Extremes of age. The elderly are sensitive to opioids and doses should be reduced. In neonates, especially premature infants, the clearance of opiates is prolonged, but after 3–6 months of age infants are no more susceptible to respiratory depression than adults.

Addicts. Current addicts need higher opioid doses; partial agonists and antagonists should be avoided as they can cause withdrawal symptoms. Former addicts should not be given opioids if at all possible to protect them from relapse into addiction.

10.10   a) False   b) False   c) False   d) True   e) True

EXPLANATION
See Answer 10.9, page 224.

10.11   a) False   b) True   c) False   d) False   e) True

EXPLANATION

Anaesthetic deaths
In the 1980s when pulse oximetry and capnography were introduced, the incidence of anaesthetic mortality fell, but it has not altered appreciably in the 1990s. Lately, the cause of anaesthetic mortality is more likely to be respiratory, i.e. hypoventilation (50% of deaths) than cardiovascular (about 30%). The number of maternal anaesthetic deaths has reduced from 4.3% to 2.7% in the last 30 years. 90% of maternal deaths are associated with general anaesthesia and the increased use of regional anaesthesia (50% of caesarean sections are currently performed under local anaesthesia) is probably the main reason for the reduction of maternal mortality.

At present anaesthetic mortality is about 0.05%; death in the recovery period is about 0.1%; and 0.6% occur in the first postoperative week. The mortality incidence while in hospital is about 1% in healthy patients. This 1% incidence is increased with pre-existing disease or reduced in certain situations as follows (Pederson 1994):

- Sex: males 2.2%, females 0.7%
- Age: below 50 0.3%; 70–80 3%
- Ischaemic heart disease 3%; myocardial infarction over 1 year previously 4%, less than 1 year 7.7%; chronic heart failure 9%
- Blood pressure: hypertension 1.3%; hypotension below 90 mmHg 9.4%
- Chronic obstructive lung disease 5%
- Renal failure 6%
- Diabetes 2%
- Neurological disease 3%
- Emergency surgery 3%
- Extent of surgery: minor surgery 0.3%, major 3%
- Duration of surgery: mortality increases from 1% for surgery lasting 1 hour to 5% if it lasts 5 hours.

Causes of anaesthetic mortality/morbidity
  Respiratory. As stated above, 50% of anaesthetic mortality/morbidity is due to respiratory problems, i.e. hypoventilation and hypoxaemia leading to cerebral ischaemia. Causes of hypoxaemia are many:

- Reduced FiO_2 – hypoxic mixtures administered either inadvertently or faulty pipe connections; faulty flow meter bobbin reading (leaks or bobbins sticking due to dirt or static electricity); addition of other gases, e.g. CO_2; low oxygen flows; leaks in anaesthetic circuits.
- Postoperative hypoxaemia accounts for about 15% of anaesthetic morbidity/mortality. This is usually associated with respiratory depression from the anaesthetic agent, intravenous opioids or relaxants; or local anaesthetics or opioids injected epidurally or intrathecally.
- Complications of tracheal intubation account for 18% of all causes – oesophageal intubation (often difficult to detect especially with preoxygenation when oxygen saturation can take up to 10 minutes to start falling); ventilator disconnection; endotracheal tube obstruction (7% of anaesthetic mortality) either due to kinking or cuff herniation or a foreign body in the lumen.
- Airway obstruction (6% of anaesthetic mortality):
  - upper airway: inhalation of food or vomit, laryngospasm
  - lower airway: bronchospasm due to asthma, aspiration, anaphylaxis.
- Aspiration, regurgitation often during induction or emergence – 3% of anaesthetic mortality.
- Inadequate pulmonary ventilation during anaesthesia (5%), e.g. pulmonary ventilation not possible because of inadequate muscle relaxation or inadequate anaesthesia causing bronchospasm and vagal cardiac arrest.
- Pre-existing pulmonary disease, higher inspired oxygen concentrations required.
- Other causes of hypoxaemia – one-lung anaesthesia; steep head-down tilt; distended abdomen (e.g. laparoscopy); pneumothorax especially in thoracic anaesthesia/trauma.

Cardiac. 30% of anaesthetic mortality/morbidity is due primarily to cardiac causes.

- Myocardial depression – anaesthetic agents; high total spinals; intravenous injection of local anaesthetics.
- Arrhythmias – sinus bradycardia caused by increased vagal tone due to surgical stimulation; suxamethonium; halothane; atrial/ventricular dysrhythmias especially with pre-existing disease; electrolytic abnormalities.
- Cardiac arrest due to hypovolaemia, profound bradycardia, ventricular fibrillation (embolus, adrenaline with halothane); electrolyte abnormalities, especially potassium; pulmonary embolism.
- Hypotension – cerebral blood flow is reduced when blood pressure falls below level of autoregulation (60 mmHg but higher in hypertensive patients). Hypotension-associated vasoconstriction (e.g. shock) is more serious than with vasodilatation (e.g. induced), where cerebral vasodilatation is maintained. Causes: hypovolaemia, anaesthetic agents, high spinals, induced hypotension especially with pre-existing disease.

Embolism. Pulmonary embolism (more likely postoperatively); air venous embolism especially in neurosurgery or cardiac surgery, arterial thrombi in heart or great vessels. Massive venous embolism causes a reduction of cardiac output; arterial emboli cause generalized or focal cerebral lesions.

Awareness during anaesthesia. (Incidence 0.2–0.9% – 0.2% in non-obstetric/non-cardiac surgery.) It is usually due to faulty anaesthetic technique (e.g. inadequate anaesthetic drugs in a paralysed patient; empty vaporizers) and is most common in obstetric general anaesthesia (25% of all cases), occurring also in cardiac surgery; endoscopies; difficult intubation; total intravenous anaesthesia.

Regional anaesthesia:

- Spinal cord and nerve root damage with epidurals or spinal anaesthesia. Causes are:
  - neurotoxic agents, e.g. inadvertent injection of neurotoxic agents such as potassium or calcium chloride; preservatives in local anaesthetics or opioids; steroids (especially depomedrone)
  - ischaemia, hypotension or local reduction in blood supply
  - unknown – vast majority of cases.
- Pain during regional anaesthesia – the effectiveness of a block should be tested thoroughly before surgery starts and if inadequate appropriate action taken.
- Backache – relatively common after epidurals/spinals in obstetric patients.

Peripheral nerve injuries (15% of claims against anaesthetists). These are usually due to compression or stretching of a nerve, rarely to direct damage from needles or extravasated drugs. Recovery usually occurs within 6–8 weeks but in a few cases the damage is permanent. Nerve damage is more likely in patients with pre-existing neuropathy. Most common nerve injuries are to the ulnar nerve because of its superficial position near a bony promontory; to the radial nerve especially with a pneumatic cuff; to the brachial plexus especially if the arm is abducted (especially if more than 90%) and externally rotated, or by shoulder braces when a patient is in a steep head-down posture; to the sciatic nerve especially in a thin patient lying on a hard table in a prolonged operation or in the lithotomy position; and lumbosacral injuries associated with regional anaesthesia.

Anaphylaxis. The incidence is about 0.01%. History of previous exposure to the drug is not necessary. Patients should be asked about allergic reactions to anaesthetic or other drugs.

Dental damage. The incidence is 0.1% in cases involving tracheal intubation of which 50% are difficult intubations. Dental damage can occur during extubation and can be caused by oral airways.

Eye injuries (3% of claims against anaesthetists). They include corneal abrasions due to eyes being kept open and drying out; or from trauma by face mask; eye trauma in prone position; eye trauma from movement (e.g. coughing) during eye surgery.

Other injuries/complaints. Dry mouth (over 50%), vomiting (22%), bruises (14%), sore throat (slight 10%, severe 2%, loss of voice 1.5%). Suxamethonium pains (patient should be warned of this possibility); post-spinal headaches; extravasation of injected drugs; superficial thrombophlebitis; fall from table; foreign bodies (needles, epidural catheter tips; lost central line catheters); burns, abrasions, lacerations, or petechiae; skin loss from adhesive tapes; skin necrosis by irritant drugs (e.g. diclofenac which should be given by deep i.m. injection); administration of wrong drugs or drug overdose; mismatched blood transfusion; halothane hepatitis which has a high mortality; fetal damage (complaint aimed mainly at obstetricians); airway damage – perforation of trachea, bronchus, oesophagus usually associated with difficult intubations, vocal cord paralysis, arytenoid dislocation, granuloma formation, injuries to temperomandibular joint, pneumothorax usually associated with intercostal or brachial plexus blocks or insertion of central venous pressure catheters.

Reference

Pederson T 1994 Mortality associated with anaesthesia. In: Clinical anaesthesiology: quality assurance and risk management in anaesthesia. ch 1

10.12   a) True   b) False   c) False   d) True   e) False

EXPLANATION

Definition. Occlusion of the glottis by action of intrinsic laryngeal muscles.
Incidence. The overall incidence is about 1%.

Predisposing factors

1. *Age.* Laryngospasm is more likely in children aged between 0 and 9 years with a peak incidence between 1 and 3 months where the incidence is about 3%.

2. *Inhalational agents.* The respiratory tract is hypersensitive to stimuli during light anaesthesia, but some inhalational agents are more irritant than others. Sevoflurane is probably the least irritant, followed by halothane, isoflurane and desflurane. When desflurane is used for inhalational induction the incidence of breath holding, coughing and laryngospasm is about 40%.

3. *Intravenous induction agents.* The induction agents most studied are thiopentone and propofol. Pharyngeal and laryngeal activity is depressed more following propofol, and therefore the incidence of laryngospasm is higher with thiopentone. Moreover, insertion of airways and laryngeal masks is much less traumatic with propofol. The cords are much more relaxed with propofol, therefore laryngoscopy and intubation is easier compared with thiopentone if no relaxant drugs are administered.

4. *Asthma and upper respiratory tract infections.* The incidence of laryngospasm is increased in asthmatic patients and in patients with upper respiratory tract infections. Children with upper respiratory tract infections undergoing general anaesthesia have an incidence of laryngospasm of about 10%. Viral infections cause mucosal oedema and shedding of epithelial cells, thus increasing the exposure of subepithelial sensory receptors to inhaled irritants. These epithelial changes persist for about 15 days. There is thus the ongoing controversy over whether non-urgent cases should be postponed in the presence of upper respiratory tract infections.

5. *Cigarette smoking.* Anaesthetists are aware that smokers have a higher incidence of coughing and laryngospasm both at induction and during recovery. As with respiratory infections, cigarette smoke causes varying loss of ciliated epithelium, thus disrupting the protective epithelial barrier. Cessation of smoking is accompanied by restoration of epithelial permeability over a period of 9–10 days.

10.13   a) False   b) False   c) True   d) True   e) True

EXPLANATION

Indications for a temporary pacemaker before surgery are:

- Sinoatrial node dysfunction causing brady- or tachyarrhythmias
- Left bundle branch block and first degree heart block
- Second degree atrioventricular (AV) block: type I – progressive PR lengthening until a beat is dropped (Wenckebach); type II – intermittent failure in AV conduction without PR prolongation
- Third degree heart block – complete dissociation between atria and ventricles.

Types of pacemakers

1. Ventricular (VVI). This is the most common type. The ventricle is paced on demand and the pacemaker is inhibited by spontaneous ventricular activity. Cardiac output may be reduced.
2. Atrial (AAI). An atrial demand pacemaker is useful in sick sinus syndrome when AV conduction is intact. Cardiac output may be improved.
3. Dual (DDD). Dual chamber pacemakers can stimulate both chambers in sequence.
4. Anti-tachycardia pacemaker. These detect tachycardias and terminate them by breaking the re-entrant circuit.
5. Programmable pacemakers. Rate, sensitivity, output and refractory period can be changed non-invasively with a programmer.

Problems

1. *Pacemaker threshold.* The threshold is the minimum voltage necessary for pacing. Pacemaker function is not only dependent on electrical function. Acidosis, hypoxia, potassium and drugs (e.g. halothane) increase the pacing threshold. If the threshold decreases there is a risk of ventricular fibrillation.
2. *Pacemaker dysfunction.* Battery failure can be detected by bradycardia and possibly fainting.
3. *Diathermy.* Although modern pacemakers are usually safe, problems do arise and diathermy should be avoided, if possible. If diathermy has to be used, the indifferent electrode should be placed on the same side as the operating site as far away from the pacemaker as possible; its frequency, duration of use and current kept to a minimum; and bipolar used preferably to monopolar diathermy.
4. *Pacemaker failure.* This can occur on induction of anaesthesia especially with suxamethonium. The pacemaker may fail during surgery because of loose connections, change in pacemaker threshold, battery failure, etc. Atropine, adrenaline, etc. should be available in case of this eventuality.

10.14   a) True   b) True   c) True   d) False   e) False

EXPLANATION

The three main reasons for difficulty in intubation are: temperomandibular joint dysfunction; reduced mobility of the cervical spine and narrowing of the airway.

A difficult intubation may be due to factors in any part of the upper airway, i.e. mouth, teeth, tongue, pharynx, larynx, neck. There are also a number of congenital syndromes associated with difficult intubation.

Mouth

- Trismus (spasms of masseter and medial pterygoid muscle) which only allows limited opening of mouth, e.g. tetanus, fractured mandible. If the mouth opening is less than 20 mm difficulty should be anticipated.
- Fibrosis: scleroderma; burns; radiotherapy; chemical burns.
- Small mouth, e.g. Down syndrome, Marfan's syndrome, Möbius' syndrome, but especially Freeman–Sheldon syndrome (whistling face).
- Temperomandibular joint causes: rheumatoid arthritis; Still's disease; ankylosing spondylitis; osteoarthritis.

- Mandibular and maxillary causes: maxillary protrusion; maxillary trauma; surgical wiring of jaw; mandibular injuries; mandibular coronal hyperplasia; micrognathia, i.e. receding mandible either on its own or part of a syndrome (e.g. Pierre Robin). If the distance between the tip of the chin and the thyroid cartilage is less than 6 cm, intubation is likely to be difficult.
- Palate: high arched palate; cleft palate.

Teeth
Absence of teeth usually makes intubation easier. Prominent upper incisors (buck teeth) can make intubation difficult. Teeth following extensive work are never as strong as normal teeth and dental damage during intubation is therefore more likely.

Tongue
Large tongue, e.g. in Down syndrome; congenital hypothyroidism; hypertrophy, e.g. acromegaly or oedema (infection, allergy); tumours – squamous cell carcinoma; haemangiomas; tongue trauma.

Pharynx

- Nasopharynx: enlarged adenoids; nasopharyngeal carcinoma.
- Oropharynx: tonsillar abscess (quinsy); Ludwig's angina (infection and oedema of the submandibular area usually due to poor dental hygiene); squamous cell carcinoma; carcinoma of the tonsils; cystic hygromas in submandibular region.
- Laryngopharynx: epiglottitis (bacterial infection causing oedema of the epiglottis presenting with stridor); epiglottic tears; croup; diphtheria; leprosy; acromegaly (because the mucosa can be hypertrophic); carcinoma of the laryngopharynx; laryngocele; laryngeal cyst.

Larynx
Laryngeal oedema in the subglottic region is easier to develop than in the supraglottic area. Laryngeal causes of difficult intubation include carcinomas; rheumatoid arthritis (due to possible cricoarytenoid arthritis and rotation of larynx); acromegaly (thickened cords and laryngeal stenosis); laryngeal papillomatosis in early childhood; subglottic stenosis (prolonged intubation; traumatic or repeated intubation; infection; Wegener's granulomatosis); recurrent laryngeal nerve lesions (carcinomas of bronchus, thyroid, oesophagus; mediastinal tumours; following thyroidectomy or pharyngeal pouch excision).

Neck

- Anatomical: short muscular neck (bull neck).
- Trauma: trauma to cervical spine.
- Deep neck abscesses: above the hyoid (submandibular, parotid, parapharyngeal, peritonsillar); below the hyoid (anterior); or in the entire length of the neck (retropharyngeal, prevertebral).
- Neck deformities: ankylosing spondylitis (fusion of cervical spine); osteoarthritis (fusion of cervical vertebrae); Still's disease (fusion of cervical vertebrae); Turner's syndrome (fusion of cervical vertebrae); rheumatoid arthritis (atlantoaxial subluxation); diabetes (atlantoaxial joint stiffness); Down syndrome (atlantoaxial subluxation); mucopolysaccharidoses (atlantoaxial instability); Paget's disease (atlantoaxial instability); osteogenesis imperfecta (cervical spine rigidity or fracture).

One can anticipate difficulty in intubation by testing cervical spine mobility. If the angle between maximal flexion and extension is less than 90° one can predict difficulty. The same applies if the atlanto-occipital extension is less than 35°.

- Burns: causing contractures at front of neck.
- Others: gross obesity; large breasts; late pregnancy (nine times more likely for intubation to be difficult compared to surgical patients because of weight gain, enlarged breasts, neck and chest and possible laryngeal oedema, especially in the presence of pre-eclampsia).

Congenital

- Achondroplasia: small mouth; large head.
- Apert's syndrome: narrow or cleft palate; small maxilla; craniosynostosis.
- Arthrogryposis congenita: small mandible; cleft palate; torticollis.
- Crouzon's syndrome: small maxilla; large tongue; craniosynostosis.
- Down syndrome: large tongue; small mouth; small mandible.
- Congenital hypothyroidism: large tongue.
- Freeman–Sheldon (whistling face): very small mouth, high palate.
- Marfan's syndrome: narrow face and palate.
- Möbius' syndrome: small mandible and mouth.
- Mucopolysaccharidoses: large tongue; limited mouth opening; neck instability.
- Pierre Robin syndrome: micrognathia; possible cleft palate.
- Treacher Collins' syndrome: facial hypoplasia including mandible and maxilla; cervical vertebral anomalies; cleft palate.
- Turner's syndrome: small narrow maxilla and mandible; short neck.

Prediction of difficult intubation

Cormack and Lahane classification. This is based on the extent of laryngeal structures that can be seen with a laryngoscope.

Grade I   Full view of cords (99% of patients)
Grade II View of posterior commisure only (1%)
Grade III View of epiglottis only (1 in 2000)
Grade IV No view of laryngeal structure (1 in 100 000)

Mallampati classification. Preoperatively, the mouth is opened as wide as possible and the tongue fully protruded.

Class I   View of fauces, pillars, soft palate, uvula
Class II View of fauces, pillars, soft palate
Class III View of soft palate only – intubation likely to be difficult
Class IV No view of soft palate – intubation likely to be difficult

The Mallampati classification is not very reliable.

10.15   a) False   b) True   c) False   d) False   e) True

EXPLANATION

Metabolic changes. If insulin is absent there is increased lipid metabolism with excess ketone production. There is also increased gluconeogenesis and

235

glycogenolysis. The results are: metabolic acidosis; hyperglycaemia; polyuria with excessive urinary loss of sodium, potassium, calcium, magnesium and ketones.

Metabolic control. Non-insulin-dependent outnumber insulin-dependent diabetics by nine to one. The former tend to be older, obese and are less likely to develop ketoacidosis but more prone to hyperglycaemia and hyperosmosis. Fewer patients are now on long-acting oral antidiabetic drugs such as chlorpropamide and it is rarely necessary to stop these drugs for a number of days before surgery. For minimal procedures it is sufficient to omit the antidiabetic drug on the morning of the operation and monitor blood sugar levels closely. With major surgery these patients often become insulin dependent, but it is usually acceptable to start the insulin/glucose infusion during surgery and continue it postoperatively until required. As regards insulin-dependent diabetics it is unnecessary to start glucose/sliding scale insulin infusions many days before surgery. One should start this regime a few hours preoperatively when the patient would normally eat, and monitor blood glucose and potassium levels closely. Provided they are well controlled and understand their disease, insulin-dependent diabetic patients should not be excluded from day case anaesthesia.

Autonomic neuropathy. About 30% of long-standing diabetics suffer from autonomic neuropathy which is a cause of significant morbidity and mortality. This is often associated with renal failure, hypertension, gastric stasis, lack of sweating, painless myocardial infarctions and impotence. These patients do not compensate for anaesthetic effects on venous return and myocardial depression. They are therefore more likely to develop bradycardias and hypotension which may not respond to atropine or ephedrine and often need adrenaline to correct these problems. They are also prone to QT prolongation on the ECG which is likely to cause arrhythmias. The 'sudden death syndrome' seen in diabetics may be due to these factors.

Cardiovascular disease. Both large and small vessels are affected by atherosclerosis and microangiopathy leading to peripheral vascular and myocardial disease, while renal and retinal vessel disease causes renal damage and possible blindness.

Renal disease. Renal failure is a common problem, often leading to hypertension. Mortality from renal transplantation in diabetics is about three times higher than in non-diabetic patients.

Respiratory problems. Diabetics have decreased sensitivity to hypoxia and impaired airway protective reflexes. Pulmonary function tests are often abnormal – usually a restrictive defect from reduced lung elasticity.

Stiff joint syndrome. About 30% of long-standing insulin-dependent diabetics develop 'stiff joint syndrome', again probably due to reduced elasticity of connective tissues. The atlanto-occipital joint may be involved and the incidence of difficult intubation is thus increased in diabetics.

Peripheral nerve damage. Peripheral nerves are more susceptible to compression injuries.

Infection. This is more likely in diabetics as is impaired wound healing.

10.16   a) False   b) False   c) True   d) False   e) True

EXPLANATION

Definition. Adult (or acute) respiratory distress syndrome (ARDS) can be defined as severe low pressure permeability pulmonary oedema with four criteria: (1) acute onset; (2) PaO_2/FiO_2 ratio less than 200 mmHg (26.6 kPa) when no positive end-expiratory pressure (PEEP) is applied; (3) bilateral infiltrates seen on a frontal chest X-ray; (4) pulmonary wedge pressures less than 18 mmHg (2.4 kPa) so long as there is no cardiac involvement.

Aetiology:

- Pulmonary causes – aspiration; lung contusion; pneumonia and other infections; radiation; inhalation of toxic gases; near drowning.
- Non-pulmonary causes – shock; sepsis; trauma; drug overdose; pancreatitis; eclampsia; CNS pathology; burns; emboli; massive transfusions.

Pathology. Unlike cardiogenic pulmonary oedema, where the oedema is mainly intra-alveolar the pulmonary oedema in ARDS is mainly interstitial. Initially the alveolar cells are damaged and endothelial permeability increased causing interstitial oedema, while the alveoli are filled with a thick exudate. After a week or so, the exudate organizes into hyaline membranes which are characteristic of ARDS and destroy the structure of the alveoli. This pulmonary oedema is accompanied by hypoxaemia due to right-to-left shunting (often above 40%) because of continued perfusion of non-ventilated alveoli. Pulmonary compliance is low, while airway resistance is high.

Clinical features. A catastrophic event precedes ARDS. First clinical symptoms include cyanosis, dyspnoea and hyperventilation; blood analysis reveals hypocarbia and hypoxaemia, which does not improve significantly with added oxygen. The classical chest X-ray signs appears 12–24 hours after presentation – alveolar infiltrations in both lung fields similar to pulmonary oedema but without the cardiac enlargement; pulmonary vascular redistribution, or pleural effusions. Eventually the infiltrates increase to the typical 'white-out' picture. Mortality is 50–80%.

Treatment:

1. *IPPV.* The best type is pressure-controlled ventilation where 'square' waves of pressure are applied. The type of pressure ventilation for these patients is pressure-controlled inverse ratio ventilation (pcCMV-IRV). In pcCMV-IRV the inspiratory time is prolonged. The shortened expiratory time prevents alveoli from collapsing below their closing volume. Thus one should start with an inspiratory to expiratory ratio of 1 : 1 and increase to 2 : 1 if oxygenation does not improve. Airway pressures should be maintained between 30–35 cmH$_2$O (2.9–3.4 kPa). High airway pressures should be avoided because of barotrauma, including a higher incidence of pneumothoraces. Since high FiO$_2$ damages healthy lungs, the inspired oxygen level is aimed to achieve a PaO_2 between 55–60 mmHg (7.3–8 kPa). The respiratory rate is set between 12 and 16 breaths/minute. PEEP can have beneficial effects on functional respiratory capacity, preventing alveolar collapse and arterial deoxygenation, and if required should be set between 8–15 cmH$_2$0. In the presence of asymmetrical distribution of lung lesions, ventilation of each lung via a double-lumen tube can improve prognosis because of the differences in compliance and airway resistances in the two lungs.

2. *Permissive hypercapnia.* There is evidence to suggest that IPPV with hypercapnia reduces mortality in ARDS patients. Acute hypercapnia leads to intracellular acidosis, pulmonary hypertension and increased cerebral blood flow and sympathetic activation; but a gradual increase in $PaCO_2$ allows compensatory mechanisms to be activated and is usually well tolerated. Thus the tidal volumes are reduced gradually to 5–6 ml/kg to allow $PaCO_2$ to rise to 70–80 mmHg

(9.3–10.7 kPa). Arterial pH should not be allowed to drop below 7.28. Contraindications to this technique include heart disease; hypertension; increased intracranial pressure.

3. *Position.* Oxygenation tends to improve if the 'healthier' lung is in the dependent position, probably because this position allows perfusion to reach the dependent lung while less of the pulmonary blood flow gets to the uppermost lung, thus reducing ventilation/perfusion mismatching. The prone posture also helps oxygenation because in ARDS the main pathology is in the dependent parts of the lung and in the prone position ventilation/perfusion mismatching is again diminished. If PaO_2 improves and shunting is reduced in these positions, positional manoeuvres should be performed twice a day for 4 hours.

4. *Treatment of pulmonary oedema.* Aim for a negative fluid balance with fluid restriction and the use of diuretics (frusemide); if these fail to establish a negative balance, haemofiltration and/or haemodialysis should be instituted. With these measures one should aim to keep haemoglobin levels between 14–15 g/100 ml; pulmonary wedge pressures below 10 mmHg (1.3 kPa); central venous pressure between 5–8 mmHg (0.7–1.1 kPa); colloid osmotic pressure between 25–29 mmHg (3.3–3.9 kPa); and urine output at 1 ml/kg/h.

5. *Extracorporeal membrane oxygenation (ECMO).* In the past, maintaining oxygenation with venoarterial ECMO was associated with a high mortality, because the necessity to anticoagulate the patient was associated with a high incidence of bleeding. However, it is now possible to employ heparin-coated extracorporeal oxygenators with minimal or no systemic heparinzation and bleeding complications are very much diminished. Rather than using full ECMO, some centres use partial ECMO, i.e. oxygenation is applied through a few ventilator breaths with low tidal volumes (apnoeic oxygenation) while carbon dioxide is removed through an extracorporeal CO_2 remover. With this technique low extracorporeal blood flow (20–30% of cardiac output) from a venovenous bypass is sufficient. The efficacy of ECMO in ARDS is still under investigation.

6. *Nitric oxide (NO).* ARDS is accompanied by pulmonary arterial vasoconstriction primarily associated with hypoxia. Inhaled nitric oxide (0.1–20 parts per million) has been shown to dilate the pulmonary vessels, improve perfusion in ventilated lungs and significantly improve oxygenation without affecting haemodynamics.

10.17   a) False   b) False   c) True   d) False   e) True

EXPLANATION

Incidence. Overall incidence is 0.2–0.9%. Procedures and circumstances with the highest incidence are: obstetric (28% of all cases of awareness) because of fear of anaesthetic agents harming the neonate; cardiac (especially on bypass); dental endoscopies (especially bronchoscopies where oxygen is insufflated via a Venturi injector and anaesthesia maintained by intravenous agents); total intravenous anaesthesia (inadequate supply of drug, due either to low dose or mechanical failure of pump, e.g. line obstruction); difficult intubation (initial induction dose of anaesthetic not supplemented); increases in FiO_2, thus reducing FiN_2O, without corresponding increase in vapour concentration.

Causes of awareness:

- Faulty anaesthetic technique (70%)
- Failure to check equipment (20%)
- Justified risks (2.5%), e.g. severe trauma
- Apparatus failure (2.5%)
- Spurious claims (2.5%)
- Unknown cause (2.5%)

Awareness is related to memory and stages of anaesthesia can be classified according to the extent of memory loss.

1. Conscious awareness, with explicit memory (explicit or episodic memory, e.g. what I did today).
2. Conscious awareness without explicit memory.
3. Subconscious awareness without explicit but with implicit memory (implicit or acquired memory, e.g. $7 \times 7 = 49$).
4. No awareness.

There is a wide range of awareness and not all of it is harmful:

1. Conscious awareness without amnesia. This is the one we have to avoid, i.e. pain or words overheard and remembered. The modality most likely to be remembered is auditory; the next one is pain.
2. Conscious awareness with amnesia, i.e. response to command during surgery, which is not remembered afterwards (e.g. procedures performed under benzodiazepine sedation).
3. Subconscious awareness, e.g. purposeful limb movements but no response to command. Subconscious awareness is unlikely to cause a problem.
4. Pseudoawareness, e.g. when patients are conscious of sounds in the recovery area which they assume to be occurring during surgery.

Clinical signs of awareness. In an unparalysed patient these are: movement, hyperventilation, signs of sympathetic activity; in a paralysed patient: signs of sympathetic activity, i.e. sweating, dilated pupils, hypertension, tachycardia, lacrimation.

Measurement of depth of anaesthesia:

- *Auditory evoked responses.* Auditory responses during anaesthesia are abolished by volatile agents, thiopentone and propofol, but not with benzodiazepines, nitrous oxide and especially opiates. Therefore awareness is much less likely if the former agents are used.
- *Cerebral metabolism.* Again volatile agents and thiopentone have been shown to reduce cerebral metabolism more so than opioid drugs.
- *Electroencephalogram.* EEG activity is greater under enflurane and ketamine anaesthesia than with isoflurane or halothane.
- *Frontalis electromyogram.* As anaesthesia deepens, there is a reduction in frontalis muscle tone measured by EMG.

Prevention of awareness. Avoid N_2O/opioid/relaxant anaesthesia without vapour. As stated above, thiopentone, propofol, 1 MAC vapour (beware of empty vaporizers) all prevent awareness. Benzodiazepines reduce auditory sensitivity, while atropine increases it.

Effects of awareness on patients. Patient response to awareness is as follows:

Fear of anaesthesia	42%
Sleep disturbances	19%
Anxiety	4%
Prolonged mental disorders	4%
No effect at all	31%

In some patients awareness leads to post-traumatic stress disorder, i.e. recurrent recollections and dreams of the event; persistent avoidance of stimuli associated with trauma; and persistent symptoms of increased arousal, e.g. difficulty with going to sleep; increased muscle jerkiness.

10.18   a) False   b) False   c) True   d) False   e) False

EXPLANATION

Unlike dopamine, dobutamine does not act on the dopaminergic receptors and therefore does not selectively increase renal and mesenteric blood flow. At low infusion doses (up to 7 µg/kg/min) dopamine has beneficial dopaminergic and beta effects. At higher doses intense unwanted vasoconstriction occurs with dopamine,

Table 10.5   Actions of sympathomimetic drugs

Drug	Dose	Alpha-1	Alpha-2
	miVdmi (←	Vasoconstriction; constriction of muscles of iris and ureter sphincters. Relaxation of gut muscle; increased salivary and sweat gland secretions	Peripheral vasoconstriction; dilatation of coronary arteries; bradycardia; platelet aggregation; inhibition of lipolysis
Adrenaline	Low	+/–	+/–
	Moderate	+	+
	High	+++	+++
Noradrenaline	Low	+	+
	Moderate	++	++
	High	+++	+++
Dopamine	Low	Nil	Nil
	Moderate	+	+/–
	High	++	+
Dopexamine		Nil	Nil
Ephedrine		+	+
Isoprenaline		Nil	Nil

but even high-dosage dobutamine infusion does not significantly alter the peripheral resistance, and pulmonary capillary wedge pressures are reduced with dobutamine, even at high dose.

Noradrenaline has strong alpha actions and weak beta actions, and when given in small doses can produce increases in cardiac output and blood pressure (BP) as a result of beta action. However, in large doses alpha action takes over, causing intense vasoconstriction with possible renal failure and tissue necrosis.

Methoxamine has pure alpha and no beta actions and although it does elevate the blood pressure by vasoconstriction, the increased peripheral resistance without beta inotropic action means that the heart has to pump against an increased peripheral resistance, increasing cardiac work, which some patients, especially those with cardiac problems, may not tolerate. Ephedrine would be more logical to use to elevate BP after spinals because it has mixed alpha (vasoconstriction) and beta (increased inotropism) actions, and does not increase cardiac work.

The actions of sympathomimetic drugs are summarized in Table 10.5.

Beta-1	Beta-2	Dopamine receptors
Increased heart rate and contractility	Bronchodilatation; vasodilatation; lipolysis; glycogenolysis; gluconeogenesis	
+	+	
++	++	
++	++	
+	Minimal	
+	Minimal	
+	Minimal	
+/−	+/−	+++
++	+	+++
++		
Minimal	+++	++
+	+	
+++	+++	

10.19   a) False   b) True   c) False   d) True   e) False

EXPLANATION

The liver is the second largest organ in the body and receives 25% of cardiac output. The portal vein is responsible for 75% of the blood supply and 50% of the hepatic oxygen delivery; the hepatic artery supplies 25% of the blood supply and 50% of the hepatic oxygen.

Severity of liver disease has been classified by Childs as shown in Table 10.6.

Liver disease causes widespread systemic problems, which affects anaesthetic management.

Cardiovascular. Possible cardiomyopathy especially if liver damage is alcohol induced leading to cardiac depression and arrhythmias; there may be a hyperdynamic response with increased cardiac output and blood volume; arteriovenous shunts and vasodilatation which is resistant to the action of catecholamines; ascites may decrease venous return.

Pulmonary. The dissociation curve is shifted to the right because of increased cardiac output. There may be restrictive lung disease (ascites); ventilation/perfusion imbalance due to shunts causing hypoxaemia; increased closing volume and reduced functional residual capacity. Pulmonary hypertension may also be present.

Kidney. Renal impairment (hepatorenal syndrome). Blood urea may be low (decreased synthesis), and creatinine level may also be reduced (reduced muscle mass); salt and water retention.

Blood. Haematocrit reduced (increased blood volume), bone marrow depression especially with alcohol causing anaemia; increased bleeding tendencies and increased prothrombin time (decreased vitamin K absorption and decreased synthesis of clotting factors); disseminated intravascular coagulation is possible; the immune system is depressed.

Neurological. Dementia (alcohol); hepatic encephalopathy ranging from confusion to coma.

Gut. Gastritis; oesophageal varices; risk of full stomach; splenic enlargement.

Endocrine. Glucose intolerance; malnutrition; low albumin.

Drugs. Drug clearance is reduced (low albumin levels; reduced metabolic enzymes; reduced hepatic blood flow; possible renal dysfunction), therefore lower doses are usually required. Portal blood flow is reduced by all intravenous induction agents and anaesthetic vapours but hepatic flow is increased by thiopentone, etomidate, propofol and all the anaesthetic vapours except halothane, which reduces hepatic flow. Thus hepatic oxygen delivery is reduced by halothane but not

Table 10.6 Classification of severity of liver disease

	Mild	Moderate	Severe
Bilirubin	< 2	2–3	> 3
Albumin	> 3.5	3–3.5	< 3
Prothrombin time	Normal	INR 1.2–2	INR > 2
Neurological state	Normal	Confused	Coma
Ascites	None	Easy to control	Difficult to control
Nutrition	Excellent	Good	Wasting

242   *Key:* INR = international normalized ratio

unduly affected by the other vapours and induction agents. The actions of suxamethonium and mivacurium may be prolonged owing to low cholinesterase levels. Atracurium is probably the best long-acting relaxant to use as its elimination is not organ dependent; Curare and pancuronium rely heavily on liver elimination and should be avoided in liver impairment, while vecuronium and rocuronium may have a slightly prolonged action.

10.20   a) False   b) True   c) False   d) False   e) True

EXPLANATION

Absence of spinal tendon reflexes is not invariable, nor is an EEG necessary for diagnosing brain death, although the presence of a flat EEG is usual with brain death. Pupils do not have to be widely dilated for brain death to be diagnosed; for example if opioid drugs were administered pupils would be constricted. Irrigation of the ear with cold water should cause nystagmus, not pupil reaction. Hypothermia depresses metabolism of brain, heart, etc. and body temperature must be normal for brain death to be diagnosed. In a normal patient consciousness is lost at 25°C and EEG activity disappears at 15–20°C. Apart from hypothermia, other potentially reversible causes should be excluded, i.e. depressant drugs, neuromuscular drugs and endocrine or metabolic disorders.

Certification of brain death should be done by two doctors with expertise in brain death criteria. One doctor should be a consultant, the other at least an experienced specialist. The brain death criteria should be assessed on two separate occasions. Tests for brain stem function include:

- Pupils – fixed, usually dilated, and do not react to light.
- Absence of corneal reflex.
- No eye movement on caloric testing – 20 ml ice-cold water injected slowly, and in turn, into each auditory canal, which is free of blood or wax.
- No motor responses in cranial nerve distribution (face, limbs or trunk), e.g. firm supraorbital pressure produces no motor response.
- No gag reflex – no cough reflex on passage of a suction catheter down the endotracheal tube.
- No respiratory movements after apnoea testing. The patient is preoxygenated for 15 minutes with 100% oxygen, then disconnected from the ventilator and insufflated with 6 litres of oxygen using a suction catheter down the endotracheal tube. When the $PaCO_2$ reaches 6.66 kPa (blood gas analysis), the patient is observed for any respiratory movements for a period of 10 minutes.

11.1 Comparing atropine, hyoscine and glycopyrolate:

a) Glycopyrolate is a quaternary ammonium compound
b) Atropine and hyoscine are less likely to cause central nervous system effects than glycopyrolate
c) Atropine has a longer duration of action than glycopyrolate
d) Tachycardia and arrhythmias are more common with atropine than with glycopyrolate
e) Glycopyrolate reduces gastric volume and acidity more so than atropine

11.2 With regard to peripheral opioid receptors:

a) Mu, kappa and delta opioid receptors are located at peripheral nerve sites
b) Intra-articular morphine produces side-effects comparable to systemic morphine
c) Analgesia produced by intra-articular morphine is more effective in the presence of inflammation
d) Naloxone injection into a knee following surgery does not increase pain
e) Tolerance to morphine after repeated intra-articular injections occurs more rapidly than after repeated systemic or oral use

11.3 With regard to air embolism:

a) Venous air embolism causes a rise in end-tidal CO_2
b) Doppler ultrasonography is more sensitive than end-tidal CO_2 in detecting air embolism
c) Transoesophageal echocardiography is more reliable at detecting paradoxical air embolus than Doppler
d) Clinical problems are likely only when the amount of air exceeds 3 ml/kg
e) The volume is increased by nitrous oxide

11.4 Properties of ketamine include:

a) Acts on GABA (gamma-aminobutyric acid) receptors
b) 'S' isomer is a better analgesic than the 'R' isomer
c) Markedly increases antidiuretic hormone secretion
d) Anticholinergic actions
e) Local anaesthetic action

11.5 Reperfusion of ischaemic tissues with oxygenated blood can cause:

a) Metabolic acidosis
b) Hyperkalaemia
c) Myoglobinaemia
d) Lung damage
e) Accumulation of free oxygen radicals

11.6 Enoximone:

a) Is a phosphodiesterase inhibitor
b) Is a bypiridine
c) Stimulates beta receptors
d) Increases calcium entry level into cardiac muscle cells
e) Can be given orally

11.7 With regard to the monitoring of neuromuscular block:

a) The diaphragm and laryngeal muscles are more sensitive to relaxants than the abductor pollicis muscle
b) The diaphragm and laryngeal muscles recover more quickly than the abductor pollicis muscle from a non-depolarizing block
c) The nerve stimulator used to monitor neuromuscular block delivers a biphasic wave
d) Double burst 'fade' is more readily detectable by visual means than train of four fade
e) Depolarizing block is characterized by post-tetanic potentiation

11.8 With regard to capnography:

a) In a normal capnograph trace (Fig. 11.1) stage IV indicates expiratory downstroke
b) The capnograph trace in Figure 11.2 is indicative of respiratory obstruction
c) It is a more useful indicator of disconnection and oesophageal intubation than pulse oximetry
d) A typical capnograph works on the absorption of CO_2 in the ultraviolet region of the spectrum
e) Regular monitoring with capnography and pulse oximetry has not significantly reduced the incidence of anaesthetic mishaps

11.9 Platelet:

a) Reproduction is rapid
b) Formation is in bone marrow from megakaryocytes
c) Synthesis is stimulated by erythropoietin
d) Half-life is 8–14 weeks
e) Aggregation is stimulated by the enzyme thromboxane synthetase

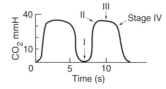

Fig. 11.1   Capnograph trace.

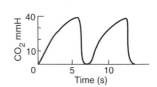

Fig. 11.2   Capnograph trace.

11.10 With regard to anaesthetic vapour hepatotoxicity:

a) Hepatotoxicity is more likely with sevoflurane than with desflurane
b) 'Halothane hepatitis' is less common in children than in adults
c) Mortality from 'halothane hepatitis' is relatively low
d) A significant proportion of 'halothane hepatitis' occurs after a single exposure to the agent
e) Halothane hepatitis is an immunologically mediated response

11.11 Stridor in children can be due to:

a) Unilateral choanal atresia
b) Unilateral vocal cord paralysis
c) Tracheal-oesophageal fistula
d) Adenotonsillar hypertrophy
e) Laryngomalacia in a 10-year-old

11.12 With regard to the hazards of blood transfusion:

a) 'O' rhesus-negative blood is as safe as 'group and type specific' blood, when required in an emergency
b) Screening eliminates the possibility of transmitting the HIV virus
c) Although not uncommon, transmission of hepatitis C is of little consequence, because it is usually asymptomatic
d) The P_{50} of haemoglobin is decreased in stored blood
e) Immunological reactions are always triggered by antigens in red blood cells

11.13 Amniotic fluid embolism:

a) Usually occurs during delivery
b) Often presents with widespread haemorrhage
c) Is often associated with a short labour with very strong contractions
d) Is caused by the entry of amniotic fluid into the maternal circulation
e) Is typified by pulmonary hypertension and right ventricular failure

11.14 In Down syndrome:

a) Cardiac defects are more likely to involve the valves than the arteriovenous canals
b) Cervical skeletal anomalies may be a feature
c) The incidence of obstructive sleep apnoea is higher than in the normal population
d) The mandible and maxilla tend to be larger than normal
e) There is a missing chromosome in the 21 position

11.15 **With regard to tetanus:**

a) The neurotoxin produced by the clostridium bacillus stimulates the inhibitory synapses in the central nervous system
b) A patient who has contracted tetanus develops lifelong immunity to subsequent infection
c) Both sympathetic and parasympathetic systems may be affected
d) Muscle hypertonicity is improved with gamma-aminobenzoic acid (GABA) agonist drugs
e) In established tetanus, tetanus vaccine and anti-tetanus immunoglobulin are not indicated

11.16 **Electrolyte facts of anaesthetic interest include:**

a) Patients with a chronic hypokalaemia of 3 mEq/litre usually develop cardiac arrhythmias
b) Cardiac arrhythmias are more likely in a patient with hypokalaemia and metabolic alkalosis, than in one with uncomplicated hypokalaemia
c) The acute hyperkalaemia caused by suxamethonium in a patient with a spinal cord injury is markedly attenuated by pretreatment with a non-depolarizing relaxant
d) Failure to defibrillate following a cardiopulmonary bypass may be due to hypomagnesaemia
e) Neuromuscular block caused by lithium can be reversed by administration of an anticholinesterase drug

11.17 **Cerebrospinal fluid (CSF):**

a) Tends to be more acidic than plasma
b) Is produced by arachnoid villi
c) Pressure is increased by aortic cross-clamping
d) Volume is reduced by glucocorticoids
e) Volume should be reduced by drainage from the lumbar subarachnoid space in patients with obstruction of CSF circulation

11.18 **Cardioversion:**

a) Using alternating current is safer than with direct current
b) Requires one paddle to be placed over the sternum, the second anterolaterally or anteroposteriorly
c) Energy required for ventricular arrhythmias is higher than for atrial arrhythmias
d) Is unlikely to be successful in patients with chronic atrial fibrillation of over 1 year's duration
e) Is contraindicated during pregnancy

11.19 **Insulin:**

a) Is synthesized in the alpha cells of the islets of Langerhans
b) Secretion is increased by somatostatin
c) Secretion is reduced by sympathetic stimulation
d) Stimulates both protein and fat synthesis
e) Allergic reactions are usually due to the impurities in animal preparations

11.20 **At high altitude:**

a) Initially, the oxyhaemoglobin dissociation curve is shifted to the right; while during acclimatization it is shifted to the left

b) Respiratory alkalosis persists throughout acclimatization

c) The amount of anaesthetic vapour delivered at a given setting is not significantly altered

d) Nitrous oxide is a less potent anaesthetic

e) The fall in barometric pressure significantly affects gas cylinder pressures

11.1   a) True   b) False   c) False   d) True   e) True

EXPLANATION
See Table 11.1.

11.2   a) True   b) False   c) True   d) False   e) False

EXPLANATION
Opioid receptors are not only located in the central nervous system but are also present and functionally active in peripheral tissues. All receptors, i.e. mu, kappa and delta, have been found at peripheral nerve sites. In the presence of inflammation, endogenous opioids (such as encephalins and endorphins) are present on immune cells, such as T and B lymphocytes, monocytes and macrophages. The immune cells migrate to the area of inflammation and, under the influence of corticotrophin-releasing factor (CRF), the endogenous opioids are released to produce analgesia. Opioid receptors are also transported to the inflammatory site. In the absence of inflammation, opioid peptides and receptors are absent; similarly, locally administered opioids are not detectable in normal tissue, but appear within minutes of the inflammatory response. As stated above, inflammation encourages the transport of opioid-carrying immune cells and opioid receptors to the affected area; moreover, the perineurium sheath surrounding the peripheral nerve is disrupted by the inflammatory process exposing the opioid receptors and therefore allowing the endogenous or locally administered opioids to attach to them. Opioids administered in the vicinity of a nerve trunk are much less effective than at the nerve terminal (e.g. intra-articularly where the inflammatory response is active).

The presence of endogenous opioids and opioid receptors in inflamed tissues has led to the intra-articular administration of opioids for postoperative analgesia after orthopaedic surgery. It has been found that small systemically inactive doses of intra-articular morphine (2–5 mg) produce postoperative analgesia without any of the side-effects of morphine. Moreover, the analgesia is very prolonged – up to 48 hours – probably because morphine is poorly lipid soluble and also because of low joint blood supply, delaying morphine clearance. The intra-articular injection of naloxone reverses the analgesia. There is also evidence suggesting that tolerance when opiates are injected onto the peripheral nervous system is much less likely to develop than when administered centrally.

11.3   a) False   b) True   c) True   d) False   e) True

EXPLANATION
Small bubbles of air do not cause problems; they either dissolve in the blood or pass into the pulmonary capillaries and are absorbed. Amounts of between 0.5–1 ml/kg can cause complications.

Types:

- Venous air embolism. Venous air embolism can occur when the pressure within an open blood vessel is below atmospheric; in practice embolism is unlikely if the surgical site is not elevated by more than 20–40 cm.
- Paradoxical (arterial) air embolism, i.e. the passage of air from the right side of the heart to the left with eventual entry to coronary or cerebral circulation. Paradoxical air embolism is likely in patients with a patent foramen ovale, which is present in about 25% of the population.

Causes of air embolism:

1. Neurosurgery, especially in the sitting position where the incidence can be over 50%. Head, neck and back surgery with open veins and a head-up tilt is also another likely source.
2. Hip surgery, usually following insertion of femoral cement.
3. Caesarean sections. Air may enter the uterine sinuses, but is rarely a problem.
4. Cardiac surgery.
5. Laparoscopic cholecystectomy.
6. Central venous catheter insertion. It is important to have the patient in a head-down position when inserting a central venous line.

Clinical features:

- Venous air embolism – hissing sound from wound, hypotension, arrhythmias, cyanosis, respiratory impairment.
- Paradoxical (arterial) air embolism – circulatory collapse, increased central venous pressure, increased bleeding, marbling of skin, presence of air in retinal vessels. ECG shows ST depression or elevation, mill-wheel murmur may be present. May be missed at post-mortem because air disappears a few hours after death.

Diagnosis:

- End-tidal CO_2 – fall in end-tidal PCO_2 precedes clinical signs with venous air embolism, but is not reliable for paradoxical air embolism.
- Doppler ultrasonography – a precordial Doppler is extremely sensitive at detecting even very small amounts of air well before any symptoms occur, but again is not as reliable with an arterial embolus.
- Transoesophageal echocardiography – this is the only reliable way of detecting paradoxical arterial embolism, but it requires constant visual attention, and detection requires considerable operator skill.

Treatment. Nitrous oxide increases the volume of the air embolus – 50% N_2O produces an increase of 200%. Therefore when a major venous embolism is diagnosed, nitrous oxide is discontinued, and the surgeon is asked to flood the wound or pack it with wet gauze. Other measures include aspiration of air through a right atrial catheter; increasing the jugular venous pressure by reducing the head-up tilt and bilateral jugular compression; application of positive end-expiratory pressure. In severe cases, cardiopulmonary resuscitation is required.

Table 11.1 Pharmacological differences between atropine/hyoscine/glycopyrolate

	Atropine
Structure	Esters formed by union of benzyl alcohol, tropic acid and tropine. Parasympatholytic anticholinergic actions
Mode of action	Parasympatholytic anticholinergic actions. Competes with acetylcholine (ACh) for muscarinic receptors. Does not inhibit nicotinic effects of ACh
Central nervous system	CNS stimulant. Stimulates respiratory centre and causes auditory hyperacusis. May cause restlessness and delirium, but possible sedation in the elderly. Antiemetic. Rarely can cause 'anticholinergic syndrome': excitement, drowsiness, memory disturbances, hallucinations, ataxia, coma. Treat with physostigmine an anticholinesterase which crosses the blood-brain barrier
Eye	Dilated pupils due to paralysis of iris sphincter
Respiration	Mild respiratory stimulant. Bronchodilatation
Glands	Bronchial, sweat and salivary glands paralysed reducing secretions from these glands
Cardiovascular system	Vagal inhibition causes tachycardia and possible arrhythmias. Raises blood pressure dropped by bradycardia (e.g. spinals). Used to prevent or treat vagal bradycardia – neostigmine/suxamethonium/halothane spinals/vagal surgical stimuli/oculocardiac reflex
Gut	Tone of gut and urinary tract reduced. Lowers gastro-oesophageal sphincter pressure; thus incidence of regurgitation increased; reduces gastric volume and secretion. Used to prevent or treat increased gastrointestinal mobility, e.g. gastroscopies and colonoscopies
Onset time (i.v.)	1 min
Duration	3 h
Dose	5–20 µg/kg

Hyoscine	Glycopyrolate
Esters formed by union of benzyl alcohol tropic acid and scopine	Quaternary ammonium compound
Same as atropine	Anticholinergic actions, but unlike atropine and hyoscine does not cross placenta or blood-brain barrier; thus it does not cause CNS actions
Unlike atropine, hyoscine is a central sedative, causing drowsiness, sedation, amnesia, but can also cause restlessness and agitation in the elderly. Better antiemetic than atropine – transdermal patch effective in nausea/vomiting caused by intrathecal/epidural opioids. Can cause 'anticholinergic syndrome'	Since it does not cross the blood-brain barrier, CNS effects and 'anticholinergic syndrome' do not occur
Action on iris sphincter stronger than atropine	Dilated pupil
Mild respiratory stimulant. Less bronchodilatation than atropine	No respiratory stimulation as central actions are absent. Bronchodilatation
Suppression of salivary, sweat and bronchial glands stronger than with atropine	Effects on gland secretion similar to hyoscine
Less tachycardia and arrhythmias than with atropine	Less tachycardia and arrhythmias than with atropine or hyoscine
Tone of gut and urinary tract reduced less than with atropine	Reduces gastric volume and secretion more so than atropine and hyoscine; thus less incidence of regurgitation

1 min	1 min
2 h	6 h
5–10 µg/kg	3–10 µg/kg

253

EXPLANATION

Ketamine

Mode of action. Ketamine is an arylocyclohexylamine available in 1%, 5% and 10% solution. It forms a precipitate with barbiturates. Unlike other general anaesthetics, ketamine does not interact with GABA receptors, but produces anaesthesia by antagonism at NMDA (*N*-methyl-D-aspartate) receptors. Stimulation of NMDA receptors causes excitatory activity.

Central nervous system effects:

- Produces dissociative anaesthesia – anaesthesia associated with involuntary limb and eye movements. Anaesthesia is often accompanied by unpleasant dreams or hallucinations during and after surgery – incidence 5% under 5 years of age, 50% in adults. The incidence of dreams can be reduced by supplementing ketamine with small amounts of sedatives. The 'S' isomer is associated with less delirium than the 'R' form.

- Cerebral and ocular. Ketamine increases pulse rate and blood pressure (BP), which is associated with increase in cerebral blood flow. There is a rise in intracranial and perhaps intraocular pressure; this latter effect has recently been questioned. It should thus not be used in neurosurgery or open eye injuries.

- Analgesia. Ketamine produces marked analgesia possibly by agonist action on kappa receptors. It is probably antagonistic at mu receptors. Analgesia may also be due to stimulation of 5-hydroxytryptamine (serotonin), which inhibits descending nerve pathways in the spinal cord. Ketamine also has local anaesthetic actions and, like all other local anaesthetics, it blocks sodium channels. Because of its analgesic action, ketamine has been employed for intravenous regional analgesia, and also for pain relief via the intravenous; intrathecal and extradural routes. These uses are unlikely to become widespread because they are often associated with marked systemic effects including general anaesthesia. The 'S' isomer is two to three times more potent as an analgesic than 'R' ketamine.

Cardiovascular effects. Ketamine causes tachycardia and a rise in blood pressure. There are a number of mechanisms to account for these changes: inhibition of catecholamine uptake; direct stimulant action on the myocardium (blocked by calcium blockers); and anticholinergic actions by its interaction with muscarinic receptors.

Respiratory effects. Respiration is not depressed by ketamine, while pharyngeal and laryngeal reflexes are well maintained, but not sufficiently to guard against aspiration. Ketamine causes marked bronchodilatation (increase in catecholamine levels, atropine-like actions) and has been used successfully in the treatment of status asthmaticus.

Effects on the gut. Increased salivation due to acetylcholine release; nausea and vomiting are common.

Metabolism. Ketamine is broken down in the liver into norketamine by demethylation and hydroxylation, and then excreted renally.

Dose. 1–2 mg/kg i.v. produces anaesthesia in 1 minute and supplementary doses of 0.5 mg/kg keep the patient anaesthetized. 10 mg/kg i.m. produces anaesthesia in 10 minutes with a duration of 10–20 minutes.

Uses:

1. Anaesthesia – induction agent; sole agent for minor procedures (e.g. burns dressings); useful in the presence of a difficult airway. The availability of the

intramuscular route is advantageous when intravenous access is difficult (e.g. in children). Because of its wide margin of safety (increasing BP), maintenance of pharyngeal and laryngeal reflexes and ease of use by the intramuscular route, it has been used widely in third world countries especially when anaesthetists are unavailable.

   2. Shock – septic or haemorrhagic.

   3. Asthma.

Strengths:

- No venous irritation
- Not painful on injection
- Bronchodilatation
- Good analgesic
- Increased BP and cardiac output
- Relative protection of pharyngolaryngeal reflexes
- Minimal hormonal effects
- Only anaesthetic which does not increase antidiuretic hormone
- Can be administered by intramuscular route.

Weaknesses:

- Dreams and hallucinations
- Nausea and vomiting common
- Increase in cerebral blood flow, intracranial pressure and ? intraocular pressure; thus unsafe in patients with high intracranial pressure and with open eye injuries
- Increased salivation
- Occasional skin rashes.

11.5   a) True   b) True   c) True   d) True   e) True

EXPLANATION

A tissue becomes ischaemic when oxygen demand exceeds supply. Tissue hypoxia leads to anaerobic metabolism, lactic acidosis, reduced production of energy (ATP), failure of cellular homeostasis, loss of ion gradients across cell membranes and eventual cell death.

   Reperfusion of the ischaemic tissue restores blood and oxygen supply and toxic metabolites are removed, but the return of toxic metabolites into the systemic circulation causes metabolic derangements, while reperfusion can also induce further local tissue injury.

Systemic effects:

- *Metabolic acidosis.* The pH of the venous effluent from reperfused ischaemic tissue is less than 7.2 and may take over 15 minutes to return to normal.
- *Hyperkalaemia.* Potassium leaks from cells because of acidosis and altered membrane permeability. Cardiac arrhythmias are possible on reperfusion especially in the presence of renal failure.
- *Myoglobinaemia.* Muscle breakdown causes the release of myoglobin, which can collect in the collecting tubules of the kidney and cause acute renal failure.
- *Lung injury.* Non-cardiogenic pulmonary oedema may occur because of increased microvascular permeability. There is also an accumulation of neutrophils

which are eventually broken down in the lung and other organs; this process is an important precursor of multisystem organ failure.

Local effects. The local damage caused by reperfusion is due to the return of oxygenated blood and specifically due to the presence of oxygen free radicals. A free radical is a molecule containing one or more unpaired electrons and is inherently unstable. Small amounts of free radicals are normally produced from the mitochondrial electron transport chain; in pathological states free radicals are derived from:

- xanthine oxidase metabolism (main source)
- activated neutrophils
- catecholamine oxidation
- endothelial cells
- prostaglandins.

Xanthine oxidase metabolism. The enzyme xanthine oxidase is the major source of oxygen free radicals in post-ischaemic tissue. Xanthine oxidase is formed in ischaemia and the rate of formation differs in different tissues, i.e. 10 seconds after onset of ischaemia in the intestine; 8 minutes in cardiac muscle and 30 minutes in liver, spleen, kidney and lungs. This probably explains the different susceptibility of these organs to ischaemic-reperfusion injury. Xanthine oxidase (together with oxygen) is required for the conversion of hypoxanthine into xanthine and superoxide (i.e. hypoxanthine $\rightarrow$ xanthine + superoxide in the presence of oxygen and xanthine oxidase). Superoxide is the precursor of hydrogen peroxide and the highly reactive hydroxyl radical. Ferritin in the presence of superoxide produces iron; then hydrogen peroxide + iron $\rightarrow$ hydroxyl radicals. The hydroxyl radical is the most damaging free oxygen radical in biological systems and causes lipid peroxidation (which causes cell damage), inactivation of cytochrome enzymes, and altered membrane transport of proteins. Thus the level of xanthine oxidase is increased during ischaemia and, when reperfusion occurs, the presence of oxygen allows the above reaction to occur causing a dramatic increase in hydroxyl radicals.

Activated neutrophils. Local ischaemic damage is associated with neutrophil accumulation in the microvasculature. The neutrophils are then activated by oxygen radicals and platelet-aggregating factor to become more adhesive. Hence the adhesive neutrophils become attached to endothelium, migrate across it and cause destruction by releasing free radicals and proteolytic enzymes and peroxidases (which cause cell damage).

Endothelial cells and some prostaglandins can also release oxygen free radicals.

Therapies to reduce reperfusion damage. Although no single approach has been consistently effective in limiting damage, possible therapies include.

- Free radical scavengers, e.g. mannitol; histidine; catalase.
- Free radical production inhibitors, e.g. allopurinol which inhibits xanthine oxidase; desferrioxamine which chelates iron and thus prevents the reaction hydrogen peroxide + iron $\rightarrow$ hydroxyl radicals.
- Neutrophil inhibitors to prevent free radical production and neutrophil adhesion – adenosine; monoclonal antibodies; perfluorochemicals; antiproteases.
- Antioxidants, which interrupt peroxidation, e.g. vitamin E, beta blockers (propranolol), calcium channel blockers, ACE inhibitors (e.g. captopril).
- Ischaemic preconditioning – a series of short episodes of ischaemia followed by reperfusion can reduce damage in prolonged ischaemia.
- Hypothermia – reduces limb ischaemic damage after tourniquet application. Tourniquet time can be prolonged to 3–4 hours. Post-ischaemic hypothermia has

also been shown to reduce damage if started immediately after a period of ischaemia.

11.6   a) **True**   b) **False**   c) **False**   d) **True**   e) **True**

EXPLANATION

Phosphodiesterase inhibitors (Table 11.2)
   Mode of action. These agents are thought to act by inhibition of type III phosphodiesterase which is found predominantly in cardiac muscle. This inhibition causes an increase in cyclic monophosphate (cAMP) which increases cell entry of calcium. This leads to a positive inotropic action, thus increasing cardiac output, as well as systemic and pulmonary vasodilatation. These agents do not act on beta receptors and therefore positive inotropism is obtained even in beta-blocked patients. Moreover they appear to increase cardiac index without increasing myocardial oxygen consumption.
   Uses. These agents have been used to improve cardiac performance in patients with congestive heart failure; in patients awaiting and after cardiac transplantation and following cardiopulmonary bypass.
   Side-effects. Arrhythmias and hypotension especially with high infusion doses; other side-effects include thrombocytopenia; nausea, vomiting, diarrhoea, insomnia, headaches.

11.7   a) **False**   b) **True**   c) **False**   d) **True**   e) **False**

EXPLANATION

Features of depolarizing/non depolarizing block
   Non-depolarizing block. This is reversed with increasing level of acetylcholine

Table 11.2   Phosphodiesterase inhibitors

Drug	Class	Half-life	Dose	Comments
Amrinone	Bypiridine	3½–4 h	Loading dose 0.75–2 mg/kg Infusion 10 µg/kg/min	
Milrinone	Bypiridine	50 min	Loading dose 50 µg/kg/min Infusion 0.5 µg/kg/min	12–15 times more inotropic than amrinone
Enoximone	Imidazole	1–2 h	Loading dose 90 µg/kg/min Infusion 2–20 mg/kg/min	Available as oral preparation

(i.e. anticholinesterase – neostigmine). Neuromuscular monitoring shows 'fade', and post-tetanic facilitation (potentiation) in response to tetanic stimulation. 'Fade' is noted at lower doses of relaxants and lower relaxant plasma concentrations than depression of 'single twitch'.

Depolarizing block. As with acetylcholine, depolarizing agents depolarize the membrane by binding to postsynaptic receptors, but unlike acetylcholine depolarization at the neuromuscular junction is prolonged. Depolarizing agents produce muscle fasciculations; neuromuscular monitoring shows depression of muscle twitch; but no fade or post-tetanic potentiation following tetanic stimulation.

Nerve stimulator

A nerve stimulator delivers a sufficient current to activate all fibres in a nerve to produce an action potential. Since I = V/R (Ohm's Law), the current delivered is dependent on the skin resistance and the voltage. Thus if the skin resistance is increased, the voltage of the stimulator must be higher to achieve the same current. The voltage on the stimulator is usually 9 volts and since the skin resistance achieved by needle electrodes or electrolytic coated surface electrodes varies between 500–2000 ohms, the current delivered by the stimulator should vary between 10–70 milliamps. The duration of the current (pulse width) should be less than 0.5 milliseconds (usually between 0.1–0.3 msec) to avoid repetitive nerve stimulation. The stimulus should be rectangular (square wave) because a biphasic wave may cause repetitive action potentials. The simulator must also be able to deliver different stimuli, i.e. single twitch, train of four, double burst, tetanic and post-tetanic count (see Table 11.3). Finally the stimulator must be portable and battery operated.

The nerve usually stimulated is the ulnar nerve to cause contractions of the abductor pollicis of the thumb with one electrode positioned on the radial side of the flexor carpi ulnaris 1 cm proximal to the wrist skin crease, and the other 3–4 cm proximally. Other nerves which are readily accessible for stimulation include: the posterior tibial behind the medial malleolus causing plantar flexion of the big toe and foot; the facial nerve 3 cm posterior to the lateral border of the orbit to stimulate the orbicularis oculi muscle or below the lip to monitor contractions of the orbicularis oris.

Apart from visual and tactile assessment, the extent of neuromuscular block can be measured by mechanomyography and electromyography. With mechanomyography the muscle contraction is converted via a transducer into an electrical signal. Electromyography (EMG) records the electrical activity of the muscle with one electrode placed over the muscle belly and the other over the tendon insertion.

Different muscles vary in sensitivity to muscle relaxants. The diaphragm and the laryngeal muscles are more resistant to both depolarizing and non-depolarizing relaxants than the abductor pollicis and require about twice the amount of agent to achieve the same amount of relaxation. On the other hand, the diaphragm and laryngeal muscles recover more quickly from the block than does the abductor pollicis. The cause of these differences is probably the higher blood supply of the diaphragm. The sensitivity to relaxants and recovery from block are much more similar between the airway muscles and the orbicularis oculi muscle which is stimulated by the facial nerve.

EXPLANATION

Use of capnography
Waveform analysis. The normal waveform is shown in Figure 11.3.

Stage 1: Inspiratory baseline. Here fresh gas drives away the CO_2 from the sampling line so CO_2 should be zero. An elevated inspiratory baseline ($FiCO_2$) indicates rebreathing (Fig. 11.4) which may be due to exhausted soda lime; low fresh gas flow; or incompetent expiratory or inspiratory valves.

Stage II: Expiratory upstroke. During expiration, CO_2 is washed out from the perfused portions of the lung and thus rises at the sampling site. The slope is rapid and steep. Prolongation or slanting of the slope (Fig. 11.5) indicates expiratory obstruction (e.g. kinked tube, bronchospasm, etc.).

Stage III: Expiratory plateau. This stage is nearly horizontal and indicates a mixed alveolar gas sample. A dip in the expiratory plateau (Fig. 11.6) indicates spontaneous respiration either because of light anaesthesia or inadequate muscle relaxation.

Stage IV: Inspiratory downstroke. As inspiration draws in fresh gas the CO_2 is washed away from the sampling site. The slope is brisk and steep.

Ventilation monitor. If the capnograph is flat, i.e. end tidal CO_2 is zero, one should assume failure of ventilation due to oesophageal intubation; tracheal extubation or disconnection; ventilator failure; or respiratory depression in a spontaneously breathing patient (e.g. opioid drugs). The other cause is a malfunctioning capnograph which can easily be diagnosed by disconnecting the CO_2 sampling line and breathing into it. If the capnograph registers CO_2, the problem must be failure to ventilate the patient. Carbon dioxide can accumulate in the stomach during manual ventilation before intubation and a small amount of CO_2 may register on the capnograph as a characteristic stepwise decrease in CO_2 (oesophageal capnograph).

Sidestream capnographs may be used to monitor ventilation in spontaneously breathing patients with face masks, nasal cannulae, etc.

Detection of hypo- and hypercapnia:

- Hypercapnia – inadequate ventilation. Low set respiratory minute volumes; leaks or obstructions in circuits; CO_2 rebreathing – low gas flows; exhausted soda lime; excessive CO_2 production, e.g. malignant hyperpyrexia; toxaemia; insufflation of CO_2 during laparoscopic insufflation.

- Hypocapnia – alveolar hypoventilation – excessive tidal volumes or rates during intermittent positive-pressure ventilation. Decreased CO_2 delivery, e.g. decreased cardiac output; decreased metabolism in a hypothermic patient; increased arterial-to-exhaled CO_2 difference (see below).

Estimation of adequacy of ventilation. In healthy subjects the difference between $PaCO_2$ and P_ECO_2 is 3–5 mmHg. This difference increases with ventilation/perfusion mismatching, e.g. in general anaesthesia, chronic obstructive lung disease, pulmonary embolus, low cardiac output, shock.

NB: A typical capnograph is an infrared spectrometer where the sample CO_2 absorbs infrared radiation in an analysis cell, and the strength of the radiation impinging on the detector is therefore less than that impinging on the detector in the reference cell.

Table 11.3 Patterns of nerve stimulation

	Stimulator settings	Response in unblocked muscle
Single twitch	Supramaximal stimulus lasting 0.2 ms at 0.1 Hz frequency repeated every 10 s	Muscle twitch
Train of four	Four supramaximal stimuli at 2 Hz frequency – amplitude of fourth response compared to first – T4/T1 ratio	T4/T1 ratio approximates 1
Tetanic stimulation	High-frequency, stimulation usually 50 Hz for 5 s	Large amounts of acetylcholine released – repetitive muscle action potentials resulting in a sustained contraction
Post-tetanic twitch count	50 Hz for 5 s (tetanic stimulus) followed 3 s later by single supramaximal stimuli delivered every second at 1 Hz frequency	Not applicable as can only be applied during PTP
Double burst stimulation	Two mini bursts of tetanic stimuli. First burst of three impulses at 50 Hz; after a pause of 0.75 s there is a second burst of three impulses at 50 Hz	D2/D1 ratio approximates 1

Response in non-depolarizing block	Response in depolarizing block	Comments
Depression of twitch amplitude, but amplitude not reduced until 75–80% of receptors are occupied; thus test not very sensitive	Depression of twitch amplitude	Not sensitive enough for practical use
T4 amplitude decreases when 70–75% receptors are occupied. T4 disappears completely when 80% are blocked; T3 disappears at 85% occupancy; T2 at 85–90%; T1 at 90–98% occupancy	Twitch height reduced but no fade. T4/T1 = 1	Not painful; thus can be applied in an awake patient. Degree of block correlates well with clinical recovery
Muscle contraction reduced compared to unblocked muscle. Fade – degree of fade depends on receptor occupancy and can be used to establish depth of block as with T4/T1 ratio. Fade greater with higher frequencies and with longer duration of stimuli. A further stimulus 60–120 s following tetanus causes an enhanced subsequent contraction – post-tetanic potentiation (facilitation)	Muscle contraction reduced compared to unblocked muscle but can be sustained for 5 s, i.e. no fade. Also no post-tetanic potentiation (PTP)	Painful during period of PTP which can last for several min. During PTP single twitch or train of four does not evoke any neuromuscular response
Number of twitches inversely proportional to extent of block (post-tetanic twitch count). Each non-depolarizing relaxant has its own time course until re-establishment of first response to train of four	Not applicable as post-tetanic twitch count (PTTC) can only be applied during PTP, which does not occur with depolarizing blocks	Applied during period of PTP to estimate extent of block. Train of four stimulation produces no response during this phase
Fade similar to train of four. As with train of four, D2/D1 ratio indicates extent of block	Twitch height reduced but no fade	Not painful. Double burst fade is more readily detectable by visual means than that of train of four

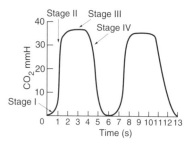

Fig. 11.3   *Capnograph trace: normal waveform.*

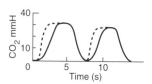

Fig. 11.4   *Capnograph trace showing an elevated inspiratory baseline.*

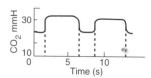

Fig. 11.5   *Capnograph trace showing slanting of the slope.*

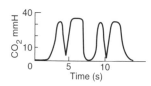

Fig. 11.6   *Capnograph trace showing a dip in the expiratory plateau.*

11.9   **a) False**   **b) True**   **c) False**   **d) False**   **e) True**

EXPLANATION

Platelets are non-nucleated (therefore cannot reproduce), round or oval discs 2–4 micrometers in diameter. They are formed in the bone marrow from large precursor cells called megakaryocytes, which fragment into platelets in the bone marrow itself, or soon after entering the blood circulation, especially in the pulmonary capillaries. Maturation of megakaryocytes, and therefore platelet formation, is controlled by a feedback mechanism, involving the hormone thrombopoietin. The normal platelet count is between 150 000–300 000 per ml, 10–20% of which lie within the spleen. The half-life is 8–12 days, while the normal life span is 8–14 weeks. When platelets reach the end of their life span, they are eliminated from the circulation by tissue macrophages; 33% of platelets are sequestrated by this process in the spleen.

Platelet functions
Platelets contain cytoplasmic granules, which release many active substances, all of which are involved in some way in the coagulation process.

- Actin, myosin, thrombostenin. All of these are contractile proteins, which allow platelets to contract.
- Adenosine diphosphate (ADP), adenosine triphosphate (ATP), 5-hydroxytryptamine (5-HT), adrenaline, calcium, fibrinogen, beta-thromboglobulin, fibrin stabilizing factor. These mediators promote platelet aggregation (ADP), vasoconstriction (adrenaline), coagulation (calcium, fibrinogen, fibrin stabilizing factor, etc.), eventually resulting in plug formation.
- Growth factor. Encourages multiplication of vascular endothelial cells, vascular smooth muscle cells and fibroblasts, helping to repair the damaged vessel wall.
- Thromboxane synthetase. This is an enzyme which is released when platelets contact damaged vascular endothelium, and stimulates platelet aggregation. On the other hand, prostacyclin is present in the vascular endothelium; it stimulates the production of platelet adenosine 3',5'-cyclic monophosphate (cAMP) which reduces release of ADP thus inhibiting aggregation. There is a fine balance between the two processes.
- Platelet cell membrane. The cell membrane contains glycoproteins, whose function is to avoid adherence to normal endothelium, but to encourage adherence to damaged areas of vessel wall. The cell membrane also contains phospholipids, which contain a lipoprotein called platelet factor 3, which activates the clotting process.

When platelets come into contact with a damaged vessel, they swell, protrude pseudopods, become sticky and their contractile elements contract to release granules which contain the active coagulation factors. ADP and thromboxane act on nearby platelets to activate them as well. As more and more platelets bunch up together, a loose platelet plug is formed. This is sufficient to stop blood loss if the vascular hole is small; if the vascular opening is large, blood coagulation progresses further, so that fibrin strands form in the platelet plug to make it tight and unyielding. Eventually, the clot either dissolves, or is invaded by fibroblasts to form connective tissue through the clot.

Assessment of platelet function:

- *Platelet number.* Bleeding time increases proportionally to the reduction in platelet numbers. Clinical bleeding is likely if the count is below 100 000/ml.
- *Bleeding time.* A small cut is made to start bleeding; the blood is blotted away with a filter paper every 30 seconds until a clot appears. Normal bleeding time is between 2–10 minutes.

Thrombocytopenia (platelet count below 150 000/ml)
Causes:

1. Platelet function disorders: either inherited, e.g. von Willebrand's disease, or acquired, e.g. renal failure, hepatic failure, autoimmune disease.

2. Inadequate platelet production in bone marrow: bone marrow infiltrated with malignant cells such as leukaemias, multiple myelomas, lymphomas; bone marrow damaged by irradiation or cytotoxic drugs; megaloblastic anaemia, aplastic anaemia, viral infections.

3. Increased platelet consumption: hypersplenism – as the spleen enlarges, platelet sequestration increases, e.g. in liver cirrhosis; massive tissue damage, e.g. burns, severe trauma; disseminated intravascular coagulation (DIC); presence of platelet antibodies either primary, e.g. idiopathic thrombocytopenic purpura, or acquired by autoimmune disease such as systemic lupus erythematosus (SLE), haemolytic anaemias, rheumatoid arthritis, or by infections, e.g. septicaemia.

4. Dilution from massive transfusion. With large transfusions, the majority of platelets are non-functional, as platelets lose their clotting action after 48–72 hours' storage.

5. Drugs:
- Platelet inhibitors: aspirin, NSAIDs, betalactam antibiotics, calcium blockers, beta blockers, quinidine, vasodilators (e.g. nitroprusside, nitroglycerine), anticoagulants, antifibrinolytics (dipyridamole), local anaesthetics, psychotropic drugs.
- Drugs causing thrombocytopenia: antibiotics, diuretics, gold salts, heparin, protamine, quinidine.

Correction of thrombocytopenia. Each unit of platelets increases the platelet count by 7500–10 000/ml. Platelets should be transfused when their level reaches 10 000/ml in idiopathic thrombocytopenic purpura; 20 000/ml in bone marrow dysplasia; 40 000/ml when caused by massive transfusions; 100 000/ml during cardiopulmonary surgery or surgery in patients with drug-related thrombocytopenia.

11.10   a) False   b) True   c) False   d) False   e) True

EXPLANATION

Before identifying halothane or other vapour as the offending agent, one must exclude other causes of postoperative jaundice, i.e. blood transfusion; excessive surgical tissue bleeding causing an increased liver bilirubin load; shock caused by hypovolaemia, sepsis or cardiac failure; hypoxaemia during surgery (especially after cardiac surgery); extrahepatic obstruction; liver metastasis; hepatotoxic drugs.

The first case of halothane hepatitis was reported in the 1960s. There are two types of hepatotoxicity associated with halothane exposure. The first type is mild hepatic damage occurring in 20% of adults who received halothane, causing mild elevation of alanine aminotransferase (ALT) and aspartate aminotransferase (AST). The second type is the fulminant, so-called 'halothane hepatitis'. This occurs in 1 in 10 000 adult patients; but in children the incidence is much lower, i.e. 1 in 200 000; hence halothane is still widely used in children. 95% of sufferers have a previous halothane exposure; other predisposing factors include female sex, obesity, middle age and high alcohol intake. Halothane hepatitis is characterized by massive hepatic necrosis with very high ALT, AST, bilirubin and alkaline phosphatase levels, and a mortality of 50–75%. It is an immunological phenomenon, wherein the halothane metabolite trifluoroacetate binds to liver proteins to form trifluoroacetylated proteins, which stimulate the formation of antifluoroacetylated protein antibodies in susceptible individuals. On subsequent halothane exposure these antibodies cause massive hepatic necrosis. Therefore, the diagnostic feature of 'halothane hepatitis' is the detection of serum antibodies against halothane metabolites.

Hepatotoxicity of other vapours
Since liver toxicity is caused by vapour metabolites, the incidence of toxicity is directly related to extent of metabolism. Methoxyflurane undergoes significant metabolism (50%), followed by halothane (25% – several hundreds of cases reported), enflurane (2.5% – 100 cases reported), isoflurane (0.2% – 6 cases reported); desflurane (0.01%). Recently the first case of desflurane hepatitis has been discovered. Although sevoflurane is metabolized (6%) to a greater extent than isoflurane, sevoflurane hepatitis should not occur, because sevoflurane metabolism does not result in trifluoroacetylated liver proteins. It is now thought that cross-sensitization can occur between different anaesthetic vapours, i.e. a patient may develop liver damage when exposed to different fluorinated anaesthetics on separate occasions.

11.11	a) False	b) True	c) True	d) True	e) False

EXPLANATION

Causes of stridor:

1. Infections: especially laryngotracheobronchitis, epiglottitis.
2. Foreign body aspiration: aspiration of a foreign body (e.g. peanut) should be suspected with a history of coughing, stridor and cyanosis while eating. Refractory wheezing is common, as well as decreased breath sounds, tachypnoea and fever. This is an emergency situation, and the foreign body should be removed as soon as possible under general anaesthesia. If the child has recently eaten, intravenous induction with cricoid pressure should be instituted, intubation carried out, and the stomach emptied with an orogastric tube; the child is then extubated and passed over to the surgeon for bronchoscopy. If the child is starved, intravenous or inhalational induction may be employed. Nitrous oxide should be avoided to reduce air trapping distal to the obstruction. Spontaneous ventilation should be maintained until the location and nature of the foreign body is determined. Close observation is required postoperatively for any signs of respiratory distress, which may be due to airway oedema or infection.
3. Congenital non-neurological causes:
- Laryngomalacia: this condition is due to incomplete development of laryngeal cartilages. Apart from post-intubation stridor, laryngomalacia is the commonest cause of stridor in an infant, and accounts for 50% of cases. The stridor is worse with agitation and in the supine position, and often better in the prone posture. Feeding is not usually a problem. It improves after 18 months , but may persist to age 4–5.
- Pierre Robin syndrome: hypoplastic mandible, glossoptosis, small epiglottis.
- Tracheo-oesophageal fistula.
4. Congenital neurological causes (i.e. vocal cord paralysis): not common.
- Unilateral cord paralysis: birth trauma, cardiac malformation affecting left recurrent laryngeal nerve, peripheral lesions.

- Bilateral cord paralysis: hydrocephalus, Arnold-Chiari malformation, posterior fossa haemangiomas; child abuse.
5. Choanal atresia: usually posterior. If bilateral, the infant must be allowed to breathe through the mouth with an oral airway until surgery is performed.
6. Upper airway (supraglottic) obstruction: laryngeal cysts, haemangiomas, laryngoceles, papillomas, adenotonsillar hypertrophy. Inspiratory stridor is usually a feature of upper airway obstruction.
7. Lower airway (subglottic) obstruction: cysts, haemangiomas, foreign bodies, vascular rings. Expiratory stridor is characteristic of subglottic obstruction.
8. Tracheal obstruction: tracheal stenosis following tracheostomy or intubation; neoplasms, tracheomalacia. Biphasic stridor (i.e. in inspiration and expiration) is characteristic of mid-tracheal obstruction.
9. Subglottic oedema: the commonest cause of this is post-intubation oedema, especially at the cricoid area which is the narrowest part of the airway. Oedema is more likely with a tight endotracheal tube, or prolonged or traumatic intubation. Oedema is reduced with steroid administration. Other causes of subglottic oedema include burns inhalation and allergic reactions.

Diagnosis. Respiratory obstruction is characterized by inspiratory stridor in supraglottic obstruction and expiratory stridor with subglottic obstruction; in severe cases stridor becomes biphasic. Stridor is accompanied by cyanosis, and nasal flaring and suprasternal retractions; in severe cases cyanosis persists even with oxygen administration, while retractions involve also the subcostal and intercostal muscles. Inspiratory wheezing is also characteristic.

11.12   a) False   b) False   c) False   d) True   e) False

EXPLANATION

Hazards of blood transfusion
  Hazards to donor. A donor should not be bled:

- if haemoglobin is less than 13.5 g/dl in a male and 12.5 g/dl in a female
- during pregnancy, and for 1 year after pregnancy
- more than two to three times a year.

  Hazards to recipient:
  Mortality. This is 0.1–1% – comparable with appendicitis.
  Transmission of disease:

- AIDS. Incidence: 1 in 225 000 units of transfusion.
  Screening: enzyme-linked immunosorbent antibody assay (ELISA) detects the presence of HIV antibodies; however HIV antibodies in carriers may not develop for weeks following exposure, therefore false negatives are possible. To avoid this, antigen screening is more reliable; even so false negatives may still occur.
- Hepatitis B. Incidence: 1 in 200 000 units transfused.
  Screening: screening is for hepatitis B surface antigen HbSAg, which appears early following exposure and persists in hepatitis B carriers. Thus, with proper screening the incidence of transmission should be very low; moreover immunization for hepatitis B reduces further the risk of infection.

- Hepatitis C. Incidence: <1 in 3000 transfusions.
90% of post-transfusion hepatitis is due to hepatitis C (non-A, non-B hepatitis). 70% of hepatitis C is asymptomatic, but it can progress to chronic hepatitis or hepatic carcinoma, and the risk of these latter complications is about 2 for every 10 000 patients who have received transfusion.
Screening: antibody screening for hepatitis C is available, and therefore should reduce the incidence of hepatitis C transmitted by blood transfusion. Unfortunately, hepatitis C is not solely transmitted by blood transfusion, and therefore its occurrence is still high.
- Cytomegalovirus (CMV). This causes a viral illness which is of no consequence to healthy individuals, but the leucocytes of an infected individual carry the virus for many years. The risk of transmitting CMV by blood transfusion is 2–3%; even so, 75% of the infected individuals remain asymptomatic; the rest develop fatigue and lethargy starting 2 weeks after the transfusion, and lasting about 2–3 weeks. The gravest risk is CMV transmission to immunocompromised patients (e.g. AIDS, transplanted patients, patients on cytotoxics), where serious disseminated infections may occur.
Screening: antibody screening for CMV infection is possible, and immunocompromised patients should be transfused with blood that is CMV free or leucocyte free.
- Bacterial/protozoal. Blood banks routinely screen donors for syphilis; most other bacterial or protozoal diseases (e.g. malaria) can be excluded by history of travel to endemic areas.
Bacterial contamination. Blood is stored at 4–6°C, and bacterial contamination, especially with Gram-negative bacteria, is possible, especially when blood is left at room temperature for over 30 minutes. Such blood should therefore be discarded.
Haemolytic reactions to red blood cells. Haemolytic transfusion reactions are triggered by antigens present in red blood cells. Although there are over 400 antigens, the principal ones are A, B, and Rh (see Table 11.4).
A Rh-negative (Rh–) recipient transfused with Rh-positive (Rh+) blood has a 70% chance of becoming sensitized to the D antigen on the red cells. Except in an emergency, Rh+ blood should not be administered to a premenopausal female, because of the risk of haemolytic disease of the newborn.
If immediate blood is required, an alternative to 'group and cross-match' is to transfuse with O Rh– blood. However, if many units of O Rh– blood are administered, the A and B antibodies in the blood may lead to the development of

Table 11.4

Group	Red Cell	Serum	Frequency
'O'	No antigens	'A' and 'B' antibodies	45%
'A'	'A' antigen	'B' antibodies	40%
'B'	'B' antigen	'A' antibodies	18%
'AB'	'AB' antigen	No antibodies	3%
Rh+	'D' antigen	No antibodies	85%
Rh–	No 'D' antigen	No antibodies before sensitization	15%

enough anti-A and anti-B antibodies to cause haemolysis of the recipient's cells. It is therefore preferable to use 'group and type specific' blood in these situations, as the test takes less than 10 minutes to perform.

Antibody formation to donor antigens occurs in less than 1% of transfusions and is usually due to human, often clerical, errors. Haemolytic reactions are either extravascular or intravascular. The latter are mediated by complement and may be fatal; the former are milder, delayed reactions (48–72 hours after transfusion), which are often undetected. Non-immunological haemolytic reactions are also possible, e.g. caused by incorrectly stored blood, time-expired blood, or blood already haemolyzed by overheating or freezing.

Haemolysis during surgery is usually detected by the presence of red or pink urine, owing to the presence of free haemoglobin. Hypotension and bronchospasm triggered by complement activation may follow. Other complications include coagulopathy and disseminated intravascular coagulation (DIC), because the lysed cells act like thromboplastin; and renal impairment due to renal vasoconstriction caused by release of vasoactive substances. Once a haemolytic reaction is diagnosed by the presence of free haemoglobin in urine and blood, the transfusion should be stopped immediately, followed by circulatory support and maintenance of renal perfusion with dopamine, frusemide, osmotic diuretics; and treatment of any coagulopathy.

Immunological reactions to blood elements other than red blood cells. Apart from reactions to red blood cells (RBCs), immunological reactions are also possible with other blood elements including platelets, leucocytes and coagulation factors. When leucocytes are transfused to a sensitized patient, an antigen-antibody reaction can occur causing flushing, hypotension, fever and even bronchospasm and pulmonary oedema. These reactions are partially relieved with antihistamines. Platelet antibodies can form in patients who require repeated platelet infusions (post-transfusion purpura), while in a haemophiliac, the development of factor VIII antibodies is a major problem.

Isoimmunization. Donor antigen causes antibody formation in the recipient that complicates future cross-matching.

Febrile reactions. The donor leucocyte or platelet antigens can cause non-haemolytic febrile reactions in recipients. Febrile reactions may also be due to products of bacterial metabolism in the container or anticoagulant. The incidence of febrile reactions has reduced considerably with the widespread use of disposable transfusion sets.

Graft-versus-host (GVH) disease. The complications mentioned above are associated with immunological disorders; at the other end of the spectrum some patients are unable to reject foreign cells, and donor lymphocytes survive in the recipient to cause chronic rejection manifest in skin, lung and kidney. Patients who are likely to develop GVH reactions are those with immunodeficiency syndromes, bone marrow transplant recipients, those with Hodgkin's disease and neonates. This possibly fatal complication can be prevented by irradiating the blood before transfusion to limit the mitotic activity of lymphocytes, with minimal effects on other blood elements.

Incompatibility. In a compatible blood transfusion the donated red cells survive as long as the host red cells, i.e. 21–35 days; in an incompatible blood transfusion, the survival time of RBCs is reduced, often to 14–16 days. This problem occurs in about 30% of transfusions, and is more likely with multiple transfusions.

Allergic reactions. Incidence: 1% of all transfusions. Reactions range from skin rashes and urticaria to anaphylactic shock with hypotension and bronchospasm, where the transfusion has to be terminated and adrenaline administered. In most cases, the transfusion can progress with antihistamine cover.

Volume overload. Over-transfusion of blood components can lead to pulmonary oedema or cardiac arrhythmias. The incidence has diminished lately with use of potent diuretics and reduced, rather than whole blood.

Citrate toxicity. Large volumes of citrate, present in stored blood as acid citrate dextrose (ACD) or citrate phosphate dextrose (CPD) cause chelation of calcium leading to hypocalcaemia – tremors, cardiac arrhythmias. Since sodium citrate is normally metabolized in the liver to sodium bicarbonate, this problem is more likely in patients with liver disease and in severe shock, in neonates and in cases of hypothermia. It may be wise to administer calcium gluconate if large volumes of blood are transfused.

Acidosis. Lactic acid is produced by red cells during storage, and multiple transfusions can cause a metabolic acidosis. This is more likely with ACD than CPD, as the pH of the ACD-stored blood is about 6.6 compared to 7.3 of CPD-stored blood.

Decreased P_{50} of haemoglobin. Stored blood has reduced 2,3-diphosphoglycerate (2,3-DPG) levels shifting the oxyhaemoglobin curve to the left, thus reducing oxygen availability to the tissues. With CPD blood, the 2,3-DPG levels fall less rapidly than with ACD blood.

Hyperkalaemia. Fresh stored blood contains 4–5 mmol/l of plasma potassium; by the expiratory date this may rise to 30 mmol/l owing to release of potassium by cells during storage.

Hypothermia. Anaesthetized patients have impaired temperature regulation, and transfusion with large volumes of blood components stored at low temperature can aggravate the hypothermia. Children are most vulnerable; increases in oxygen consumption, bradycardia and arrhythmias are possible. Therefore blood should be transfused at body temperature (but not above 4°C).

Haemosiderosis. Iron overload results from repeated transfusions of red blood cells.

Microaggregates. Blood storage leads to the formation of microaggregates.

Possible diminished immune responses. Blood transfusions may lead to decreased immune activity. It has therefore been suggested that there is an increased recurrence of malignancy in patients who require perioperative blood transfusions; on the other hand, renal transplants are less likely to be rejected following blood transfusions. There is some doubt about the validity of these observations.

11.13   a) False   b) False   c) True   d) True   e) True

EXPLANATION

Amniotic fluid embolism
   Incidence. About 1 in 40 000 pregnancies.
   Mortality. Very high – about 85% for both mother and fetus.
   Predisposing factors:

● Advanced maternal age
● Multiple pregnancies

- Short duration of labour
- Intense contractions perhaps aggravated by oxytocin
- Placental abruption present in 50% of cases
- Placenta praevia
- Ruptured uterus
- Caesarean section
- Amniotomy or amniocentesis especially if amniotic fluid is meconium stained
- Intra-amniotic injections of fluid, e.g. saline, urea
- Large babies.

Amniotic fluid embolism is caused by the entry of amniotic fluid into the maternal circulation. Three conditions must exist for this to occur: amniotomy (e.g. amniocentesis); laceration of cervical or uterine vessels (e.g. damaged uterine vessels during a caesarean section, retained placenta, placental abruption, uterine rupture); and a high pressure gradient to force the fluid into the mother's circulation (e.g. intra-amniotic injections of hypertonic saline).

Pathophysiology. Two major problems occur:

1. cardiopulmonary failure
2. disseminated intravascular coagulation (DIC).

Cardiopulmonary failure:

- Cardiac: there is raised pulmonary pressure causing right ventricular failure, decreased left ventricular output and cardiovascular collapse.
- Lungs: characteristically, the small pulmonary arterioles show evidence of embolization with amniotic fluid material; vessels of other organs – brain, kidneys, liver – are also affected. Amniotic fluid is also found in the right side of the heart. The lungs show evidence of pulmonary oedema and haemorrhage.

Disseminated intravascular coagulation. The infused amniotic fluid with its thromboplastin action causes widespread deposition of fibrin, and activates the fibrinolytic system resulting in afibrinoginaemia, coagulopathy and severe haemorrhage.

Clinical features. Presentation is usually in the first stage of labour; more rarely during delivery or postpartum. Initial symptoms include shivering, sweating and coughing. These are followed by respiratory problems – cyanosis, tachypnoea, bronchospasm and pulmonary oedema. Cardiovascular collapse follows – hypotension, arrhythmias, possible cardiac arrest. If the patient survives these stages, bleeding secondary to DIC follows. Therefore the usual course of events is as follows: prodromal symptoms – respiratory failure – cardiovascular collapse – DIC. Chest X-ray shows right ventricular enlargement, a prominent pulmonary artery, and pulmonary oedema. Lung scans reveal ventilation/perfusion abnormalities, while central venous pressure/Swan-Ganz catheters reveal pulmonary hypertension. A coagulation profile is essential.

Management. Predisposing factors should be avoided, such as accidental incision of the placenta during caesarean section, while labour with very strong contractions should be controlled with beta-adrenergic drugs or magnesium sulphate. There is no specific therapy for this condition; management is mainly supportive. Respiratory failure is treated with intermittent positive-pressure ventilation (IPPV) with 100% oxygen and positive end-expiratory pressure (PEEP); bronchospasm with sympathomimetic drugs and hydrocortisone; pulmonary oedema with diuretics; pulmonary hypertension with steroids, indomethacin or isoprenaline;

cardiovascular collapse with fluid resuscitation, digoxin, inotropes, preferably ephedrine, which does not reduce uterine perfusion. Ideally, the coagulopathy should be treated with fresh whole blood; otherwise fresh frozen plasma, cryoprecipitate and platelets are required. Postpartum uterine bleeding should be controlled with massage and intravenous oxytocin; if this is not effective, exploration for retained placenta or uterine lacerations may be required. Obviously the anaesthetic is very hazardous, and the choice of anaesthetic agents will depend on the patient's condition

11.14   a) **False**   b) **True**   c) **True**   d) **False**   e) **False**

EXPLANATION

Down syndrome is due to a chromosomal abnormality; there is an extra chromosome in the 21 position (trisomy 21), causing mental retardation. The overall incidence is 1 in 660; between the ages of 15 and 19 the chances of having a Down syndrome child are 1 in 1050, but increase to 1 in 50 over the age of 45. Apart from mental retardation, other characteristic features are: small head, epicanthic folds, short stature, short broad hands and feet. Males are usually sterile while females are not. Although mortality during childhood is increased, better medical and nursing care means that 65% are surviving beyond the age of 10.

Anaesthetic considerations

Cardiac. Cardiac anomalies occur in about 50% of Down syndrome patients, especially atrial septal defect, ventricular septal defect, Fallot's tetralogy and patent ductus arteriosus. Echocardiography is required before any surgery in the newborn. The anaesthetic must take into account any cardiac lesions, while antibiotics may be required for endocarditis prophylaxis.

Respiratory. There may be abnormalities of the upper respiratory tract, chest wall recession and hypotonia of the pharyngeal muscles. Compared to normal children, respiratory complications are therefore more common – postoperative desaturation and stridor.

Obstructive sleep apnoea is also more frequent in Down syndrome patients, and in severe cases prolonged hypoxaemia can lead to pulmonary hypertension and right-sided heart failure.

Skeletal. Cervical instability is not uncommon, possibly due to hypotonia of muscles and ligaments. There may be subluxation at C1–C2, or abnormalities of the odontoid peg. Intubation may therefore be complicated by atlantoaxial subluxation and possible cord compression. Preoperatively, lateral X-rays should be taken in flexion and extension to detect any atlantoaxial instability, in which case neck immobilization is required during intubation and muscle relaxation.

Intubation. Intubation may be difficult because of atlantoaxial anomalies, large tongue, small mouth, small mandible and maxilla, narrow nasopharynx, and irregular teeth. The endotracheal tube should be smaller in diameter than that predicted by age.

Intestinal obstruction. The incidence is increased.

Immune system. Immunity is often defective, causing an increased incidence of infections.

Biochemical. Biochemical abnormalities involving 5-hydroxytryptamine (5-HT), amino acid and catecholamine metabolism are possible.

Hormonal. Thyroid hypofunction has been reported. Males are usually sterile; females are usually fertile.

11.15   a) False   b) False   c) True   d) True   e) False

EXPLANATION

Aetiology. Tetanus is caused by an anaerobic bacillus, *Clostridium tetani*, which is present in soil and gut. In an anaerobic environment, it multiplies and produces a potent neurotoxin, which prevents transmission at inhibitory synapses in the spinal cord and medulla, causing overactivity of the motor system. The incubation period is 3–21 days, and in 65% of cases there is a history of a wound, often penetrating, but this may be of a trivial nature.

Clinical features. A small number of patients have localized tetanus, e.g. cephalic tetanus, which follows a wound in the neck or head, and causes cranial nerve palsies. In most cases it is generalized, and characterized by widespread muscle hypertonicity, resulting in trismus (lockjaw), rigidity of the facial muscles (risus sardonicus), neck stiffness and arching of back (opisthotonos). Intermittent muscle spasms are superimposed on the muscle hypertonicity, and these spasms can be precipitated by a strong external stimulus. Spasms of the laryngeal and intercostal muscles can cause respiratory failure, with greatly increased oxygen consumption. Sometimes, dysphagia is the major symptom, causing pooling of saliva and fits of pharyngeal spasm. A toxic myocarditis is also possible, causing ST and T changes on the ECG. The autonomic system may be involved, affecting both the parasympathetic and especially (in 25–60% cases) the sympathetic system. Sympathetic involvement is accompanied by increased catecholamine levels, causing tachycardia, hypertension, arrhythmias, vasoconstriction, sweating, salivation and pyrexia. Parasympathetic dysfunction can lead to hypotension and bradycardia. Mortality is around 10%. An attack of tetanus does not give lifelong immunity, possibly because the toxin travels up the nerves, and does not come into direct contact with gamma globulin.

Anaesthetic considerations

Specific treatment. In established cases: anti-tetanus immunoglobulin 30 mg/kg i.m.; tetanus toxoid; antibiotics, e.g. benzylpenicillin or any other appropriate antibiotic; the wound should be cleaned and excised, and tissue sent for culture.

Prophylaxis against tetanus in patients who are at risk. Active immunization (tetanus vaccine) is indicated in patients who have never had a complete immunization course; tetanus immunoglobulin should be given in addition to the vaccine in patients with severely contaminated wounds. The latter precaution is probably not necessary if a patient has an established immunity; in this case, further protection can be achieved by a booster dose of vaccine.

Muscle hypertonicity/spasms. In mild cases, diazepam or midazolam; in severe cases, intermittent positive-pressure ventilation (IPPV) with tracheostomy, nasogastric or parenteral feeding because of gastrointestinal stasis, sedatives, muscle relaxants. Suxamethonium should be avoided, because of possible hyperkalaemia; pancuronium should also not be administered because of sympathetic stimulation. The relaxants of choice are atracurium or vecuronium. Other drugs which have been used for control of spasms include: propofol infusions, continuous extradural anaesthesia, sodium valproate, dantrolene, and intrathecal baclofen – an antispasmodic agent which acts on GABA receptors resulting in sedation, hypotonia, and central depression, which if severe can be reversed with flumazenil.

Autonomic disturbances. Sympathetic overactivity can be treated with beta blockers, but bradycardia and hypotension may be the result. Infusions with short-acting beta blockers such as esmolol may be associated with fewer problems. Opioid infusions have also been used for the treatment of hypertension and tachycardia.

Fluids/nutrition. Fluid losses may be severe because of excessive sweating, salivation, and losses from the gut. 6–8 litres of fluid may be required daily. Nutrition is also mandatory, and may have to be given parenterally in the presence of gastrointestinal stasis.

Anticoagulation. Low-dose heparin should be administered, because the risk of deep vein thrombosis is high.

11.16   a) False   b) True   c) False   d) True   e) False

EXPLANATION

Potassium. Since serum potassium represents only 1/40th of the intracellular potassium concentration, it is important to distinguish between acute hypokalaemia, where a low potassium is accompanied by normal body potassium level, and chronic hypokalaemia, where body levels are reduced. Serum potassium level is not a reliable reflection of total body potassium.

Acute hypokalaemia. Anaesthetists cause acute, usually harmless hypokalaemia by hyperventilation. Alkalosis causes intracellular shift of potassium in exchange for extracellular hydrogen to bring the serum pH towards normal.. For each 0.1 pH increase, there is an intracellular potassium shift of 0.5–1 mEq/litre.

Chronic hypokalaemia. Common causes include persistent diarrhoea, nasogastric aspiration, diuretics, digoxin. Acceptable serum potassium levels before elective surgery are 3.0–3.5 mEq/litre. The decision to administer preoperative potassium will depend upon a number of factors – physical status of the patient, rate and magnitude of potassium loss, and the presence of other factors affecting potassium levels. Hypokalaemia occurring over hours or days is much more debilitating than if it occurs over weeks or months. Moreover, patients on long-standing potassium-losing diuretics, patients with metabolic alkalosis or patients on digoxin therapy are more likely to develop cardiac arrhythmias, than if the hypokalaemia was uncomplicated by these factors.

Patients with chronic hypokalaemia do not usually develop cardiac arrhythmias, and the only ECG changes may be low T waves.

Acute hyperkalaemia. The most common causes of acute hyperkalaemia encountered by an anaesthetist are related to suxamethonium administration in acute burns, severe trauma, cord injuries and chronic neuromuscular wasting diseases. Use of a non-depolarizing agent before administration of suxamethonium is not a reliable method of preventing rise in potassium levels.

Chronic hyperkalaemia. The most common cause of chronic hyperkalaemia is chronic renal failure. These patients often have potassium levels above 6 mEq/litre without any cardiovascular effects.

Sodium. *Hyponatraemia.* Sodium imbalance is often associated with potassium imbalance. The most common cause of acute hyponatraemia of anaesthetic relevance is TURP syndrome. Chronic hyponatraemia with a decreased extracellular volume is often due to replacement of lost fluid with salt-free solutions. Hyponatraemia with increased extracellular volume occurs in oedematous patients with cardiac, hepatic or renal insufficiency. Allowing free fluids and restricting sodium to these patients increases the oedema and the hyponatraemia.

Calcium. Contractility of cardiac and skeletal muscle is closely dependent upon extracellular calcium concentration. When a patient is being given massive transfusions of acid-citrate-dextrose (ACD) blood, the citrate binds to the ionized calcium, producing a reduction in calcium concentration and myocardial depression. One should therefore administer calcium when large volumes of blood are transfused.

Magnesium. Magnesium is often overlooked; it plays an important role in calcium ion movement. Magnesium sulphate causes vasodilatation and neuromuscular depression, and is used in the treatment of eclampsia.

Hypomagnesaemia. This may be due to chronic diarrhoea, diuretics, diabetes mellitus, renal failure, haemodialysis, cardiopulmonary bypass. It causes cardiac arrhythmias and increased neuromuscular activity such as fits, and tremors. Magnesium sulphate may be indicated in arrhythmias associated with hypocalcaemia and hypokalaemia, while patients who fail to defibrillate after cardiopulmonary bypass may do so after administration of magnesium sulphate.

Hypermagnesaemia. This is usually due to renal impairment; it is characterized by muscle weakness, sedation, confusion and treated with i.v. calcium chloride.

Electrolytes and muscle relaxants. Non-depolarizing neuromuscular block is enhanced by hypokalaemia, hyperkalaemia, hyponatraemia, hypermagnesaemia, hypocalcaemia, and lithium administration. Lithium, used in the treatment of a number of psychiatric disorders, reduces the synthesis and release of acetylcholine, and potentiates both depolarizing and non-depolarizing muscle relaxants. There is no reversal drug for neuromuscular block caused by lithium, and therefore such patients have to be ventilated until the lithium is renally excreted.

11.17   a) False   b) False   c) True   d) True   e) False

EXPLANATION

Physiology

The volume of CSF is 150 ml. CSF production is 15–36 ml per hour. 90% of CSF is formed by the choroid plexuses in the lateral and fourth ventricles. The remaining 10% arises from the brain itself. From the lateral ventricles, it passes along the aqueduct of Sylvius to join the CSF in the fourth ventricle. It leaves the fourth ventricle through the foramina of Luschka and Magendie to enter a large space behind the medulla – the cisterna magna – which is continuous with the subarachnoid space that surrounds the brain and spinal cord. The CSF is removed by arachnoid villi, which project into the subarachnoid space close to the major dural venous sinuses. When CSF pressure is greater than the venous sinus pressure, CSF flows into the sinuses; when the venous sinus pressure is greater than the CSF pressure, the villi close to prevent reverse flow. The normal CSF pressure is 10–15 mmHg, with zero level taken either as base of skull, or external auditory meatus. It can be measured by an intraventricular catheter, which can be inserted via a burr hole, or using a subdural or extradural transducer. CSF has a specific gravity of 1003–1009, and a pH of 7.39–7.50. The contents are 90% water, with glucose (40–80 mg/100 ml), protein (14–45 mg/100 ml), 3–5 mononuclear cells per ml, 138 mEq/l sodium, 2.8 mEq/l potassium, 2.4 mEq/l calcium, 2.7 mEq/l magnesium, and 1.4 mEq/l chloride. The CSF contents differ from blood contents; moreover there is a blood-brain and blood-CSF barrier in the choroid epithelium. Thus only water, oxygen and carbon dioxide enter the brain with ease; lipid-soluble agents (most anaesthetics) and electrolytes diffuse more slowly, while lipid-insoluble substances and plasma proteins hardly reach the CSF or brain from blood.

CSF functions
The CSF ensures a stable metabolic and biochemical environment for the brain and spinal cord, and provides buoyancy thus protecting the brain against injury. It also distributes local anaesthetics and narcotics during spinal anaesthesia. Without the protection of the meninges and CSF, the brain would be very vulnerable even to minor trauma. The brain is most likely to be damaged by a skull fracture when bone penetrates brain tissue, by vascular trauma, or when a blow on the head drives the brain onto the skull at a point opposite to where the blow was delivered (contracoup injury). Thus, a frontal blow is likely to cause occipital brain trauma.

Abnormal CSF volumes
Increased CSF volume can occur from obstructed flow or obstructed reabsorption, or rarely from excessive CSF production. The dura of the brain extends as a sheath around the optic nerve; therefore, a rise in CSF pressure is reflected inside the optic nerve sheath causing papilloedema. In external hydrocephalus, the reabsorption capacity of the arachnoid villi is decreased; in internal hydrocephalus, there is obstruction within the ventricular system. A large brain tumour reduces the upward flow of CSF through the subarachnoid space, thus reducing absorption by the cerebral arachnoid villi and causing a rise in intracranial pressure. Intracranial pressure haemorrhage or infections are accompanied by the appearance of numerous cells in the CSF causing blockage of the arachnoid villi and again reducing CSF absorption. CSF pressure also increases with aortic cross-clamping. The cause of this CSF pressure rise is not known, but several vascular surgeons drain spinal fluid during aortic occlusion.

Reduction of CSF volume
Surgical methods of reducing CSF volume require the insertion of a ventriculoperitoneal or ventriculointestinal shunt using a silicone rubber tube. In an emergency, the quickest way of reducing CSF volume is drainage. Before draining CSF from the lumbar region, a CT scan should be performed to determine if there is obstruction to CSF flow or a mass lesion. If this is the case, CSF should be drained by insertion of a catheter into the lateral ventricle. In other situations, drainage can be achieved either via the ventricle or the lumbar subarachnoid routes. Medical measures to decrease CSF volume are only used in mild cases or to limit damage before surgical drainage. A number of drugs reduce CSF production including mannitol, other diuretics (e.g. acetazolamide, frusemide), glucocorticoids, and digoxin; low plasma carbon dioxide levels (hyperventilation) also have this effect.

11.18   a) True   b) False   c) True   d) True   e) False

EXPLANATION

Principles

The conducting system of the heart, i.e. sinoatrial node, atrioventricular node and right and left bundle of His, is responsible for generating the cardiac rhythm. The sinoatrial node will respond to an external electrical current in the same way as to an internal impulse. When an external current is delivered to the heart, the myocardium is depolarized and contracts; the defibrillator recognizes an R wave on the ECG, and the shock is delivered to coincide with it. Once the current is removed, defibrillation occurs, and hopefully the sinoatrial node or the intrinsic pacemaker of the heart will take over, thus converting the cardiac arrhythmia into sinus rhythm. When defibrillators were first used on humans in 1947, DC current was employed; nowadays AC shock is applied as it causes fewer muscle contractions and less risk of ventricular fibrillation to patient and operator. The energy (E) delivered (in joules) equals voltage (V) multiplied by stored charge (C). $E = CV$. Thus $E = 160$ mC $\times 5000$ V $= 800$ J. Since the voltage decreases from its initial peak, the stored energy is only about half, i.e. 400 J. The 400 J energy is further reduced by the transthoracic impedance of the patient, which typically is about 50 ohms. Impedance is reduced by using large paddles, application of electrolytic gel, applying firm pressure on the paddles, avoiding placing the paddles over the sternum because bone is a poor conductor (correct placement is anteroposteriorly or anterolaterally), and by defibrillating when the lung volume is at its lowest, i.e. at the end of expiration. The paddles should not touch each other, to ensure that all the current reaches the heart. For ventricular arrhythmias (e.g. tachycardia), one should start with 200 J; for atrial arrhythmias (e.g. flutter, fibrillation) 25–100 J should be sufficient; for internal defibrillation, 10–20 J.

Indications:

- Ventricular fibrillation in emergency situations.
- Ventricular tachycardia.
- Arrhythmias (atrial tachycardia, atrial fibrillation, atrial flutter) due to Wolff–Parkinson–White syndrome.
- Supraventricular tachycardia – when other therapy has failed.
- Atrial fibrillation (AF) if:
  - onset less than 1 year
  - history of systemic embolism
  - persistent AF after cardiac surgery
  - persistent AF after thyrotoxicosis
  - AF accompanied by fast ventricular rate not responding to drugs.

There is a 90% success rate, though the incidence of relapse to AF is high.

Relative contraindications:

- Atrioventricular block.
- Digoxin therapy.
- Beta blocker therapy.
- Abnormal electrolytes especially hypokalaemia.
- Poorly controlled anticoagulation, otherwise systemic embolism likely.
- Atrial fibrillation with slow ventricular rate.

NB. Pregnancy is not a contraindication for cardioversion, though it can cause fetal arrhythmias.

Anaesthetic considerations
Since cardioversion is often conducted in areas where general anaesthesia is not frequently undertaken, one must make sure that all safety measures are in place before commencing the anaesthetic. If patients are on anticoagulants to guard against embolization, the level of anticoagulation must be adequate preoperatively. Likewise, electrolytic levels should be checked, because defibrillation may fail with abnormal levels, especially hypokalaemia. Glyceryl trinitrate patches should be removed, as there is a risk of explosion with electric sparks.

Following preoxygenation, an intravenous induction agent is administered, perhaps in conjunction with a short-acting analgesic such as fentanyl or alfentanil. All i.v. anaesthetic agents have been used, but diazepam and midazolam should probably be avoided, as amnesia is not guaranteed. Propofol is probably best, because recovery is rapid even with repeated doses; hypotension is, however, likely. Etomidate is more stable on the cardiovascular system, but recovery is more prolonged. Suxamethonium is not contraindicated, if cardioversion is required on an unstarved patient; however hyperkalaemia must be excluded prior to administration.

Complications

- Ventricular fibrillation; bradycardias; death due to synchronization failure of the defibrillator.
- Systemic embolus.
- Myocardial necrosis with excessive shocks.
- Muscle breakdown causing possible elevation in cardiac enzymes, and in rare cases rhabdomyolysis and renal failure.
- Oxygen burns if oxygen is left close to the patient during cardioversion.

11.19   a) False   b) False   c) True   d) True   e) True

EXPLANATION

Synthesis
Insulin is synthesized in pancreatic islets, which although they only constitute 2% of pancreatic mass, produce other important proteins such as glucagon and somatostatin. Insulin is formed in the beta cells, glucagon in the alpha cells and somatostatin in the delta cells. Insulin is a small protein (MW 5800), containing two peptide chains – an A chain with 21 amino acids, and a B chain with 30 amino acids. The chains are linked by disulphide bonds. Insulin is synthesized as a larger protein called proinsulin, in which the A and B chains are linked by a further fragment called C-peptide. In the presence of hyperglycaemia, proinsulin is converted into insulin by the loss of the C-peptide, and released into the hepatic portal vein to reach the liver where it has maximum effect. Insulin has a short half-life in the circulation (4–6 min), and is rapidly broken down in the liver and other tissues by insulinases.

Actions

- *Sugar.* Insulin lowers blood sugar by inhibiting output of hepatic glucose, and by facilitating uptake of glucose and fat. In the liver and muscle, it stimulates glycogen   277 synthesis and inhibits glycogen breakdown (glycogenolysis). It also stimulates glucose uptake in muscle and adipose tissue.

● *Proteins*. Insulin stimulates protein synthesis from amino acids, and inhibits protein catabolism.

● *Fat*. Lipogenesis and ketogenesis with formation of ketone bodies are increased by insulin, while lipolysis and the concentration of plasma lipids are reduced.

● *Potassium*. Insulin increases potassium uptake into cells, and is used for the treatment of hyperkalaemia.

Control of secretion

Insulin secretion is stimulated by:

● Hyperglycaemia. Hyperglycaemia causes a rapid initial increase in insulin secretion, followed by a lower sustained release.
● Amino acids, e.g. arginine.
● Gastric inhibitory peptide.
● Glucagon. Glucagon is a polypeptide secreted by the alpha cells of the pancreatic islets in response to a low level of sugar in the blood. It raises the blood sugar levels by stimulating gluconeogenesis (synthesis of glucose from lactate, amino acids and glycerol) and glycogenolysis. The ratio of insulin/glucagon is the prime factor determining blood sugar levels.
● Drugs, e.g. sulphonylureas.
● Parasympathetic activity.

Insulin secretion is reduced by:

● Somatostatin
● Adrenaline and other beta agonists
● Increased sympathetic activity.

Insulin used therapeutically

In the past, the insulin used for treatment of diabetes, was obtained from pigs (porcine insulin) or cows (bovine insulin). These agents have to be highly purified to avoid localized or generalized insulin allergy or fat atrophy. These reactions are thought to be immunological in origin, and can be reduced by the use of human insulins, which have been synthesized in the last 10 years. Insulin is broken down in the gut, and therefore cannot be given orally. Its duration of action can be prolonged by decreasing its solubility, and delaying its absorption after subcutaneous injection. This can be achieved by adding zinc or protamine to the insulin, resulting in preparations which have an immediate, intermediate or prolonged onset. Preparations with an intermediate duration are usually given twice daily, those with a long duration once daily.

Thus:

● Neutral insulin is short acting, has an onset of action within 30 minutes, and has a duration of 8 hours.

● Isophane insulin (isophane protamine insulin) or insulin zinc amorphous suspension has an intermediate onset of action, with an onset of 2 hours and 15–18 hours' duration.

● Insulin zinc crystalline suspension or protamine zinc insulin is long acting with a 5-hour onset of action and 36-hour duration. Long-acting preparations are not commonly used.

11.20   a) False   b) False   c) True   d) True   e) False

EXPLANATION

Physical changes of altitude

- *Barometric pressure.* Decreases by 50% every 5500 metres.
- *Temperature.* Decreases by 2°C every 300 metres; at 12 200 metres the temperature is –60°C.

Physiological changes of altitude
Acute changes:

- *Respiratory.* Since $P_AO_2 = FiO_2 \times P_B$, as the inspired oxygen and barometric pressure fall with altitude, the alveolar oxygen level drops. Hypoxia stimulates the respiratory centre via the peripheral chemoreceptors causing hyperventilation, hypocapnia and respiratory alkalosis. Alkalosis shifts the oxyhaemoglobin curve to the left.
- *Cardiovascular.* There is tachycardia, and increased cardiac output, while blood pressure remains more or less normal.
- *Cerebral function.* There is cerebral impairment associated with hypoxia. Coma is likely at 6000 metres without added oxygen. After 8–24 hours, newcomers to high altitude may develop acute mountain sickness which may last 4–8 days. Symptoms are probably due to cerebral oedema and include headache, dizziness, insomnia, fatigue, nausea, vomiting and breathlessness.

Chronic compensatory changes:

- *Respiratory.* Hyperventilation persists; pulmonary diffusing capacity increases owing to increased pulmonary blood flow and increased alveolar surface.
- *Cardiovascular.* Cardiac rate and output return to normal; hypoxic vasoconstriction of pulmonary arterioles causes pulmonary hypertension and right ventricular hypertrophy, which has no physiological advantage.
- *Renal.* The kidneys excrete the extra bicarbonate so that within 2–3 weeks the respiratory alkalosis is corrected.
- *Blood.* Increases in 2,3-diphosphoglycerate shift the oxyhaemoglobin curve to the right; thus oxygen becomes more readily available to the tissues. Hypoxia stimulates erythropoietin secretion, causing an increased red cell mass and polycythaemia and raised haemoglobin levels. These changes limit the fall in arterial oxygen content. The myoglobin content of skeletal muscle also increases, raising the reserve store of oxygen in myoglobin.
- *Chronic mountain sickness.* Some fully acclimatized individuals may develop chronic mountain sickness. In this condition, the compensatory mechanisms fail, pulmonary hypertension increases further causing right heart failure with cyanosis, dyspnoea and pulmonary oedema.

Anaesthetic implications

- *Oxygen.* Since inspired and arterial oxygen levels are low, the inspired oxygen should not fall below 40%.
- *Nitrous oxide.* This is of little use at altitude — apart from the inspired levels being limited to 60%, its partial pressure decreases as barometric pressure falls, and is of no value above 3000 metres.

- *Flow meters.* Because of lower gas density, flow meters read low at altitude, especially at high flows (where density of gas is more important than viscosity – at low flows, viscosity is more significant than density). At 3000 metres the under-reading is about 20%. Venturi oxygen flow meters deliver the correct concentration.
- *Vaporizers.* The vapour pressure of a liquid is unaffected by the barometric pressure. It is reduced by lower temperatures, but since vaporizers are temperature compensated, the amount of anaesthetic delivered at a given setting is not markedly affected by altitude.
- *Cylinder pressures.* Since cylinder pressures are so high, any changes in barometric pressure will not affect cylinder pressure gauges.
- *Vapour analysers.* Since these measure partial pressures, they under-read at altitude, because all measurements are calculated at sea level barometric pressures.

12.1 **With regard to alternatives to blood transfusions:**

a) Pure perfluorochemicals dissolve more oxygen than normally oxygenated blood
b) Perfluorochemicals remain in the circulation for at least 48 hours
c) Reconstituted haemoglobin solutions cause widespread vasodilatation
d) Both perfluorochemicals and reconstituted haemoglobin solutions are cleared by the reticuloendothelial system
e) Washed blood used for autotransfusion has very few platelets

12.2 **In septic shock:**

a) Lung damage is usually widespread
b) Large tidal volumes and high ventilator pressures are required to maintain normal arterial carbon dioxide levels
c) Pulmonary hypertension is a feature
d) Fluid administration should be guided by pulmonary artery pressures
e) There is reduced production of nitric oxide

12.3 **In congenital heart disease:**

a) Diastolic murmurs are more likely than systolic murmurs to be pathological
b) Cyanosis is due to a right-to-left shunt
c) Anaesthetic induction is slower in patients with a right-to-left shunt
d) Nitrous oxide causes pulmonary vasodilatation in cyanotic patients
e) Patients who have had a corrective primary repair of an atrial septal defect require life-long antibiotic prophylaxis for 'dirty' surgical procedures

12.4 **With regard to temperature measurement:**

a) Thermistors operate on the principle that the resistance of metal oxides increases with rises in temperature
b) Thermistors are very accurate and most suitable for measurement of small temperature changes
c) Thermocouples operate on the principle of the 'Seebeck effect'
d) A thermocouple tends to be more accurate than a platinum resistance thermometer
e) A rectal temperature measurement is a true reflection of 'core' temperature

12.5 **Radial nerve paralysis causes:**

a) Wrist drop
b) Claw hand
c) Sensory loss on the lateral two-thirds of the palmar aspect of the hand
d) Inability to extend fingers
e) Inability to abduct and adduct fingers

12.6 A facet (zygoapophyseal) joint:

a) Is formed from articular surfaces of two adjacent vertebrae
b) Is only present in the lumbar region
c) Is innervated by the dorsal primary spinal root
d) Pain typically radiates to leg and foot, and is worse on extension
e) Pain is almost always associated with degenerative changes in the joint

12.7 With regard to pneumonia:

a) Hospital acquired pneumonia in ventilated patients is typically caused by aerobic Gram-negative rods
b) AIDS pneumonia is often caused by cytomegalovirus infection
c) *Staphylococcus aureus* typically causes a cavitating bronchopneumonia
d) Penicillins are the antibiotics of choice for treating legionella pneumonia
e) *Haemophilus influenzae* typically causes lobar pneumonia

12.8 Signs of distress in the full-term fetus include:

a) Type 1 (early) decelerations
b) Increased fetal movement
c) Decreasing variability in fetal heart rate
d) Metabolic acidosis
e) Bradycardia or tachycardia

12.9 The following agents increase intracranial pressure:

a) Propofol
b) Fentanyl
c) Ketamine
d) Isoflurane
e) Nitrous oxide

12.10 With regard to lumbar sympathetic block:

a) The lumbar sympathetic chain lies posterior to the psoas muscle
b) Correct position of needle can be determined solely with a lateral X-ray or lateral image intensifier view
c) It can be beneficial in treating intractable pain from carcinoma of the kidney
d) It is usually of great benefit in treating phantom limb pain
e) Pre-treatment with vasoconstrictors is required to prevent hypotension

12.11 Problems in severely burnt patients include:

a) Increased sensitivity to non-depolarizing relaxants
b) Hyperthermia
c) Hypoglycaemia
d) Pulmonary oedema, which has a lower incidence if colloids rather than crystalloids are administered during resuscitation
e) Fat embolism

12.12 Methaemoglobinaemia:

a) Is due to oxidation of the iron in the haemoglobin molecule from the ferrous to the ferric form
b) Can be treated with methylene blue
c) Can be caused by methylene blue
d) Causes shift of the haemoglobin dissociation curve to the right
e) Causes low arterial oxygen levels

12.13 With regard to inherited disorders:

a) Most patients suffering from inherited hyperlipoproteinaemia eventually develop ischaemic heart disease
b) Porphyria is due to an inherited deficiency of the enzyme delta-aminolaevulinic (ALA) synthase
c) Familial periodic paralysis is associated with changes in serum potassium levels
d) Patients with inherited glycogen storage disease are typically hypoglycaemic
e) Patients with inherited myotonias and muscular dystrophies often have associated cardiac abnormalities

12.14 If a fit pregnant woman (14 weeks' gestation) undergoes general anaesthesia for an emergency appendicectomy:

a) Vasoconstrictor drugs with pure alpha actions should be avoided
b) Higher induction doses and higher vapour concentrations are required to induce and maintain anaesthesia
c) A dramatic fall in blood pressure could be due to aortocaval compression
d) Non-steroidal anti-inflammatory analgesics are contraindicated because they increase uterine tone
e) Neostigmine is likely to cause a fetal bradycardia, unless supplemented with an anticholinergic drug

12.15 With regard to maternal obstetric problems:

a) Uterine blood flow at term accounts for 5% of cardiac output
b) Fetal distress can present with tachycardia or bradycardia
c) Disseminated intravascular coagulation may be a complication of intrauterine fetal death
d) Placenta praevia usually presents with painful vaginal bleeding, abruptio placenta with painless vaginal bleeding
e) Both fetal head entrapment and cord prolapse are more likely with breech presentations

12.16 Problems in patients with chronic renal failure include:

a) Hypermagnesaemia
b) Thrombocytopenia
c) Hyperphosphataemia
d) Coagulopathy
e) Shift of oxyhaemoglobin curve to the left

12.17 Of the opioid analgesics:

a) Morphine acts primarily at mu receptors to mediate analgesia and respiratory depression
b) Pentazocine and nalbuphine are examples of analgesic drugs which are agonist at kappa receptors and antagonist at mu receptors
c) Stimulation of the kappa receptors produces more respiratory depression than stimulation of the mu receptors
d) Pentazocine causes dysphoria and cardiovascular stimulation by acting on the delta receptors
e) Naloxone is antagonist at mu, kappa and sigma receptors

12.18 With regard to laryngotracheobronchitis and epiglottitis:

a) Epiglottitis is usually caused by a viral infection
b) Laryngotracheobronchitis is usually associated with marked toxaemia and a high temperature
c) Laryngotracheobronchitis develops over a number of days and lasts about 4–5 days; epiglottitis gets established within hours and lasts about 1–2 days
d) Differential diagnosis should be made on the ward by laryngoscopy
e) If intubation is deemed necessary in a 4-year-old child with epiglottitis, a 5.5 mm diameter tube should be used

12.19 Anaesthetic pollution:

a) Presents significant health risks to theatre personnel
b) By halothane is potentially more risky than by nitrous oxide
c) Can be significant even with scavenging devices
d) Levels reaching 10% of the minimum alveolar concentration (MAC) of vapour impair the mental ability of anaesthetists
e) Contributes significantly to the greenhouse effect and depletion of the ozone layer

12.20 With regard to spinals and epidurals in children:

a) Post-spinal headaches are less common in young children than in adults
b) The dural sac ends at S3 in a baby and at S1 in an adult
c) The epidural space is relatively larger in an adult compared to an infant
d) Spinous processes are more parallel to each other in an adult than in a child
e) Haemodynamic changes (sympathetic blockade, hypotension) are more pronounced in an infant than in an adult

12.1   a) True   b) False   c) False   d) True   e) True

EXPLANATION
Alternative measures to blood transfusions are always being investigated, because there are a number of hazards with blood administration, i.e. volume overload, allergy, sepsis, transmission of disease (hepatitis C – 1 every 3000 units; hepatitis B – 1 every 200 000; HIV – 1 every 225 000), adult respiratory distress syndrome, graft-versus-host disease, immunosuppression.

Perfluorochemical emulsions
Perfluorochemicals (PFCs) are inert liquids whose capacity to dissolve oxygen is 20 times that of water. The amount of oxygen they carry is proportional to the oxygen partial pressure PaO_2 and the percentage of PFC in the blood. At 1 atmosphere (760 mmHg), 100 ml of pure PFC carries 40 ml of oxygen; twice the capacity of arterial blood (20 ml/100 ml). Unfortunately pure PFCs cause a lethal liquid embolus, and therefore 10–20% emulsions are used instead. The amount of oxygen carried by these emulsions is much less than that of arterial blood with a normal haematocrit, but in theory the oxygen transported by these PFCs is sufficient to sustain life. Since PFCs are cleared from the circulation within 24 hours, repeated daily doses would be required. This is not feasible because PFCs are not metabolized but are cleared from the vascular system by the reticuloendothelial system which cannot deal with large amounts of PFCs, and toxic effects are then likely. Ultimately PFCs collect in the liver and spleen and leave the body slowly as a vapour. In conclusion, perfluorochemicals may have a role as a blood substitute to transfer oxygen perioperatively.

Haemoglobin solutions
A second method of transporting oxygen is to use haemoglobin solutions. Haemoglobin can be purified, dried into a powder and mixed with saline. As with PFCs, it is cleared by the reticuloendothelial system within 24 hours. Again, there are a number of problems with reconstituted haemoglobin solutions.

- The residual red cell membranes are toxic especially to the kidney.
- Removing the red cell membranes causes further problems. The alpha and beta chains of haemoglobin come apart and reduce the P_{50} of Hb from 26.7 mmHg to 12–14 mmHg. This means that rather than release oxygen to tissues, the membrane-stripped Hb will actually pick up oxygen. Moreover the free Hb chains are easily filtered by the kidney and act as osmotic diuretics possibly reducing intravascular volume. The P_{50} can be increased by reacting the molecule with peridoxal-5-phosphate, while the size of the molecule can be increased to reduce renal clearance.
- Allergy. Haemoglobin solutions are ideally synthesized from expired human blood. Because this is in short supply, bovine haemoglobin has been tried which can cause allergic reactions.
- Vasoconstriction. Haemoglobin solutions produce widespread vasoconstriction. This is due to the fact that removing the red cell membrane also reduces levels of nitric oxide, which is formed from the endothelial cells and causes vasodilatation.

In conclusion, haemoglobin solutions may be useful for resuscitation in shocked patients prior to hospital admission.

Autotransfusion

Two systems are available: unwashed and washed.

Unwashed system. Here the blood is collected into a sucker into which there is a constant flow of anticoagulant, then collected into a chamber and filtered through a 40-micron filter for reinfusion. The collected blood has little or no fibrinogen, platelets or factors V or VIII.

Washed system. Again there is a similar suction device, canister and anticoagulant system; there is also a centrifuge bowl rotating at 5000 rpm which removes debris, plasma and platelets by flushing with saline, leaving a concentrate of 200–250 ml of cells at 55% haematocrit. Platelets and plasma proteins are washed into the waste.

12.2   **a) False**   **b) False**   **c) True**   **d) False**   **e) False**

EXPLANATION

Some facts about septic shock

Lungs. It was originally believed that the lung damage and adult respiratory distress syndrome (ARDS) in septic shock are uniform; in actual fact the dense infiltrates usually affect the dependent parts of the lung. The traditional method of ventilation was to use large tidal volumes and high airway pressures to maintain normal $PaCO_2$ and overcome the increased lung compliance. This method of ventilation causes barotrauma resulting in increased alveolar permeability, haemorrhage and inflammation in the normal segments of the lung. Therefore intermittent positive-pressure ventilation (IPPV) must be instituted with low tidal volumes (less than 10 ml/kg), while airway pressures should not exceed 30–35 cmH_2O. High respiratory rates may limit time in both inspiration and expiration and increase dead space. The inspiratory time should be increased, and expiration time shortened. Positive end-expiratory pressure (PEEP) may be required to improve oxygenation, while atelectasis may be prevented by occasional sigh breaths. One must accept that normal arterial blood gases are not going to be achieved; a moderate gradual hypercapnia is well tolerated, and allows compensatory mechanisms to go into operation.

Heart. Septic shock is associated with decreased myocardial contractility. Cardiac output should be maintained by optimizing fluid preload, and by administering appropriate inotropes such as adrenaline/noradrenaline, while intravenous nitrates should be avoided because they may be associated with pulmonary vasodilatation, ventilation/perfusion mismatch and hypoxaemia.

Blood vessels. Sepsis is associated with an increased production of nitric oxide which produces widespread vasodilatation. This is an attempt to increase blood flow to compensate for the reduced oxygen delivery and increased tissue oxygen demand, which is a feature of septic shock; in fact a fall in oxygen delivery during treatment is a bad prognostic sign. Blood vessel flow is reduced, including splanchnic flow (largely controlled by angiotensin and vasopressin – both of which are dependent on renal perfusion); skeletal blood flow (catecholamine controlled) and renal flow (controlled by angiotensin, vasopressin and catecholamines). Pulmonary blood flow is also reduced, and there is associated pulmonary hypertension. Inotropes are usually required to improve organ blood flow. Adrenaline may dilate skeletal muscle beds and pulmonary vasculature and constrict the splanchnic bed; noradrenaline raises blood pressure and constricts skeletal muscle and splanchnic vessels. Dopamine may improve renal and splanchnic flow, while dopexamine with its beta-2 action is most likely to increase renal and splanchnic blood flow. It is vitally important to perfuse the kidneys, not only to reduce the possibility of renal damage, but also to reduce the production of angiotensin which leads to splanchnic vasoconstriction.

Fluids. Septic shock is characterized by widespread capillary leak, which increases lung water and predisposes to the development of ARDS. Flow is more important than pressures, and an increased preload may be required to improve myocardial contractility and improve renal and splanchnic flow, even though lung water may increase further while pulmonary artery pressures rise.

12.3	a) True	b) True	c) False	d) False	e) False

EXPLANATION

Some facts about patients (usually children) with congenital heart disease
Pathophysiology. Congenital heart disease primarily causes two major problems:

- Abnormal blood flow pathway, i.e. shunting through intracardiac or extracardiac defects. Shunt lesions alter pulmonary blood flow which can be increased or decreased. An increase in pulmonary blood flow is associated with a left-to-right shunt (e.g. ventricular septal defect (VSD)), and causes increased pressure and volume in the pulmonary circulation and congestive heart failure. A reduction in pulmonary blood flow is associated with a right-to-left shunt (e.g. Fallot's tetralogy, transposition of great vessels, single ventricle) and causes cyanosis because of a reduced ability to oxygenate blood.

- Obstruction to blood flow. i.e. cardiac valvular congenital abnormalities. The prime consequence of this is increased cardiac work to overcome the obstruction and a reduced circulation distal to the obstruction.

Diagnosed case of congenital heart disease. The defect may be unrepaired, palliated or corrected. In many cases palliative surgery will have been done to minimize the cardiovascular anomalies. Corrective surgery is hardly ever completely successful; for example ventricular dysfunction often persists after correction of a Fallot's tetralogy. Moreover, further cardiac problems may arise after surgery, e.g. postoperative heart block after repair in Fallot's tetralogy or VSD.

Undiagnosed heart murmur. One may discover a murmur during preoperative assessment, and a cardiologist should be consulted to determine whether the murmur is functional (innocent) or pathological. Innocent murmurs tend to be early systolic, of short duration and low intensity, poorly transmitted and not accompanied by cardiovascular abnormalities. A pathological murmur should be suspected if it is late systolic, pansystolic or diastolic, loud and associated with cardiac anomalies.

Cyanosis. Cyanosis indicates a reduced pulmonary blood flow and a reduced ability to oxygenate blood. Cyanotic children are prone to cyanotic attacks when there is further pulmonary vasoconstriction. The child may alleviate this by squatting, which increases the systemic vascular resistance and reduces pulmonary shunting. Further pulmonary vasoconstriction may be precipitated by sympathetic stimulation (stress, anxiety), hypoxia, or falls in cardiac output. With this in mind, preanaesthetic sedation, adequate anaesthetic depth to avoid sympathetic overactivity, avoidance of hypoxia and hypovolaemia are all of prime importance. If the child is on preoperative beta blockers to reduce right ventricular obstruction, these should be continued preoperatively. Cyanotic attacks should be treated with oxygen, sedation, increasing the depth of the anaesthetic and use of an appropriate alpha agonist and perhaps a short-acting beta blocker, such as esmolol.

Other congenital anomalies. 25% of children with congenital heart disease have other congenital anomalies, and these must be excluded.

Polycythaemia. Cyanotic children are polycythaemic to increase the oxygen-carrying capacity. The increased haematocrit is associated with an increased incidence of thrombosis.

Coagulopathy. Platelet function is abnormal in these patients, and coagulopathies are likely.

Air bubbles. The introduction of air bubbles into the circulation can be disastrous in children with shunt defects. Venous bubbles can be shunted into the arterial circulation causing air embolism.

Antibiotic prophylaxis. All patients who have had palliative or corrective surgery require antibiotic prophylaxis to protect against bacterial endocarditis when they are having 'dirty' procedures including dental; ear, nose and throat; respiratory; gut; and genitourinary procedures. The only exceptions are patent ductus arteriosus and atrial septal defect, where antibiotic protection is only required for 6 months after the surgical correction.

Anaesthetic agents. Induction may be more rapid or delayed depending on the lesion. With a right-to-left shunt, intravenous induction is shortened because the pulmonary circulation is bypassed. Overdose of volatile agents should be avoided, because myocardial depression will reduce cardiac output and pulmonary blood flow and aggravate hypoxaemia. Halothane with its negative inotropic and chronotropic effects may improve pulmonary blood flow in patients with outflow obstruction, e.g. Fallot's tetralogy, pulmonary stenosis, aortic stenosis. Nitrous oxide should probably be avoided in cyanotic children. Apart from limiting the inspired FiO_2, and the risk of air bubble enlargement, it causes pulmonary vasoconstriction. Ketamine, on the other hand has not been associated with increased pulmonary vascular resistance.

12.4   a) False   b) True   c) True   d) False   e) False

EXPLANATION

Types of thermometer

Mercury clinical thermometer. This is satisfactory for routine use, with an accuracy of $\pm 0.1°C$. Unfortunately it can easily be broken, has a slow response because of high thermal capacity, and is unsuitable for measurements from many sites.

Dial thermometers. In one type, movement of a bimetallic strip (a strip made of two different metals, which unwinds or winds on heating owing to differential expansion of the two metals) is transferred to a pointer. A 'pressure' dial thermometer consists of a hollow metal strip, which unwinds as the pressure inside it alters with temperature changes. Dial thermometers are relatively inaccurate – $\pm 0.25°C$.

Table 12.1 Sites of temperature measurement

Site	Advantages	Disadvantages
Tympanic/nasopharyngeal	Close to hypothalamus which regulates temperature	Tympanic perforation possible; probe affected by temperature of inspired gas
Oesophageal	Close to heart and great vessels	Must be placed in lower oesophagus to avoid cooling by inspired gas
Rectal	Convenient	May not be an accurate measurement of core temperature; affected by faeces
Axillary	Convenient	Must be placed over axillary artery; affected by blood pressure cuff and i.v. fluids
Skin	Skin temperature correlates well with peripheral resistance	Correlates poorly with core temperature
Pulmonary artery	Reflects temperature of mixed venous blood	Probe can be affected by temperature of inspired gas

Thermocouples. These operate on the principle of the Seebeck effect – when a circuit of two dissimilar metals (often nickel-chrome and constantan, an alloy of copper and nickel) has two junctions at different temperatures an electromotive force is produced. One junction is maintained at a reference ice-cold temperature which must remain constant; the other junction is used for temperature measurement. Two probes are available; one for temperatures from 0–50°C; the other from 16–46°C. Accuracy is ± 0.1°C. These thermometers can be very small, respond rapidly because of low thermal capacity, and can be used at various sites.

Resistance thermometers. The resistance of a metal increases in a fairly linear fashion with temperature. Again, the resistance of a coil (often platinum) is measured at a reference constant ice-point temperature and at the temperature to be measured. Platinum resistance thermometers are extremely accurate up to thousandths of a degree, but small probes are difficult to produce, and have a slow response time.

Thermistors. Thermistors consist of heavy metal oxides, such as oxides of zinc, nickel, manganese, cobalt, etc. The resistance of these oxides falls as temperature rises. They can be of minute size, and a metal oxide bead can be sealed onto the tip of a hypodermic needle. Since they are so small, the response time is very rapid – within 0.2 seconds – but thermistors exhibit an increase of resistance with ageing and large temperature fluctuations, and hence require frequent recalibration. Moreover, the resistance changes exhibit considerable non-linearity with temperature changes, and therefore thermistors are most suitable for measurement of small temperature changes, such as that within the pulmonary artery for measuring cardiac output by dilution techniques.

Sites of temperature measurement
See Table 12.1.

12.5   a) True   b) False   c) False   d) True   e) False

EXPLANATION
  Radial nerve. Arises from C5, 6, 7, 8, T1. Paralysis of the radial nerve causes inability to extend the wrist and fingers causing wrist drop. About 7 cm above the wrist, the nerve passes under the brachioradialis tendon to lie subcutaneously on the extensor aspect of the wrist. It divides into branches to supply the radial side of the dorsum of the hand. The superficial position of the radial nerve makes it vulnerable to compression by bone or operating table, and even blood pressure cuffs.
  Radial nerve block. The radial nerve can be blocked at the wrist by a subcutaneous injection of 15 ml of local anaesthetic on the dorsal and lateral aspect of the wrist.
  Median nerve. Arises from C5, 6, 7, 8, T1. Median nerve paralysis causes weakness of pronators of forearms, and flexors of wrist, thumb and index finger. Therefore the hand deviates to the ulnar side, while the metacarpal bone of the thumb moves over on the same plane as the other metacarpal bones – 'ape hand'. Sensory loss affects the lateral two-thirds of the palmar aspect of the hand.
  Median nerve block. At the wrist, the median nerve lies fairly superficially radial to the palmaris longus. It can be blocked at the level of the proximal skin crease, just lateral to the palmaris longus, or if this is absent 1 cm medial to the flexor carpi radialis. 5 ml local anaesthetic are injected at a depth of about 1 cm.
  Ulnar nerve. Arises from C8, T1. Paralysis of the ulnar nerve causes weakness of flexors of the little, ring and middle fingers causing hyperextension of these fingers. There is also abductor and adductor weakness of fingers so that a piece of paper cannot be gripped between the fingers affected – 'claw hand'. Sensory innervation is to the medial third of the palmar aspect of the hand and the fifth and ring fingers; and through the dorsal nerve it supplies the medial side of the dorsum of hand. As with the radial nerve, the superficial position of the ulnar nerve makes it vulnerable to compression damage.
  Ulnar nerve block. The ulnar nerve is very superficial at the elbow, and it is easier to block it here than at the wrist. 5 ml of local anaesthetic are injected to block it behind the medial condyle, as it lies in the groove between the medial condyle of the humerus and the olecranon.

12.6   a) True   b) False   c) True   d) False   e) False

EXPLANATION
The facet joints are formed by the superior articular facet of one vertebra and the inferior articular facet of the adjacent vertebra above. The cervical facet joints lie in

the coronal plane to allow flexion and extension of the neck; the thoracic facets are at a 20° angle to the coronal plane, while the lumbar facet joints lie 45° off the sagittal plane. Facet joints are innervated by the medial branch of the dorsal primary rami. Each root sends two branches – one to the facet at its own level, the second to the one below. Therefore each posterior ramus innervates two facet joints.

Lumbar facet syndrome. Lumbar facet joints are often the cause of low back pain, and X-rays and isotope scanning are of little value in identifying patients with facet joint pain. The patient suffers from tenderness and dull back pain especially on extension, with radiation to the buttocks, hips, and posterior and lateral parts of thigh to the knee. It is unlikely that the pain extends below the knee. Decreased leg raising and depressed tendon reflexes may be present. Treatment may involve physiotherapy, NSAIDs, acupuncture, transcutaneous electrical nerve stimulation (TENS), injection into trigger points, and facet joint injections. Relief can be achieved either by intra-articular injection, or block of the medial branch of the dorsal spinal ramus – medial branch block. The patient lies prone on an X-ray table, with a pillow under the abdomen. A 22-gauge spinal needle is inserted vertically about 1.5 cm from the midline. The lumbar facet joints are best viewed at 45° obliquely, and this can be achieved by rotating the 'C' arm of the image intensifier from a sagittal to a more lateral plane. 2 ml of local anaesthetic and methylprednisolone are injected into the joint or local anaesthetic onto the nerve. The nerve is situated just lateral to the facet joint at the site of the 'dog's ear' appearance on the image. It is usually necessary to inject at two or three levels. 60% of patients get temporary pain relief; 25% get relief for over 6 months.

Thoracic facet syndrome. This is often caused by a sudden twisting movement resulting in paravertebral pain and tenderness radiating laterally, often round the chest wall. Thoracic medial branch block is done with the aid of image intensification. With the patient lying prone, the transverse process is identified in an anteroposterior projection. A needle is then directed onto the upper border of the medial end of the transverse process and local anaesthetic administered. Paravertebral or intercostal blocks may also be of benefit. It is difficult to inject the thoracic facet joint itself. The only important complication of this procedure is pneumothorax.

Cervical facet syndrome. This may be caused by neck injuries or degenerative joint changes. There is cervical pain and tenderness especially with neck rotation and extension, radiating to occiput, shoulder arm and scapular areas. As with lumbar facet pain, physiotherapy, NSAIDs, TENS, acupuncture and local trigger injections may help. Injection of the cervical facet joints with local anaesthetics and steroids, or medial branch block may provide pain relief for up to 6–12 months. An anterior or posterior approach can be employed, and the needle should be directed at the mid-point of the articular pillar with image intensification. Complications include subarachnoid and epidural injection, while if an anterior technique is employed, vertebral artery puncture is a possibility. Percutaneous radiofrequency coagulation or neurotomy of the medial branch can provide more prolonged pain relief in the cervical and lumbar regions.

12.7	a) True	b) True	c) True	d) False	e) False

EXPLANATION
See Table 12.2.

Table 12.2 Pneumonias

Pneumonia	Organism	Clinical features
Typical		
Pneumococcal/ streptococcal	Gram-positive diplococci	Fever, chills, cough, purulent sputum – sometimes bloodstained, tachypnoea, pleuritic pain, herpes labialis. Signs of consolidation in 50% of cases with bronchial breathing. Chest X-ray: areas of consolidation; pleural effusion in 25% of cases
Haemophilus influenzae	Gram-negative cocci	Symptoms as above. More likely to cause bronchopneumonia than lobar pneumonia
Staphylococcus	Clusters of Gram-positive cocci	As above. A common pathogen in children, the elderly and hospital patients. Often a bilateral cavitating bronchopneumonia with possible abscess formation
Legionnaire's disease	*Legionella pneumophila*	Subacute presentation with cough, headache, fever, systemic toxicity, gut symptoms, hyponatraemia – confusion, encephalopathy, hepatitis, haematuria. WBC $< 15 \times 10^9$/l, lymphopenia. Chest X-ray: diffuse picture. Prolonged course
Anaerobes	Mixed flora	Upper segments of lower lobes often involved. Cavitation and abscess formation common
Atypical		
Primary atypical pneumonia	Mycoplasma	In closed communities as an epidemic in young adults. Subacute presentation with headache, myalgia, cough. Prolonged course. WBC $< 15 \times 10^9$/l, Chest X-ray: consolidation with no characteristic features
Viral pneumonia	Influenza A/B; adenovirus; respiratory syncytial virus; varicella zoster; ECHO virus	Viral symptoms – fever, headache, myalgia. May present as pneumonia or bronchiolitis. There is often superimposed bacterial infection

Treatment	Comments
Penicillin	Usually resolves within 3–5 days; chest X-ray lags behind clinical symptoms and may take 6 weeks to resolve
Ampicillin/amoxycillin; second generation cephalosporins	Beta-lactamase in 25% of cases
Methicillin; vancomycin	Often associated with influenza epidemics and drug addicts
Erythromycin; vancomycin as second drug	Occurs especially in hotels and hospitals owing to contaminated water or air conditioning. Mortality: < 10%
Penicillin; clindamycin; third generation cephalosporins	Often follows aspiration
Erythromycin; tetracyclines	Very high erythrocyte sedimentation rate with cold agglutinins; rise in antibody titres over 10–14 days
No specific therapy	Difficult to make a diagnosis other than from rises in viral antibody titres

Table 12.2 *(Cont'd)*

Pneumonia	Organism	Clinical features
AIDS related		
Pneumocystis carinii	Opportunistic infections with atypical microorganisms	Cough and dyspnoea for weeks, progressing to respiratory failure. Chest X-ray: diffuse infiltrates/ consolidations, cavitation possible
Cytomegalovirus pneumonia	Cytomegalovirus	Similar to *Pneumocystis carinii*, there may be associated encephalitis, colitis, retinitis
Nosocomial pneumonia, i.e. hospital-acquired pneumonia	Aerobic Gram-negative rods – pseudomonas, klebsiella enterobacter, proteus, *Escherichia coli*, staphylococcus	Fever, purulent secretions, leucocytosis. Chest X-ray: infiltrates

12.8 a) False   b) False   c) True   d) True   e) True

EXPLANATION

Fetal distress can be detected by:

1. *Fetal history.* A fetal history will determine whether predisposing conditions for fetal distress are present, e.g. complicated pregnancy; fetal prematurity; inadequate fetal growth; abnormal amount of amniotic fluid or meconium-stained amniotic fluid.

2. *Fetal heart tracing:*

- Heart rate. The normal heart rate in a mature infant varies between 120–160 beats per minute. If the fetus has a normal rate of 120 beats per minute, an increase to 160 is suspicious. The stroke volume in a fetus is relatively fixed, and the increase in rate may be an attempt to increase the cardiac output.

- Heart rate variability. The heart rate may be observed over a long period by a fetal scalp electrode. The heart rate in a normal mature fetus is not fixed at say 140 beats per minute, but varies from time to time. As the fetus matures, the autonomic system matures, sleep cycles are more apparent, and breathing and fetal movements more frequent; all these factors cause beat-to-beat heart rate variability. External factors can also alter the rate, e.g. tachycardia can be caused by fetal scalp stimulation or by acoustic stimulation. The absence of this variability suggests lack of fetal movement or fetal CNS depression by sleep, which is normal, or by hypoxaemia, acidosis, narcotics and other CNS-depressant drugs, which is ominous. Therefore, sustained lack of rate variability is a sign of fetal distress, and if the cause cannot be corrected, delivery of the fetus may be required.

- Decelerations. These are of three types:
  - Type 1 or early decelerations: reductions in rate of 10–30 beats per minute seen during uterine contractions. These decelerations are vagal reflexes during contractions, and recover after the contraction.
  - Type 2 or late decelerations: reductions in rate of around 5 beats per minute seen after a uterine contraction. These decelerations are chemoreceptor reflexes caused by falls in fetal PO_2. If sustained they indicate fetal hypoxaemia.
  - Type 3 or variable decelerations: reductions in rate of over 30 beats per minute caused by umbilical cord compression. Baroreceptors are

Treatment	Comments
High-dose co-trimoxazole; pentamidine	Non-specific pneumonias are common in AIDS; they are often associated with Kaposi's sarcoma and adult respiratory distress syndrome; both can be difficult to distinguish from pneumonias
No effective therapy	
Initially empirical, until culture/sensitivity available, e.g. third generation cephalosporin – ceftazidime. Pseudomonas: ceftazidime and gentamicin	Common in ventilated patients from inhalation of airborne bacteria, contaminated equipment, aspiration, or more rarely from extension from contaminated site or blood-borne

responsible for these decelerations and, although the rate can fall below 70 beats per minute, recovery is prompt.

3. *Fetal capillary blood sampling.* When there is doubt about fetal heart rate tracing, fetal capillary blood sampling is indicated. A full set of blood gas determinations can be done with a 0.25-ml blood sample. With smaller volumes only pH can be determined; in such a case one cannot distinguish between types of acidosis. This may be important, because metabolic acidosis requires immediate delivery, while respiratory acidosis should respond to treatment. The pH of capillary blood correlates well with fetal heart rate patterns and also with the Apgar score. A pH above 7.25 is associated with an Apgar score above 7, and a pH below 7.15 with a score below 6 in most cases.

12.9   a) False   b) False   c) True   d) True   e) True

EXPLANATION

Intracranial pressure. Normal range: 5–15 mmHg. If the pressure is sustained above 20 mmHg, intracranial hypertension may be present; if it is sustained above 40 mmHg, there is definite intracranial hypertension.

Anaesthetic factors affecting intracranial pressure

Intravenous agents. See Table 12.3.

Volatile agents. See Table 12.3.

Relaxants. Suxamethonium increases intracranial pressure (ICP) (muscle fasciculations). All non-depolarizing agents are suitable for intubation and maintenance of patients with raised ICP.

Fluids. Since increasing blood sugar aggravates cerebral ischaemia, glucose-free isotonic electrolyte solutions should be used for fluid replacement in neurosurgical patients. Hypotonic solutions should be avoided, while hypertonic saline may have a place in reducing cerebral oedema and lowering intracranial pressure.

Anaesthetic induction. A number of techniques can be employed to limit rise in intracranial pressure. Some anaesthetists favour pre-induction hyperventilation to help reduce ICP. Thiopentone is probably the best induction agent to use, as besides

Table 12.3   Effects of intravenous and volatile agents on cerebral blood flow and intracranial pressure

	Cerebral blood flow	Intracranial pressure
Intravenous agents		
Thiopentone	–	–
Methohexitone	–	–
Etomidate	–	– (possible myoclonus)
Propofol	–	–
Ketamine	++	+
Benzodiazepines	Minimal effects	+
Fentanyl	–	–
Volatile agents		
Nitrous oxide	+	+
Halothane	+++	+++
Isoflurane	+	+
Sevoflurane	+	+
Desflurane	+	+

lowering ICP it also has a cerebral protective effect by reducing cerebral metabolism. When the long-acting relaxant takes effect, the stress and blood pressure rise of intubation can be reduced by fentanyl, further doses of thiopentone, a short-acting beta blocker or lignocaine.

Measures to reduce high intracranial pressure:

● *Decrease cerebrospinal fluid volume.* Cerebrospinal fluid (CSF) can be drained by ventricular catheter, which, however, can cause direct brain injury and infection; or via a lumbar catheter which may result in a downward herniation if a brain mass is present. Another method of decreasing CSF volume is to decrease its production with acetazolamide but the response from this is limited and slow.

● *Decrease blood volume.* Blood volume can be reduced by appropriate posture to reduce venous return; hypoventilation (not below 3.5 kPa as the intense vasoconstriction can reduce the cerebral oxygen delivery); maintenance of PaO_2 above 13 kPa (both high PaO_2 and low $PaCO_2$ cause cerebral vasoconstriction); decrease in cerebral metabolism with barbiturates or hypothermia; prevention of fits with anticonvulsant agents.

● *Decrease brain volume.* Diuretics; osmotic diuresis which, however, may transiently increase intracranial volume and intracranial pressure; steroids – only effective in patients with brain tumours.

12.10   a) False   b) False   c) True   d) False   e) False

EXPLANATION

Anatomy. The lumbar sympathetic chain lies at the anterolateral border of the vertebral bodies. The aorta lies anteriorly and medially on the left side; while the inferior vena cava is anterior to the chain on the right side. The psoas muscle is posterior and lateral to the sympathetic chain; the genitofemoral nerve lies laterally on the psoas. The chain is formed from preganglionic nerves leaving T11 to L2. The preganglionic axons leave the spinal cord and join the anterior spinal nerves, and then enter the chain as white communicating ramus and synapse in the ganglia. Postganglionic axons leave the chain as grey communicating rami to join the spinal nerves of the lumber and sacral plexuses. Most of the fibres travel through the second, third and fourth lumbar ganglia, and blockage of these ganglia results in sympathetic denervation to the lower limb. The lumbar sympathetic afferent fibres carry pain sensations from the distal portion of the transverse colon, the descending colon, rectum, kidney, ureter, bladder, prostate, testicle, cervix and uterus.

Indications:

1. Peripheral vascular disease. Diffuse peripheral vascular disease is more amenable to sympathetic blocks than proximal disease.

2. Sympathetic dystrophy and causalgia. Pain relief even with a local anaesthetic sympathetic block can be long-lasting.

3. Acute herpes or early post-herpetic neuralgia. By improving the circulation, a sympathetic block can reduce inflammation and prevent further nerve damage by the herpes virus.

4. Deafferent pain syndromes, e.g. phantom limb pain, though results are not often satisfactory.

5. Cancer pain, i.e. pain originating from the organs innervated by the lumbar sympathetic chain – lower limb, large intestine distal to transverse colon or pelvic organs.

Technique. The patient lies laterally, with the back absolutely vertical. One, two or three needles need to be placed anterior to L2, L3, L4 lumbar vertebrae. After local infiltration, a 15-cm 20-gauge needle is inserted 7–10 cm lateral to the spinous process of L3 at an angle of 60 degrees until contact is made with the vertebral body. Image intensification should be used to confirm position. The needle is then withdrawn slightly, and redirected more anteriorly to walk past the vertebra to lie anterior to it. If the needle is in the correct position, contrast dye will spread longitudinally. If the needle is in the psoas muscle the contrast will spread downwards and laterally away from the vertebra in a 'fan-like' fashion. Correct position of the needle should be checked in both lateral and anteroposterior image or X-ray views. If local anaesthetic solution is being used, 5–10 ml of 0.5% bupivacaine is injected at each level. For a neurolytic block, 3–5 ml of 6% phenol, or a higher concentration, is usually employed. When the neurolytic agent is injected, the needle should be flushed with local anaesthetic before withdrawal to avoid leaving a track of phenol in the superficial tissues.

Complications:

1. Complications caused by the needle:
   - Backache: usually transient and due to soft tissue damage by the needle.
   - Damage to kidney, ureter (if the needle is inserted too laterally), or intervertebral disc – all rare.
2. Complications caused by the injection:
   - Intravascular injection of local anaesthetic can cause serious toxic reactions, and should be avoided by careful aspiration before injection.
   - Inadvertent intrathecal injection causing total spinal blocks with local anaesthetics, or disastrous widespread paralysis with neurolytic agents. Again, this can be avoided with careful aspiration before injection.

- Nerve damage. Destruction of the sympathetic nerves can cause a burning pain in the anterior thigh. A more specific neuritis is genitofemoral neuritis, which is due to spread of the neurolytic agent onto the genitofemoral nerve. The incidence is about 6% and it presents with a burning pain and dysaesthesia in the groin. Treatment: transcutaneous electrical nerve stimulation (TENS); antiepileptics; antidepressants. The condition usually resolves over several weeks.
3. Hypotension. Hypotension is possible from vasodilatation, especially in the elderly, and after bilateral blocks. It is rarely a problem.

12.11   a) False   b) False   c) False   d) False   e) True

EXPLANATION

Skin burns

- First degree (superficial) – reversible damage.
- Second degree (partial thickness) – partial destruction of skin and its appendages (hair follicles, sweat glands, nerves); very painful because nerve endings are exposed. Healing is from epithelial elements.
- Third degree (full thickness) – full destruction of skin and appendages; not painful. Dead skin will separate in 2–3 weeks revealing a red granulating surface, which is prone to infection. Healing is from the edge, causing contractures; thus burn requires grafting.

Causes:

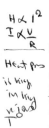

- Thermal
- Chemical
- Electrical: usually causes full thickness burns because the heat generated (H) is proportional to the square of the current flow ($H \propto I^2$). High-voltage tensions (over 1000 volts) are especially dangerous, because current is proportional to voltage ($I = V/R$), so the heat produced is proportional to the square of the voltage. Heat production is highest in tissues with high electrical resistances (i.e. skin; internal organs offer low resistances). Electrical injury can also cause myocardial damage if the current passes through the heart, and renal failure from myoglobinuria secondary to muscle damage.

Effects:

- *Skin.* An inflammatory response occurs soon after the injury – increase in local blood flow, increase in white blood cells, complement, prostaglandins and cytokines – all designed to combat infection and promote healing. Burns cause a significant increase in vascular permeability, from the burn itself and from release of oxygen free radicals, histamine, prostaglandins, serotonin, etc. This increased permeability causes significant plasma and fluid loss.
- *Metabolic effects.* Increased metabolism starts 1 week after injury; the increase in basic metabolic rate (BMR) is related to the size of burn. Oxygen consumption is increased, together with heat production and body temperature (owing to raised catecholamine levels). Protein catabolism is also increased leading to a fall in body proteins. The levels of the hormones released in stress are all raised –

catecholamines, cortisol, glucagon, insulin, growth hormone. This leads to increased gluconeogenesis and hyperglycaemia.

- *Cardiovascular system*. Fluid loss is maximal in the first 6 hours and lasts 24–36 hours, after which reabsorption of fluid begins and fluid requirements decrease. There is often myocardial depression in the first 24 hours because of fluid loss but also owing to circulating myocardial depressant factors (? oxygen free radicals).
- *Kidney*. High catecholamine levels cause renal vasoconstriction, reduced glomerular filtration rate and oliguria. Renin and aldosterone are released to initiate compensatory sodium and water retention.
- *Liver*. Liver function is impaired because of fatty changes and oedema.
- *Brain*. Hyperaemia, oedema and possible fat embolism.
- *Lung*. Pulmonary injury can be divided into:
  - carbon monoxide poisoning
  - airway injuries
  - pulmonary damage.

Carbon monoxide poisoning. This is likely in closed-space fires. Carbon monoxide causes tissue hypoxia, because it binds to haemoglobin 200 times more readily than does oxygen, leading to decrease in oxygen delivery. Clinical signs are headache, dyspnoea without cyanosis, nausea, angina, and mental changes. Pulse oximetry does not distinguish between carboxy- and oxyhaemoglobin. Carboxyhaemoglobin levels above 15% are toxic, and above 50% usually fatal. Treatment is 100% oxygen; ? hyperbaric oxygen.

Airway injury. Damage to the lower respiratory tract (below vocal cords) is rare, because the upper airway dissipates the hot air. Initially there is erythema, blistering and necrosis of the upper airway, and in severe cases within 4–48 hours there may be considerable swelling of the epiglottis and laryngeal structures, which may necessitate intubation for a few days.

Pulmonary damage. Pulmonary damage is due to inhalation of toxic irritant products of combustion. Complications may be early, intermediate or late:

- Early: non-cardiogenic pulmonary oedema
- Intermediate: adult respiratory distress syndrome (ARDS) is a possibility within 2–5 days and may be due to cytokines or oxygen free radicals
- Late: patients who survive into the second week are susceptible to pneumonia and atelectasis and pulmonary emboli (due to immobilization and hypercoagulable state).

A burn over 15% of the surface area in an adult, or over 10% in a child, requires fluid replacement. Estimation of body surface involved can be made in an adult from the rule of nines (head 9%; upper limbs 9% each; lower limbs 18% each; front of body 18%; back 18%), and in children from the rule of tens (head 20%; limbs 10% each; front 20%; back 20%). Between 2–4 ml/kg of crystalloid fluid is required in the first 24 hours for each 1% burn. Half of this volume is given in the first 8 hours, the rest over the next 16 hours. Fluid requirements decrease after 2 days. The use of colloids is controversial. Colloids are associated with less tissue oedema than crystalloids, but the incidence of pulmonary oedema is not lower with colloids. In severe burns, red blood cells are destroyed, the patient rapidly becomes anaemic, and blood transfusion is required. Adequacy of treatment is gauged by regular checks on pulse rate, blood pressure, warm/cold extremities and especially urine output, which should be kept at 0.5–1 ml/kg per hour.

The dramatic increase in metabolism requires a daily calorific intake of between 3000–6000 kilocalories to ensure adequate nutrition. This is achieved with continuous enteral feeding if the patient's oral intake is inadequate.

Anaesthetic considerations

Burns patients may require numerous surgical procedures – wound debridement, escharotomies, tracheostomies, skin grafts, etc. There are a number of problems:

- Blood loss: can be considerable especially during wound debridement and escharotomies.
- Practical problems: positioning of patient especially with extensive burns; difficulty in establishing venous access and difficulty with placement of monitors. Hypothermia is likely because of loss of the protective skin layer; therefore measures to maintain an adequate body temperature should be instituted.
- Airway management: with facial and neck burns, airtight application of a face mask can be difficult, while contractures of neck and mouth can make laryngoscopy difficult. In these situations gas induction is preferable to ensure the ability to control the airway; if the contractures are severe, awake intubation with a fibreoptic laryngoscope is required under appropriate sedation and local anaesthesia.
- Anaesthetic agents: ketamine has been used widely for burn surgery, because of its ease of administration by the intramuscular route, and because laryngeal and pharyngeal reflexes are partially maintained, making airway control easier. The major concern with burnt patients is the complications associated with suxamethonium. Suxamethonium is contraindicated from 10 days after injury until complete closure of the wound, usually at about 6 weeks. In these patients suxamethonium has been associated with ventricular arrhythmias and cardiac arrest, because of hyperkalaemia probably caused by the spread of acetylcholine receptors over the muscle. Although probably safe in the first 8–12 hours following the burn, suxamethonium should be avoided if at all possible. Burnt patients are also resistant to non-depolarizing muscle relaxants, and very large doses are often required.
- Intermittent positive-pressure ventilation (IPPV): if IPPV is required, high minute volumes are often required, because of increased oxygen consumption and increased carbon dioxide production. Intensive care ventilators may be needed to meet these criteria.

12.12   a) **True**   b) **True**   c) **True**   d) **False**   e) **False**

EXPLANATION

Definition. Methaemoglobin is produced when iron in the haem of haemoglobin is oxidized from the ferrous to the ferric form. Under normal circumstances the methaemoglobin concentration does not exceed 1%; methaemoglobinaemia exists when the concentration is above 1%, but symptoms do not appear until the level is 20%.

Causes:

- *Congenital.* There are at least five types of methaemoglobinaemia. The defect is in the histidine residue near the haem ring which stabilizes the haem iron in the ferric state which cannot transport oxygen. The homozygous condition is often incompatible with life. Heterozygote sufferers are often asymptomatic, but may suffer a haemolytic crisis when administered oxidant drugs

● *Drugs.* There are a number of agents which can oxidize haemoglobin: aniline; benzenes; benzocaine; prilocaine (when dose exceeds 8 mg/kg) – it is broken down into orthotoluidine which oxidizes haemoglobin causing methaemoglobinaemia, until it is excreted within 2–6 hours; nitroprusside; antimalarials; antileprosy drugs, e.g. dapsone; high doses of methylene blue, e.g. when used as an infusion to locate the parathyroid glands during parathyroidectomy.

Clinical picture. In mild cases there is cyanosis with possibly low oxygen saturation readings, but normal arterial oxygen levels. The oxygen dissociation curve is shifted to the left, so that tissue delivery of oxygen is impaired. In more severe cases there is giddiness, headache, dyspnoea, vascular collapse, and coma.

Treatment:

● Acute: methylene blue, 1–2 mg/kg, stimulates the synthesis of the enzymes which oxidize ferrous haemoglobin to the ferric form; exchange transfusion in severe cases.
● Chronic: ascorbic acid.

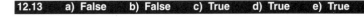

12.13　a) False　b) False　c) True　d) True　e) True

EXPLANATION

Inherited disorders of anaesthetic interest
Inherited disorders can be subdivided into groups, according to which system is affected:

1. Metabolic disorders
    ● Lipid disorders.
        – Hyperlipoproteinaemia
    ● Carbohydrate disorders
        – Galactosaemia
        – Fructosaemia
        – Glycogen storage disease
    ● Amino acid disorders
        – Cystinuria
        – Phenylketonuria
2. Blood disorders
    ● Disorders of cholinesterase
    ● Haemoglobinopathies
        – Sickle cell disease
        – Thalassaemia
    ● Porphyrias
    ● Glucose 6-phosphate dehydrogenase deficiency
    ● Clotting disorders
        – Haemophilia
        – Von Willebrand's disease
3. Gland disorders
    ● Cystic fibrosis

4. Neurological disorders
   - Huntington's chorea
   - Mucopolysaccharidoses
   - Familial dysautonomia
5. Muscle disorders
   - Malignant hyperpyrexia
   - Muscular dystrophies
   - Myotonias
   - Familial periodic paralysis
6. Skin and bone disorders
   - Achondroplasia
   - Osteogenesis imperfecta
   - Neurofibromatosis

Further information about these disorders is given in Table 12.4.

12.14   a) True   b) False   c) False   d) False   e) False

EXPLANATION

Avoid teratogenic drugs
Susceptibility to teratogenic agents is highest between 15 and 90 days of gestation, which is the period of maximal organ development.
   Teratogenic drugs include:

- Alcohol: hallucinogens (e.g. lysergic acid diethylamide (LSD))
- Angiotensin-converting enzyme (ACE) inhibitors
- Antithyroid drugs
- Cytotoxic drugs
- Cocaine
- Coumadin anticoagulants
- Diethylstilboestrol
- Lead
- Lithium
- Mercury
- Phenytoin
- Streptomycin
- Thalidomide
- Trimethadione
- Valproic acid.

Nitrous oxide has been implicated in causing teratogenesis either because it interferes with folate metabolism by inactivating vitamin B_{12}, or because it reduces uterine blood flow by its sympathomimetic action. Evidence supporting these theories is not strong, and to date teratogenicity with nitrous oxide has not been demonstrated in humans. Apart from the local anaesthetic cocaine, no anaesthetic induction agent, nor any anaesthetic vapour, muscle relaxant or narcotic, has been associated with teratogenic effects.

Occupational exposure to anaesthetic agents among theatre personnel has also been implicated in increased incidences of miscarriage; congenital abnormalities;

decrease in birth weights and increase in perinatal mortality; but again there is very little evidence supporting these theories, especially if scavenging devices are used.

Avoid anaesthetic techniques which can cause fetal abnormalities or fetal distress

Although anaesthetics are not teratogenic, fetal malformations and death can be caused by anaesthetic complications: i.e. hypoxia; hypocarbia and reduced uterine blood flow due either to hypotension or uterine vasoconstriction. Normal blood sugars also help to prevent fetal problems.

- *Hypoxia.* Fetal oxygenation depends upon maternal oxygenation and uterine blood flow. Physiological changes of pregnancy include fall in functional residual capacity (FRC) and increase in oxygen consumption, which predispose to rapid falls in PaO_2, thus subjecting the fetus to risks of hypoxaemia especially during periods of apnoea, obstruction, etc. Prolonged preoxygenation before induction, and a high inspired oxygen level during anaesthesia is therefore recommended. Aspiration is another possible cause of fetal hypoxia (and maternal morbidity); thus preoperative aspiration prophylaxis, i.e. antacids, H_2 blockers and metoclopramide should be instituted.

- *Hypocarbia.* Excessive ventilation causes metabolic alkalosis and leftward shift of the oxyhaemoglobin dissociation curve, decreasing oxygen release to the fetus. Intermittent positive-pressure ventilation (IPPV) may also reduce uterine flow by up to 25% by diminishing venous return.

- *Reduced uterine blood flow.* The most likely causes of reduced blood flow is maternal hypotension. This may be due to excessive concentrations of anaesthetic vapours (minimum alveolar concentration (MAC) for inhalational agents is reduced by 30% during pregnancy); or too much local anaesthetic during a spinal or epidural (30% less local anaesthetic required during pregnancy because progesterone reduces nerve sensitivity to local agents). Hypotension should be treated with ephedrine as it preserves uterine blood flow better than other sympathomimetics, because it has both alpha and beta effects. Other causes of reduced uterine flow include aortocaval compression, especially after 24 weeks' gestation; hyperventilation; administration of vasoconstrictor drugs; increased uterine activity (reduced by indomethacin suppositories – by prostaglandin inhibition); pain and anxiety which increase circulating catecholamines and cause uterine vasoconstriction. The latter can be prevented with adequate sedative premedication, and adequate postoperative pain control. (NB: neostigmine is a quarternary compound and does not cross the placenta or cause fetal bradycardia.)

- *Hypoglycaemia/hyperglycaemia.* Diabetic patients have a 4–10% incidence of congenital abnormalities; this risk can be reduced to about 1% with strict control of blood sugar. It therefore follows that blood sugars should be kept at normal levels especially during pregnancy.

Conclusion

If possible, surgery should be postponed until the second trimester; if this is not feasible, there is no evidence that anaesthetic drugs cause any teratogenic effects, but fetal anomalies and death can be caused by a faulty anaesthetic, and specifically by the four 'H's, i.e. hypoxia, hypocarbia, hypotension, hypo/hyperglycaemia.

Table 12.4 Common inherited disorders

	Type of disorder
Metabolic disorders	
Lipids	
Hyperlipoproteinaemia	Familial disorders where there is an increase in blood concentration of lipids, cholesterol or triglycerides
Carbohydrates	
Galactosaemia	Deficiency of galactinase causes an inability to convert galactose to glucose, leading to hypoglycaemia
Fructosaemia	Deficiency of fructose-1,6-diphosphatase leads to inability to convert fructose and amino acids to glucose
Glycogen storage diseases	Hereditary enzyme defect causing a disturbance in formation of glycogen from glucose
Amino acids	There are many autosomal recessive disorders of amino acid metabolism; most are rare – the best known are cystinuria and phenylketonuria
Blood disorders	
Plasma cholinesterase	Autosomal recessive disorder of inadequate cholinesterase synthesis

Clinical picture	Anaesthetic considerations
Increased incidence of ischaemic heart disease, if cholesterol or lipids are elevated	Possible presence of ischaemic heart disease
Mild: no symptoms Severe: hypoglycaemia; hepatic failure	Look for possible hypoglycaemia; hepatic impairment
Hepatomegaly; muscle hypotonia; hypoglycaemia; metabolic acidosis	Hypoglycaemia may require preoperative glucose; metabolic acidosis treated with Hartmann's; hepatic impairment
Von Gierke's: hypoglycaemia; hepatomegaly; possible platelet dysfunction Pompe's: hypoglycaemia; glycogen deposits in skeletal/cardiac muscle causing hypotonia and cardiac failure McArdle's: mainly affecting muscle causing myoglobinuria and renal failure	Hypoglycaemia; hepatic/renal dysfunction; possible platelet abnormalities; increased bleeding; hypotonia; suxamethonium should be avoided if there is myoglobinuria
Mental retardation; fits; aminoaciduria; metabolic acidoses; hepatic failure; thromboembolism. With cystinuria, there is a prevention of formation of cysteine which is a collagen constituent, causing symptoms of weakened collagen – osteoporosis; kyphoscoliosis; lens abnormalities	Maintain adequate hydration to prevent thrombosis; treat acid-base abnormalities; avoid enflurane in presence of fits
Diagnosed by dibucaine or fluoride inhibition of cholinesterase. Homozygous individuals with the normal gene have a dibucaine inhibition number (DN) of 80; heterozygous (one normal, one abnormal gene) – DN = 60; homozygous with two abnormal genes – DN about 20. Fluoride inhibition is similar. Some individuals have silent genes with very little enzyme activity	Incidence about 1 in 1800. Normally cholinesterase hydrolyses suxamethonium, terminating its action within 1–5 min. If plasma cholinesterase levels are low, muscle paralysis lasts between 10 and 120 min.

Table 12.4 (*Cont'd*)

	Type of disorder
Haemoglobinopathies Sickle cell anaemia	Inherited structural alteration of one or more of the globin chains in haemoglobin
Thalassaemia	Inherited impaired structural synthesis of one or more of the globin chains in haemoglobin
Porphyrias	Autosomal dominant condition interfering with haem (present in haemoglobin) synthesis. Haem inhibits delta-aminolaevulinic (ALA) synthase; since haem levels are low ALA synthase levels are high, causing accumulation of porphyrins
Glucose-6-phosphate dehydrogenase (G6PD) deficiency	Inherited disorder where G6PD enzyme activity is diminished. G6PD is required for glucose and methaemoglobin metabolism in RBCs; its absence increases RBC destruction causing haemolytic anaemia
Clotting disorders Haemophilia	Sex-linked recessive inherited coagulation disorder due to reduced levels of factor VIII. Males are affected; females are carriers

Clinical picture	Anaesthetic considerations
Heterozygous: no symptoms Homozygous: haemolytic anaemia due to premature destruction of red blood cells (RBCs). Sickle cell disease affects 0.25% of UK blacks; trait 10%. Low O_2 levels cause cells to become sickle shaped, increasing blood viscosity and obstructing blood vessels to cause organ infarctions in bone – osteomyelitis; bone marrow – aplastic anaemia; liver; kidney – papillary necrosis; spleen; brain; lung – chest pain, lung infiltrates; gallstones	Sickling precipitated by hypoxia – the amount of sickling is proportional to the PaO_2; stasis; dehydration; acidosis; cold. Thus maintain adequate hydration and oxygenation; avoid cold, tourniquets. Prone to thromboembolism; increased cardiac output due to chronic anaemia
Alpha (heterozygous): no symptoms Beta (homozygous): haemolytic anaemia leading to tissue hypoxia which stimulates erythropoietin production causing marrow hyperplasia and iron deposits in heart/liver – hepatosplenomegaly and iron overload	Chronic haemolytic anaemia with raised cardiac output; possible difficult intubation because marrow hyperplasia causes enlarged frontal and maxillary bones
Nausea; abdominal pains; motor/sensory neuropathies; fits; psychiatric symptoms; tachycardia; high blood pressure; red urine due to porphyrins	Precipitated by barbiturates; sulphonamides; anticonvulsants; alcohol. Ketamine/propofol are safe; there is doubt about etomidate
Haemolytic anaemia and methaemoglobinaemia; usually precipitated by drugs including prilocaine, antimalarials, sulphonamides, nitrates, tolbutamide, high-dose aspirin, vitamins C and K, fava beans	Avoid prilocaine, sodium nitroprusside; haemolytic anaemia
Spontaneous bleeding affecting joints and muscles; prolonged bleeding after trauma; clotting abnormal, increased partial thromboplastin time (PTT) but bleeding time normal	High HIV and hepatitis B and C risk; avoid i.m. injections and regional anaesthesia; factor VIII (half-life) 12 h) may be required preoperatively. Some patients have factor VIII antibodies requiring very large doses of factor VIII

307

Table 12.4   (*Cont'd*)

	Type of disorder
Von Willebrand's	Autosomal dominant coagulation disorder involving factor VIII

Gland disorders

Cystic fibrosis	Autosomal recessive systemic disorder affecting mucus-secreting glands which produce abnormal viscous fluid. Incidence: 1 in 2000 births

Neurological disorders

Huntington's chorea	Autosomal dominant disorder which causes progressive neurological degeneration
Mucopolysaccharidoses	Inherited connective tissue enzyme deficiency resulting in abnormal metabolism of polysaccharides and accumulation of metabolites in various tissues especially in cardiac and skeletal muscle
Familial dysautonomia (Riley-Day syndrome)	Autosomal recessive neurological disorder associated with autonomic and gastrointestinal dysfunction. Present mainly in Jews

Clinical picture	Anaesthetic considerations
Unlike haemophilia, bleeding tends to be mucosal – from nose, gut, mouth, lungs, etc. Bleeding time prolonged, PTT may be normal	Surgical bleeding not usually as severe as in haemophilia
May be asymptomatic, or else viscous secretions cause repeated chest infections resulting in chronic pulmonary disease with bronchiectasis, pulmonary fibrosis, emphysema and recurrent pneumothorax. Pulmonary hypertension and right heart failure follow owing to hypoxia. Pancreatic insufficiency is common, leading to malabsorption and hypoproteinaemia; less common are liver cirrhosis, nasal polyps and coagulopathy secondary to vitamin K deficiency. Sweat test: high Na and Cl levels	High incidence of preoperative respiratory problems; thus preoperative physiotherapy is required. Cardiovascular system also often affected. Electrolytic state should be assessed, especially Na since hyponatraemia is common. Vitamin K may be required if prothrombin time is prolonged. Viscosity of secretions may be reduced by keeping patient well hydrated but not overloaded
Choreiform movements; ataxia; dysarthria; dementia	These patients are usually on psychotropic drugs, which may interact with anaesthetic drugs. Abnormalities of pharyngeal/laryngeal function predispose to aspiration
Craniofacial and skeletal anomalies; respiratory problems – sleep apnoea; respiratory obstruction; excessive secretions causing infections; cardiac/coronary disease, valvular lesions; possible mental subnormality and hepatosplenomegaly, e.g. Hurler's or Hunter's syndromes	Possible difficult intubation; cardiac problems; respiratory impairment
Postural hypotension; labile blood pressure; poor temperature control; absent sweating; reduced gut motility; impaired swallowing – increased secretions causing respiratory infections due to pulmonary aspiration	Unable to respond to hypovolaemia or to drugs that cause cardiac depression; respiratory impairment; risk of aspiration

Table 12.4 (*Cont'd*)

	Type of disorder
Muscle disorders	
Malignant hyperpyrexia	Autosomal dominant condition of muscle where there is an anzyme disturbance controlling movement of calcium ions causing intense muscle contraction and heat, and triggered mainly by suxamethonium and halothane
Muscular dystrophies	Inherited muscle disorders, some dominant, some recessive. Most common and most serious is Duchenne type which is an X-linked muscle disease
Myotonia	Autosomal dominant disorder causing myotonia, i.e. sustained muscle contractions
Familial periodic paralysis	Autosomal dominant condition causing muscle weakness associated with either hyperkalaemia or hypokalaemia

Clinical picture	Anaesthetic considerations
Incidence 1 in 100 000. Cyanosis; muscle rigidity; hypercapnia; hyperventilation; arrhythmias; pyrexia; hyperkalaemia; respiratory and metabolic acidoses; hypocalcaemia; disseminated intravascular coagulation; haemolysis; myoglobinuria; renal failure; raised creatinine phosphokinase and transaminases	Hyperventilation with high FiO_2. Patient cooled with ice etc.; electrolytic disturbance corrected; high K with glucose/insulin; dantrolene 1–10 mg/kg to transfer calcium out of muscle. In patients with known history, N_2O/opioid/non-depolarizing anaesthetic is safe with preoperative oral dantrolene for 24 h – 4 mg/kg in three doses. Patients and relatives identified by muscle biopsy
Duchenne: progressive lower limb and pelvic weakness; affects heart muscle causing ECG anomalies and cardiomyopathy; eventually respiratory muscles are affected. Death is often between 10–20 years from respiratory or cardiac failure	Suxamethonium should be avoided – can cause cardiac arrest due to high K. Increased sensitivity to non-depolarizers; thus lower doses are required. Halothane should be avoided as it can cause cardiac problems. Look for associated cardiac and respiratory problems
Usually presents between the ages of 30 and 40. Progressive muscle weakness and wasting in many muscles including those of eye and mouth, affecting eye movements and swallowing. Associated features: baldness; ptosis; facial weakness; cataracts; hypogonadism; cardiomyopathy. Death is from respiratory/cardiac failure	Poor respiratory reserve owing to respiratory muscle weakness – thus increased sensitivity to respiratory depressants; increased incidence of postoperative respiratory problems; associated cardiac anomalies; suxamethonium should be avoided as it can cause prolonged contraction and high K; non-depolarizers can be used but muscle relaxation is not guaranteed. Anaesthetic drugs should be used sparingly
Attacks of muscle weakness in any muscle but not usually diaphragm or cranial muscles. With hypokalaemic form, paralysis lasts up to 48 h; with hyperkalaemic usually less than 2 h; attacks often triggered by stress, cold or factors which reduce or increase K	Suxamethonium should be avoided in hyperkalaemic form; non-depolarizers are permissible, K levels should be monitored closely perioperatively and measures to achieve normal levels instituted if required

Table 12.4 (*Cont'd*)

	Type of disorder
Skin and bone disorders	
Achondroplasia	Autosomal dominant disorder causing dwarfism
Osteogenesis imperfecta	Inherited collagen disorder resulting in bone fragility
Neurofibromatosis	Autosomal dominant inherited disorder of neural crest origin resulting in formation of nerofibromas anywhere in the body

---

12.15   a) False   b) True   c) True   d) False   e) True

EXPLANATION

See Table 12.5.

Oxygen delivery to the fetus is dependent on maternal and fetal factors:

Maternal factors. Oxygen delivery is related to the oxygen flux equation and thus dependent on haemoglobin and cardiac output, which determines uterine perfusion (reduced by aortocaval compression and vasoconstrictors; improved by drugs that suppress uterine contractions). Fetal oxygenation is also affected by alveolar oxygenation (e.g. reduced in severe asthma) and placental oxygen transfer (reduced by placental abnormalities).

Fetal factors. Fetal oxygen delivery is dependent on the fetal oxygen flux equation, i.e. fetal haemoglobin and fetal cardiac output.

12.16   a) True   b) False   c) True   d) True   e) False

EXPLANATION

Chronic renal failure causes numerous pathophysiological changes which may have anaesthetic implications:

Clinical picture	Anaesthetic considerations
Short stature; small pelvis; prominent forehead; large tongue and mandible; short maxilla; possible kyphoscoliosis	Kyphoscoliosis may cause respiratory dysfunction; sleep apnoea may be a feature; possibly difficult intubation especially with caesarean section which would be required because of small pelvis; technical difficulties with regional anaesthesia
Fractures especially in children; lax joints; tendons prone to rupture; possible dental and other skeletal anomalies, e.g. kyphoscoliosis; aortic valve incompetence and renal stones possible; sclerae may be blue	Careful positioning to avoid fractures which may be caused by violent suxamethonium fasciculations; possible respiratory impairment if kyphoscoliosis present
Light brown skin spots; iris hamartomas; dumbbell neurofibromas in vertebral foramina; possible neuroma of facial nerve – acoustic neuroma. There may be associated cerebral gliomas/meningiomas; kyphoscoliosis; pulmonary fibrosing alveolitis and rarely phaeochromocytoma	Kyphoscoliosis may be associated with respiratory impairment; airway lesions may complicate airway management; exclude presence of phaeochromocytoma

1. Fluids and electrolytes:
    - Urea: a product of protein metabolism. A high urea level leads to defective ion transport across cells causing rises in intracellular sodium and water accumulation.
    - Fluids: urea itself predisposes to water accumulation and pulmonary oedema. In patients with poor urine output, fluid elimination is dependent on dialysis, apart from insensible fluid losses of 500 ml per day. In these patients excessive sodium intake causes hypernatraemia, oedema and hypertension. Patients with adequate urine output cannot concentrate the urine, and fluid losses can cause hypovolaemia.
    - Metabolic acidosis: due to retained sulphates and phosphates. This is usually well compensated.
    - Potassium: chronic stable high potassium levels do not cause ECG or clinical changes of hyperkalaemia; these are usually due to sudden changes in potassium levels, e.g. stress from surgery, trauma, metabolic acidosis, diuretics which retain potassium (aldosterone), blood transfusions. Hypokalaemia is also possible as a result of excessive dialysis or malnutrition.
    - Phosphate and calcium: since phosphate is eliminated via the kidney, renal failure causes hyperphosphataemia which leads to hypocalcaemia and increased bone deposition of calcium. Vitamin D is synthesized by the kidney, and its lack also accounts for hypocalcaemia. The increased bony calcium

Table 12.5   Maternal obstetric emergencies

	Placenta praevia	Abruptio placentae	Uterine rupture	Coagulopathy
Definition	Placenta partially (marginal placenta praevia) or completely covering os	Placental separation before fetal delivery	Rupture of uterus	Consumptive or dilutional coagulopathy with severe blood loss
Incidence	< 1% Mortality: 1%	About 1%	0.1%	
Risk factors	Multiparity; advanced age; previous placenta praevia; previous uterine scar	High blood pressure; multiparity; uterine abnormalities; premature rupture of membranes; previous abortion; cocaine abuse	Previous caesarean section or uterine surgery; uterine anomaly; uterine manipulation; multiparity; rapid labour; placenta percreta	Pre-eclampsia; intrauterine fetal death, abruptio placentae

Placenta accreta	Uterine inversion	Uterine atony	Cord prolapse	Fetal head entrapment
Absence of decidual layer between placental villi and myometrium. Accreta: villi attached to but do not invade muscle; increta: villi invade myometrium; percreta: villi invade myometrium and surrounding structures	Uterus turned inside out	Uterus does not contract normally to stop haemostasis	Umbilical cord prolapses into vagina	Entrapment of after-coming head during vaginal delivery or caesarean section
< 0.1%	0.0001–0.0002%	2.5% of vaginal deliveries	10% in breech deliveries	
Placenta implanted in fundus; uterine atony; inadvertent uterine traction	Big baby; prolonged labour; multiparity; polyhydramnios; drugs inhibiting contractions: beta-2 agonists, alcohol	Breech delivery	Breech delivery	

Table 12.5 (Cont'd)

	Placenta praevia	Abruptio placentae	Uterine rupture	Coagulopathy
Effects on fetus Distress: early, late decelerations; tachycardia; bradycardia; respiratory and metabolic acidosis; increased catecholamines; high blood pressure; preferred flow to heart, brain, adrenal; gasping respirations	Uterine perfusion decreases if bleeding significant, causing fetal distress	Intrauterine death may occur especially with concealed haemorrhage	Fetal distress	May be secondary to intrauterine fetal death
Maternal clinical picture	Painless vaginal bleeding before or during labour	Bleeding, vaginal or concealed	Constant severe abdominal pain; breaks through epidural owing to peritoneal irritation; contractions uncoordinated; low blood pressure	Diffuse bleeding from gums, vagina, cannula sites; renal failure possible
Diagnosis	Vaginal examination; ultrasound	Vaginal examination; ultrasound	May only be noted postpartum	PT, PTT, platelet and fibrinogen levels

Placenta accreta	Uterine inversion	Uterine atony	Cord prolapse	Fetal head entrapment
		Oxygen delivery to fetus compromised very quickly	Fetal distress can be severe. Oxygenation very compromised when umbilicus delivered	
Haemorrhage at time of placental delivery	Haemorrhagic shock and abdominal pain	Soft uterus; constant vaginal bleeding	Pulsatile mass in vagina	
	Mass in vagina		Pulsatile mass in vagina	

Table 12.5 *(Cont'd)*

	Placenta praevia	Abruptio placentae	Uterine rupture	Coagulopathy
Anaesthetic problems	Acute haemorrhage: general anaesthetic; if haemorrhage is chronic and pulse/blood pressure stable, spinal or epidural probably OK	Regional technique appropriate if clotting is normal; if fetal distress severe, emergency delivery under general anaesthetic	Depends on maternal haemodynamic state and urgency of delivery	Regional technique ? contraindicated because of coagulopathy. Blood/clotting factors required
Postpartum haemorrhage Uterine flow = 10–15% cardiac output (500 ml/min); thus blood loss may be severe	May be severe if placenta accreta present	Likely if coagulopathy present	Hysterectomy may be required. Coagulopathy unlikely	Transabdominal hysterectomy may be required. Wedge resection possible
Delivery	Vaginal for marginal placenta praevia; otherwise caesarean	Vaginal if abruption small; caesarean if large or if there is fetal distress	Caesarean section usually with uterine repair	Depends on state of fetus and maternal haemodynamics

deposits cause renal osteoarthropathy – bone deformity, osteoporosis, osteomalacia. Treatment consists in vitamin D administration, calcium and phosphate restriction. Hypophosphataemia is also possible with aggressive dialysis. This can lead to muscle weakness and increased sensitivity to muscle relaxants. Phosphate is required for 2,3-diphosphoglycerate synthesis.
- Magnesium: hypermagnesaemia is often a feature of renal failure and like hypoposphataemia leads to muscle weakness and increased sensitivity to muscle relaxants.

2. *Cardiac:*
   - Congestive heart failure: due to fluid and sodium overload, chronic hypertension, coronary artery disease, hypoalbuminaemia.
   - Pericarditis and pericardial effusion.
   - Hypertension: due to excessive sodium load; increased renin levels.

Placenta accreta	Uterine inversion	Uterine atony	Cord prolapse	Fetal head entrapment
General anaesthetic preferable if blood loss is severe	Emergency general anaesthetic to provide relaxation to replace uterus; i.v. nitroglycerine helps relaxation	? general anaesthetic: causes uterine relaxation; tone increased by i.v. oxytocin/ ergot/ prostaglandin $F_{2\alpha}$	If epidural in place, it may be intensified; otherwise a general anaesthetic is required	Uterine relaxation with general anaesthetic or i.v. nitroglycerine 50–20 µg
Postpartum haemorrhage may be severe				Postpartum haemorrhage possible with cervical incisions
		Urgent to save baby; umbilical cord elevated until delivery	Cervical incision may facilitate delivery	

- Atherosclerosis: coronary artery disease is common because of hypertension and disturbed glucose and fat metabolism.
3. *Pulmonary.* Postoperative pulmonary complications are common – pulmonary oedema; pneumonia (decreased resistance to infections); reduction in functional residual capacity; abdominal distension which restricts ventilation.
4. *Haematology:*
   - Anaemia: chronic anaemia is due to reduced erythropoietin levels, decreased blood cell mass and chronic blood loss. Compensatory mechanisms include increased cardiac output and shift of oxyhaemoglobin curve to the right which facilitates oxygen tissue delivery. Preoperative blood transfusion should not be administered for a chronic anaemia because of increased risks of infection, fluid overload and shift of oxyhaemoglobin curve to the left, reducing tissue oxygen availability.

- Coagulopathy: although prothrombin time (PT) and partial thromboplastin time (PTT) are usually normal, platelet function is often abnormal because of defective factor VIII production. The coagulopathy is not corrected with platelet infusions, but with dialysis, cryoprecipitate or vasopressin which stimulates factor VIII release.
- Hepatitis: risks of transmitting hepatitis B or C are high with chronic haemodialysis.

5. *Metabolic.* Hyperglycaemia is likely owing to insulin resistance. High triglyceride levels are also possible because of reduced lipoprotein lipase activity.
6. *Nutrition.* Renal patients are on a low-protein diet; thus hypoalbuminaemia is likely, predisposing to interstitial and pulmonary oedema.
7. *Infection.* There is a reduced resistance to infection because of malnutrition, anaemia and uraemia. Therefore postoperative infections and delayed wound healing are common, and the incidence is not reduced with dialysis.
8. *Gut.* Uraemia causes anorexia, vomiting, hiccoughs. The risk of regurgitation at induction is therefore increased. Gut mucosa is often inflamed and ulcerated, causing peptic ulcers and chronic bleeding.
9. *Central nervous system.* Uraemia causes personality changes, drowsiness, fits. Symptoms are more likely if urea and creatinine levels rise rapidly. Peripheral and autonomic neuropathy are also possible.
10. *Drugs.* See Table 12.6. Doses of drugs should in general be reduced by 25–50%.

12.17   a) True   b) True   c) False   d) False   e) True

EXPLANATION

Opioid drugs act and bind to opiate receptors within the central nervous system and in peripheral nerve sites. The binding affinity differs with different opioids and relates to anaesthetic potency.

There are primarily four types of opioid receptors: mu, delta, kappa and sigma. The mu, delta and kappa receptors mediate analgesia. The mu (morphine) receptors

Table 12.6 Drugs dependent on renal function

Drugs mainly excreted renally	Drugs partially renally excreted	Drugs with increased plasma levels due to raised unbound protein fraction (e.g. low albumin, acidosis)	Metabolites of drugs excreted renally
Gallamine	Atropine	Barbiturates	Morphine – glucuronides
Penicillins	Glycopyrolate	Benzodiazepines	Pethidine – norpethidine (fits)
Cephalosporins	Neostigmine		Diazepam – oxazepam
Aminoglycosides	Pancuronium		Midazolam – hydroxymidazolam
Vancomycin	Tubocurare		Sodium nitroprusside – thiocyanate
Digoxin	Vecuronium		Sevoflurane/enflurane – fluorides
	Barbiturates		Vecuronium – deacetylvecuronium
			Pancuronium – hydroxypancuronium

are primarily located in the periaqueductal grey matter, nucleus raphe magnus and medial thalamus, and some are also located on the spinal cord. The mu receptors are essentially responsible for supraspinal analgesia. The delta and kappa receptors are mainly located in the spinal cord, and are responsible for spinal analgesia. Therefore, it would be logical to assume that if one is using the intrathecal or epidural route for analgesia, delta agonists should be more effective than mu agonists. One such delta agonist is the endogenous opioid encephalin, which has been shown to be five times more potent than morphine when injected intrathecally, but unfortunately it is unstable. Apart from being more potent, delta agonists, together with kappa agonists do not cause any respiratory depression and therefore the development of a stable delta agonist may prove very efficacious. Morphine mu receptors are divided into two subtypes, mu_1 and mu_2 – activation of mu_1 is responsible for analgesia; mu_2 for respiratory depression, bradycardia, and inhibition of gut motility. At present there are no specific mu_1 agonists. Activation of kappa receptors causes spinal analgesia and sedation but without respiratory depression. Activation of the sigma receptors (e.g. pentazocine) produces dysphoria, hallucinations, tachycardia, tachypnoea and dilated pupils.

Analgesics that produce a maximal response at a receptor are called 'agonists', e.g. morphine, which produces a maximal response at mu receptors, both mu_1 and mu_2. Agents such as naloxone prevent opioids binding to their receptors and are called 'antagonists'. In between are drugs which produce a partial response at receptors and are thus called 'partial agonists' (e.g. buprenorphine). Because partial agonists do not bind fully to receptors the analgesia and respiratory depression is less than with pure agonists. Partial agonists also show a 'ceiling effect', i.e. as the dose is increased there comes a point where increasing the dose further does not achieve greater analgesia or respiratory depression. If a partial agonist (e.g. buprenorphine) is administered at the same time as a pure agonist (e.g. morphine), it can antagonize the effect of the pure agonist. While morphine and other opioids are pure agonists at mu receptors, and buprenorphine is a partial agonist at mu receptors, other agents may be agonist at some receptors and antagonist at other receptors. These agents are called 'agonist-antagonist' drugs.

Properties of analgesics that act at opioid receptors are summarized in Table 12.7.

12.18   a) False   b) False   c) True   d) False   e) False

EXPLANATION
Laryngotracheobronchitis (croup) and epiglottitis are probably the most common causes of upper respiratory tract obstruction in children, and differential diagnosis between the two is of vital importance. Table 12.8 compares the two conditions.

Further details on treatment of epiglottitis
Under no circumstances must laryngoscopy be done by doctors outside an operating theatre to 'have a look', because laryngoscopy can make the obstruction total. The child should be oxygenated, and taken rapidly to the operating theatre. A doctor should be present and ready to undertake a quick tracheostomy if necessary. The child should be disturbed as little as possible. Ideally an intravenous access should be established immediately, but if cannulation attempts are going to upset the child, it should be done after induction of anaesthesia. Full monitoring is started

Table 12.7 Properties of analgesics that act on opioid receptors

	Mu receptors
Location	Periaqueductal grey matter; nucleus raphe magnus; medial thalamus; spinal cord. Also present in peripheral nerve sites
Effects	Supraspinal analgesia and sedation; mu_1: analgesia; mu_2: respiratory depression; bradycardia; reduced gut motility
Drug examples	
Pure agonist	
Morphine, pethidine, fentanyls, etc.	Agonist
Partial agonist	
Buprenorphine	Partial agonist
Agonist-antagonist	
Nalbuphine	Antagonist
Pentazocine	Antagonist
Antagonist	
Naloxone	Antagonist

before induction, and all required drugs, especially atropine, drawn up. Following prolonged preoxygenation, the child is given a gaseous induction preferably with nitrous oxide/oxygen/halothane (sevoflurane may be a suitable alternative). Laryngoscopy and intubation are attempted when the depth of anaesthesia is adequate. The diameter of the tube should be 1 mm smaller than that predicted for the child's age. Nasal intubation is preferable, but an oral tube should be used if nasal intubation proves difficult. If control of the airway is lost, an emergency cricothyrotomy/tracheostomy may be required. Once the airway is secure, blood cultures are taken and wide spectrum antibiotics started. The child is than transferred to the intensive care unit, and sedated appropriately to avoid accidental extubation, which can have disastrous consequences. The airway obstruction usually resolves within 12–36 hours of commencement of antibiotics, and the child can then be extubated.

12.19   a) False   b) False   c) True   d) True   e) False

In the 1960s and 1970s there were a number of articles suggesting that theatre personnel were at risk from anaesthetic pollution. The risks mentioned were short-term problems, e.g. headaches and transient impairment in performance which is likely to occur at 10% of the minimum alveolar concentration (MAC) of the vapour.

Delta receptors	Kappa receptors	Sigma receptors
Spinal cord. Also present in peripheral nerve sites	Spinal cord. Also present in peripheral nerve sites	
Spinal analgesia without respiratory depression	Spinal analgesia and sedation without respiratory depression	Dysphoria; hallucinations; tachycardia; tachypnoea; dilated pupils
Nil	Nil	Nil
Nil	Nil	Nil
Nil	Agonist *albuphin*	Agonist
Nil	Agonist *pentay*	Agonist
Antagonist	Antagonist	Antagonist

For nitrous oxide, this equates to 100 000 parts per million (p.p.m.). Suspected long-term effects were hepatotoxicity, immunological impairment, carcinogenicity especially in the reticuloendothelial system, increased incidence of female offspring, and increased incidence of miscarriages, chronic depression and other psychological problems. A recent study showed that suicide accounts for 5–10% of deaths among anaesthetists who died before retirement.

These risks were probably exaggerated, and it is now believed that there is no significant health risks amongst anaesthetists. However, because of potential problems, scavenging devices were introduced in the early 1980s, and most anaesthetists felt that the pollution problem was solved. The scavenging equipment used in most hospitals is either passive or active. In a simple passive system, a collecting device is placed over the relief valve of the anaesthetic machine, and the waste gases are then scavenged away through tubing to the outside atmosphere. With an active system, a suction device is used to remove the waste gases. A safety device is included to avoid direct suction from the patient. These scavenging devices do not eliminate anaesthetic pollution, and it was wrongly believed that they reduce it to an acceptable level.

Anaesthetic pollution still exists and the sources are usually leaks, e.g. round a patient's mask or leakage and spillage from careless filling of vaporizers, or leaving anaesthetic gases on the anaesthetic machine in the 'on' position when not connected to a patient. The amount of air pollution will then depend upon the size of the room – anaesthetic room, theatre or recovery room – and amount of ventilation in it. Another source of pollution is the failure to use, or the inefficient use of, a scavenging system.

Table 12.8 Distinguishing features between laryngotracheobronchitis and epiglottitis

	Laryngotracheobronchitis (croup)	Epiglottitis
Aetiology	Viral	Bacterial usually *Haemophilus influenzae*. Incidence may be decreasing, because of the *H. influenzae* vaccine
History	Long (days); often accompanied by upper respiratory tract infection	Hours
Clinical	Child not too ill; malaise; low pyrexia; signs of respiratory obstruction.	Child usually aged 3–5; very ill; toxaemia; high temperature; signs of respiratory obstruction. Five 'D's: drooling; dysphagia; dyspnoea; dysphonia; dehydration
Lateral X-ray	Normal	Enlarged epiglottis
Duration	4–5 days	1–2 days
Treatment	No antibiotics; intubation, tracheostomy often not required. Some centres prefer tracheostomy	Wide spectrum antibiotics; intubation/tracheostomy often necessary. Intubation preferable

Anaesthetic pollution can be measured either by sampling the air in a specified area, or preferably by sampling the gas breathed in by an individual. The former is measured by a portable infrared analyser; with personal sampling, the individual wears a charcoal or molecular sieve badge which absorbs the sample, and the analysis is then conducted by gas chromatography.

Studies have shown that level of pollution of nitrous oxide and halothane varies widely, and can alter significantly at different times. The mean levels of nitrous oxide vary from 150 to over 2000 p.p.m., and can reach high levels even with scavenging devices. Midwives are exposed to approximately 300 p.p.m. With halothane, mean levels of exposure vary between 2 and 3 p.p.m. with maximum levels of 16 p.p.m. Concern is greater with nitrous oxide than with the volatile agents because nitrous oxide appears to have a smaller margin of safety. Animal experiments indicate that nitrous oxide is a mild teratogen at very high levels, which are not achieved in the anaesthetist's environment. There were also concerns about the inhibitory effects of nitrous oxide on vitamin B_{12} leading to impairment of folate metabolism, but again in practice this is not a problem. Although studies have shown that occupational hazards from anaesthetic pollution are unlikely, more and more governments are introducing maximal exposure limits. In America and the United Kingdom, the suggested safety levels over an 8-hour exposure are as follows:

	Nitrous oxide (p.p.m.)	Halothane (p.p.m.)	Isoflurane (p.p.m.)
USA	25–50	2–50	2
UK	100	10	50

Apart from occupational hazards, there have also been studies on the effects of anaesthetic gases and vapours on the environment, i.e. whether they contributed to the greenhouse effect or to the depletion of the ozone layer. The answer is that they do, but the quantity of anaesthetics released to the environment is much less than the damaging chlorofluorocarbon (CFC) gases, and moreover the lifetime of anaesthetics in the atmosphere is very much less than that of CFCs.

12.20   a) True   b) True   c) False   d) False   e) False

EXPLANATION

There are a number of differences between adults and children which one must bear in mind when conducting caudals, epidurals or spinals.

Anatomy:

- *Sacrum.* During childhood the sacral vertebrae are separated by intervertebral discs (thus trans-sacral blocks are possible); by the age of 18 the discs are fused. The sacrum is slightly higher than in an adult and the intercristal iliac line may cross the fifth lumber vertebra in children.
- *Spinous processes.* Through the entire spine in children, the spinous processes are more parallel to each other, thus facilitating central blocks.
- *Spinal cord.* At birth the cord is at L3 level and ascends to T12–L1 in the adult. The dural sac stops at S3 in a baby and S1 in an adult. Thus in children, dural taps are possible even with caudals.
- *Epidural space.* This is larger in children owing to lack of fat; thus haemodynamic changes are less pronounced than in adults. The distance from skin to epidural space can be calculated by the formula: distance in mm = (weight in kg + 10) × 0.8.
- *Cerebrospinal fluid (CSF).* In the newborn the CSF volume is 4 ml/kg compared to an adult where it is only 2 ml/kg. The rate of production of CSF is also very high in infants. These two facts probably explain why the incidence of post-spinal headache is rare in children below the age of 8.

Physiology. Spinals and epidurals produce less pronounced haemodynamic changes than in adults especially if the child is under 8. This is because children have a low peripheral resistance; thus sympathetic blockade will not cause dramatic vasodilatation. Another reason is that the area blocked with a lumber epidural is about 35% of the total body volume while in an adult it is approximately 70%.

Pharmacology. Children have lower protein levels than adults; thus local anaesthetics are less protein bound and also have a larger level of distribution, reach a maximal effect more quickly, and are eliminated more slowly than in adults. Maximal doses are: 10 mg/kg of lignocaine; 4 mg/kg of bupivacaine. Concentrations of bupivacaine as low as 0.125% produce sufficient sensory blockade without causing motor block.

Narcotics have the same effects as in adults though urinary retention is less common. The epidural space is mainly used (50 µg/kg morphine; 2 µg/kg fentanyl).

The caudal space can also be used, in which case morphine is the drug of choice, because its poor lipid solubility ensures enough spread even for thoracic postoperative analgesia.

Equipment and technique:

● *Caudals.* A 23-gauge needle can be used. For continuous caudals, the best method is to pass a catheter through a short intravenous catheter. Caudals are suitable for surgery between T5 and S5.

● *Lumbar and thoracic epidurals.* In children below 5, a 19-gauge Tuohy needle and a 23-gauge catheter are appropriate; in older children a normal 18-gauge Tuohy needle can be used. Even in neonates, a smaller Tuohy needle than 19-gauge should not be employed because the epidural space is relatively large, and if a small needle is used misplacement of the catheter is likely. In small infants the catheter is inserted only 1 cm into the epidural space to avoid a high block. A lumbar epidural is suitable for surgery between T5 and S5.

● *Trans-sacral epidurals.* The trans-sacral route, which can be used up to the age of 18, combines the advantages of a continuous epidural catheter technique and the safety of a caudal. A line joining the posterior superior iliac joint crosses the S1 vertebra and the puncture is performed at the S1/S2 or S2/S3 space.

● *Spinals.* A short 25-gauge needle is commonly employed. In the newborn one should choose the L5/S1 interspace to avoid a high block.

INDEX